“Why wait for a heart attack? Follow Dr. Houston’s excel[illegible] health of your cardiovascular system now.”

Dr. Joe Pizzorno, Author, *The Toxin Solution* and
Co-Author, *Textbook of Natural Medicine*

“If you, or someone you know, is living with high blood pressure or heart disease, this is the book you *must* read. Evidence based and approachable, I’ll be recommending it to all my patients, as well as my colleagues.”

Tieraona Low Dog, MD

“If I had to recommend only one required reading for every American this year, it would be “What You Need to Know About High Blood Pressure” by Dr. Mark Houston and Lee Bell. Cardiovascular Disease (CVD) remains the number one killer of men and women worldwide and high blood pressure is the #1 leading MODIFIABLE risk factor for CVD. Two out of every three Americans have an unsafe elevation in blood pressure, even those that are treated with prescription medications. We know that more drugs are not the answer. This book described how YOU, each individual person, can take control of your own health and make simple changes that will save your life. Dr. Houston is a unique physician and teacher that explains complex biology in a very simple easy to understand language. Most importantly, he teaches you how to implement simple, scientifically and clinically proven changes in your diet and lifestyle that can reverse hypertension and significantly decrease your risk of dying from cardiovascular disease.”

Nathan Bryan PhD

“Hypertension is the most common and modifiable risk factor for cardiovascular disease. Rather than a disease, hypertension is a manifestation of an abnormal vascular system. Therein is both the problem and opportunity: we need a systems biology approach to address the root cause, and that’s what Dr. Mark Houston uniquely provides. He is my go-to expert on hypertension, a world-class leader in precision and personalized medicine for cardiovascular health. This book can help you meet the latest criteria for normal blood pressure with evidence-based diet, lifestyle, and nutraceutical recommendations—and limit your risk of scary downstream consequences, including stroke, heart attack, and dementia.”

Sara Gottfried MD, *New York Times* bestselling author of
The Hormone Cure, The Hormone Reset Diet, and *Younger*

Controlling High Blood Pressure through Nutrition, Nutritional Supplements, Lifestyle, and Drugs

Mark C. Houston and Lee Bell

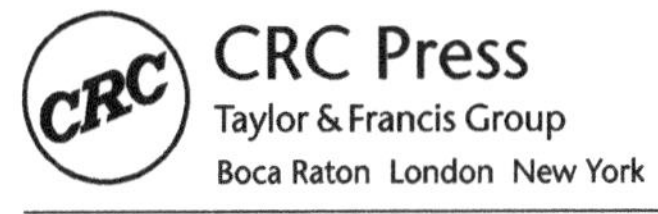

CRC Press is an imprint of the
Taylor & Francis Group, an **informa** business

First edition published 2021
by CRC Press
6000 Broken Sound Parkway NW, Suite 300, Boca Raton, FL 33487-2742

and by CRC Press
2 Park Square, Milton Park, Abingdon, Oxon, OX14 4RN

Library of Congress Cataloging-in-Publication Data

Names: Houston, Mark C., author. | Bell, Lee (Holistic nutritionist), author.
Title: Controlling high blood through nutrition, nutritional supplements, lifestyle, and drugs / Mark C. Houston, Lee Bell. Description: First edition. | Boca Raton : CRC Press, 2021. | Includes bibliographical references and index. | Summary: "High blood pressure or hypertension is the most common primary diagnosis in the United States. Despite extensive research over the past several decades, the cause of most cases of adult hypertension is still unknown and thought to be genetic. Current methods of controlling blood pressure in the general population is inadequate, high blood pressure may result in heart attack, heart failure, stroke, or kidney failure. This book provides an integrative approach on how to prevent and treat high blood pressure. It includes scientific research and clinical applications which helps patients learn easy solutions to implement and manage hypertension"-- Provided by publisher.
Identifiers: LCCN 2020056850 (print) | LCCN 2020056851 (ebook) | ISBN 9780367647797 (paperback) | ISBN 9780367653798 (hardcover) | ISBN 9781003129196 (ebook)
Subjects: LCSH: Hypertension--Nutritional aspects. | Hypertension--Alternative treatment. | Hypertension--Treatment. Classification: LCC RC685.H8 H648 2021 (print) | LCC RC685.H8 (ebook) | DDC 616.1/32--dc23 LC record available at https://lccn.loc.gov/2020056850
LC ebook record available at https://lccn.loc.gov/2020056851

ISBN: 978-0-367-65379-8 (hbk)
ISBN: 978-0-367-64779-7 (pbk)
ISBN: 978-1-003-12919-6 (ebk)

Typeset in Times
by KnowledgeWorks Global Ltd.

Contents

Preface: How to Use this Book

Welcome to the newest and most advanced scientific book on high blood pressure (hypertension) that is written for the non-medical person in terms that you can understand and knowledge that you can apply. We hope that this book will change your risk of a major cardiovascular problem like a heart attack, stroke, heart failure, or kidney failure, and save your life or the life of a family member or friend if you or they have high blood pressure. Here are some guidelines on how to read this book:

1. **All chapters** are written in an easy-to-understand manner, and terms are defined for the reader.
2. **Tables and figures** within each chapter help illustrate what is described in the text and provide concise information.
3. **All references** are numbered in the text and then listed at the end of each chapter number. If you wish to read more, the references will provide additional medical information.
4. **Summary and key takeaway points** are provided at the end of each chapter. This will give you a rapid and concise overview of the information in each respective chapter.
5. **A sources section** is listed at the end of the book to provide you with contact information for the best nutritional supplement, lab, and testing companies as well as other important sources mentioned in the text of the book.
6. **The name of a specific nutritional supplement,** if appropriate, is mentioned in the text with the name of the company that you can contact. Also, labs and testing companies are provided in the text.

About the Authors

Mark C. Houston, MD, MS, MSc, FACP, FAHA, FASH, FACN, ABAARM, FAARM, DABC

Dr. Mark Houston graduated Phi Beta Kappa and summa cum laude from Rhodes College, with a BA in chemistry and math. He graduated with highest honors and the Alpha Omega Alpha honorary society distinction from Vanderbilt Medical School. He completed his medical training at the University of California in San Francisco (UCSF) then returned to serve as Chief Resident in Medicine at Vanderbilt Medical Center where he received the Hillman Award for the Best Teacher. Dr. Houston is the Director of the Hypertension Institute and Vascular Biology, Medical Director of the Division of Human Nutrition, and Medical Director of Clinical Research at the Hypertension Institute in Nashville, Tennessee. He is on the faculty and Director of the Advanced Cardiovascular Modules 16 with A4M/MMI in the United States and Director of the Cardiovascular Module 2 for A4M/MMI. He is a Clinical Instructor in the Department of Physical Therapy and Health Care Sciences at George Washington University (GWU) School of Medicine and Health Science. Dr. Houston subsequently served as an Assistant Professor of Medicine then as an Associate Professor of Medicine from 1978–1990 at Vanderbilt University School of Medicine (VUMS) and then as Associate Clinical Professor of Medicine (1990–2012). He also served as an Adjunct Professor in Metabolic Medicine at the University of South Florida, Tampa (USF) Medical School (2014–2918).

Dr. Houston has four board certifications by the American Board of Internal Medicine (ABIM), the American Society of Hypertension (ASH) (FASH-Fellow), the American Board of Anti-Aging and Regenerative Medicine (ABAARM, FAARM), and American Board of Cardiology (ABC) Certification in Hypertensive Cardiovascular Disease (DABC). He holds two Masters of Science degrees in Human Nutrition from the University of Bridgeport, Connecticut (MS) and another in Metabolic and Nutritional Medicine (University of South Florida School of Medicine—Tampa).

He was selected as one of the top physicians in the United States in Cardiovascular Medicine in 2018 by the US Consumer Research Council. Dr. Houston was also named as one of the Top Physicians in Hypertension in the United States in 2008–2014 by the Consumer Research Council. He was twice honored by USA Today as one of the Most Influential Doctors in the United States in both Hypertension and Hyperlipidemia in 2009–2010 and was selected as The Patient's Choice Award in 2010–2012 by Consumer Reports USA. He was also selected one of the Top 100 physicians in the United States by the American Health Council in 2017 and one of the Top 50 Functional and Integrative Medical Doctors in the United States in August 2017. He was also named one of America's Best Physicians in Cardiology 2018 by the National Consumer Advisory Board. In 2019, he was elected to the Continental WHO'S WHO as a Top Doctor in the field of Medicine as the Medical Director and Founder of the Hypertension Institute.

Dr. Houston has presented over 10,000 lectures, nationally and internationally, and published over 250 medical articles, scientific abstracts in peer-reviewed medical journals, books, and book chapters. He is an author, teacher, clinician, and a researcher.

He has published nine books:

Handbook of Antihypertensive Therapy
Vascular Biology for the Clinician
What Your Doctor May Not Tell You About Hypertension
Hypertension Handbook for Students and Clinicians
The Hypertension Handbook
What Your Doctor May Not Tell You About Heart Disease
Nutrition and Integrative Strategies in Cardiovascular Medicine. Sinatra and Houston, Editors
Vascular Biology and Cardiovascular Medicine for the Clinician. Mark Houston, Joe Lamb, and Anita Hays. 2019
Personalized and Precision Integrative Cardiovascular Medicine. Houston, Mark. Editor and Contributor. Wolters Kluwer Publishers, Philadelphia and Chicago. 2020

Lee Bell, NC, BCHN, is board certified in holistic nutrition, earned a Bachelor's degree from University of Southern California, and is also a graduate of the Bauman College of Holistic Nutrition in Berkeley, California. She is a member of both the NANP, National Association of Nutrition Professionals, and the AANC, American Association of Nutrition Consultants. Lee has completed Dr. Ben Lynch's program on Methylation and Clinical Nutrigenomics as well as the Institute for Functional Medicine's Methylation Strategies in the Clinical Management of Depression and Cardiovascular Disease. She holds certification in plant-based nutrition through the T. Colin Campbell Institute at Cornell University. Lee is the former Director of Nutrition for Attune Health in Beverly Hills, California, a clinic devoted to autoimmune and inflammation care and research. Further, she has served as a nutrition consultant for CARD, the Center for Autism Related Disorders.

Introduction

Tom was a 52-year-old white male who just had a suffered a massive stroke and died. He had no idea that he had long standing high blood pressure or hypertension. Tom was like millions of other people in the United States who have hypertension, commonly known as high blood pressure, and are not aware of it. Due to their undetected hypertension, this wide-ranging group is at increased risk for complications to the heart, the blood vessels, the brain, and the kidneys.

Hypertension = High blood pressure.

Hypertension does **NOT** mean that you are overly tense or "hypertense". Let us dispel that misconception immediately.

Do you know if you have high blood pressure? Are you at risk for cardiovascular issues such as a heart attack, heart failure, stroke, kidney failure, an aneurysm (an enlarged weakened artery that can burst), loss of vision, vascular dementia (loss of memory due to diseased arteries in the brain), or death? If you have high blood pressure then you need to read this book as it can save your life! You will learn everything you need to know about what causes high blood pressure, how to prevent it, and how to treat it.

Why is this book on high blood pressure different and better from all of the other hypertension books that have been published? It is very simple. This book is based on science and fact; it is realistic, proven, you can do it, and it definitely works. As Director of the Hypertension Institute in Nashville, Tennessee and at Saint Thomas Hospital, I have reviewed the medical literature on this topic, done clinical research, published numerous articles, textbook chapters and books on hypertension, lectured around the world about hypertension, and I have been in clinical practice seeing and treating patients with hypertension for over 25 years using the Hypertension Institute program. I am board certified in Hypertension and a Fellow of the American Society of Hypertension (FASH) and a Diplomate of the American Board of Cardiology in Hypertension (DABC).

Hypertension is the most common primary diagnosis in the United States; despite extensive research over the past several decades, the cause of most cases of adult hypertension is still unknown. Control of blood pressure is inadequate in the general population. (1–19) According to the American Heart Association (AHA), approximately 86 million adults (34%) in the United States are affected by hypertension. (1, 19, 20) The statistics are staggering. Hypertension contributes to over 1000 deaths per day in the United States. (1, 19, 20) If you have uncontrolled hypertension and your blood pressure readings are not within the present blood pressure guidelines then you are already at risk of having of one or more of these health conditions! Blood pressure is the force of the blood pushing against the walls of the arteries that carry blood, nutrients, and oxygen from your heart to other parts of your body. (20) If this force is too high then the arteries become damaged, stiff, non-elastic, and constricted and can even burst or clot, which causes each of these cardiovascular problems. (20)

Physicians are very concerned about high blood pressure, as it needs to be treated early and aggressively and then followed by your doctor on a regular basis to be sure it is controlled to the recommend level of 120/80 mm Hg. (1) The top number is called the **systolic** blood pressure which is the pressure in the arteries when the heart pumps out the blood. The bottom number is the **diastolic** blood pressure which is the pressure in the arteries when the heart is relaxed, after contracting and not pumping blood. Blood pressure normally rises and falls throughout the day. (20)

For each 1-mm Hg increase in your blood pressure, there is an increased risk of a cardiovascular event. (1–5) Hypertension may be primary, also called essential or genetic, or it may be secondary which means that it is due to some other cause. (1–5, 11–15, 19) Most hypertension is genetic (about 90–95%), so you will have a family history of hypertension in a parent or grandparent. (1–5, 11–15, 19) Hypertension, known as the "silent killer", is one of the most common reasons that patients see a physician in the United States. (1–19) The drugs that treat hypertension in the United States alone generate over 20 billion dollars in revenue annually. (1–19)

Hypertension is one of the top five cardiovascular disease risk factors, along with abnormal cholesterol and other fats in the blood, diabetes mellitus, obesity, and smoking. (1–19) Cardiovascular disease, including coronary heart disease (blockage in the arteries of the heart), heart attack (myocardial infarction), and stroke (cerebrovascular accident), remains the leading cause of death in the United States. Approximately 50% of people who have hypertension do not know that they have it, and of those who know they have hypertension, only 50% are treated and controlled to a normal blood pressure level of 120/80 mm Hg. (19) There are over 100 million people in the United States with hypertension based on new hypertension guidelines. (1, 19) In numerous clinical trials, drugs will control blood pressure and reduce stroke, coronary heart disease, heart attack, congestive heart failure, and chronic kidney disease. (16, 17) Some hypertensive patients either refuse to take drugs or prefer to be treated with nutrition, nutritional supplements, and other lifestyle programs. These treatment recommendations are appropriate and safe, as they are recognized by national and international guidelines, depending on the initial blood pressure level, the need for early and aggressive treatment, and other important factors that would predict a higher risk for cardiovascular events. (1–20) This integrative approach to hypertension that includes optimizing nutrition, targeted nutritional supplements such as minerals, vitamins and antioxidants, appropriate exercise, weight management, and stress reduction is preferred in order to reduce cost, improve blood pressure control, lower side effects, allow for reduction in the total number of medications, their respective doses, and decrease cardiovascular disease. The challenge is that most physicians have not been trained in nutrition or supplement protocols for hypertension and cardiovascular disease, and thus are not up to date with current science that supports the legitimacy and efficacy of those non-medicinal interventions.

There are three finite (limited) responses of the blood vessel to injury that cause hypertension. These include *inflammation* (a process by which the body's white blood cells and other substances they produce protect us from infection with foreign organisms, such as bacteria and viruses), *oxidative stress* (similar to "rusting of the arteries"), and immune dysfunction of your arteries (which are overactive white cells and other compounds that also protect the arteries from injury and infections)

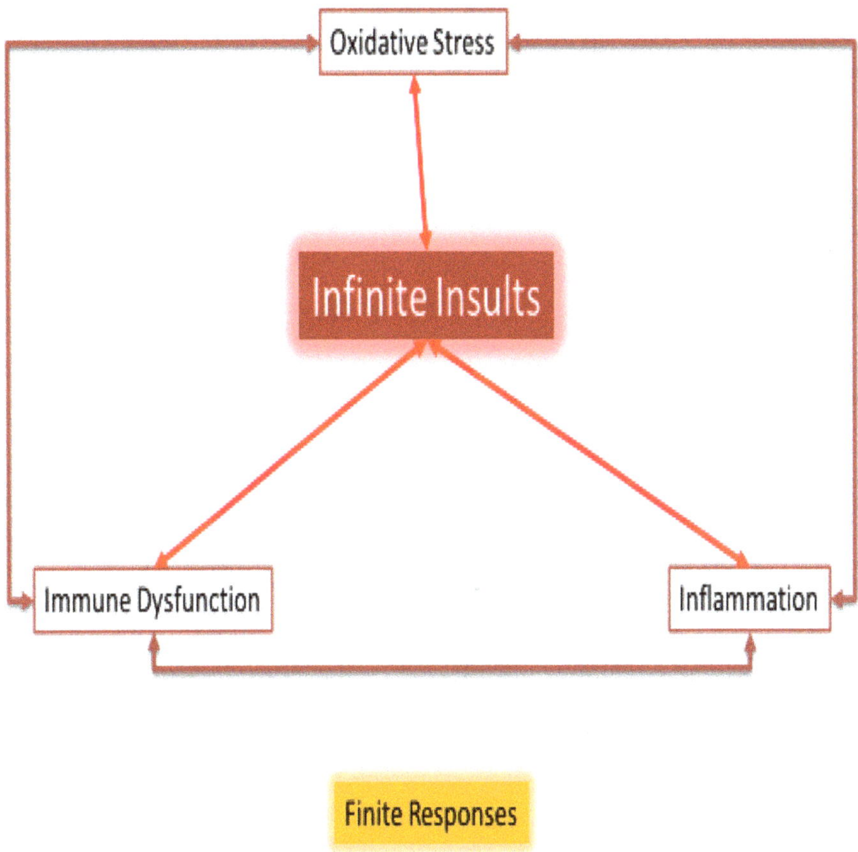

FIGURE 1 Infinite insults to the blood vessel result in only three finite responses of inflammation, oxidative stress, and vascular immune dysfunction. These three responses lay the groundwork for hypertension, especially when coupled with your genetics.

(Figure 1). (2–5, 11–14) These three finite responses of the arteries coexist and interact with your genes to increase blood pressure, heart attack, heart failure, stroke, and kidney disease (Figure 2). (2–5, 11–14) In addition, in hypertensive patients, there is a reduction in the production of an important blood vessel compound known as *nitric oxide*. (2–5) Nitric oxide is a gas that is released by the lining of the blood vessel (called the endothelium) and improves vascular health, function and structure of your arteries, lowers blood pressure, reduces atherosclerosis (plaque and fat build-up and hardening of the arteries), all of the cardiovascular diseases (heart attack, heart failure, stroke) and kidney disease, and increases life expectancy. (2–5, 11–14) The endothelium must function normally to prevent hypertension. The endothelium is the largest organ in the body, serves as a physical barrier between the blood and the arterial muscle, functions like an endocrine organ that makes many compounds that alter blood pressure and the risk for cardiovascular events. (2–5, 11–14) The

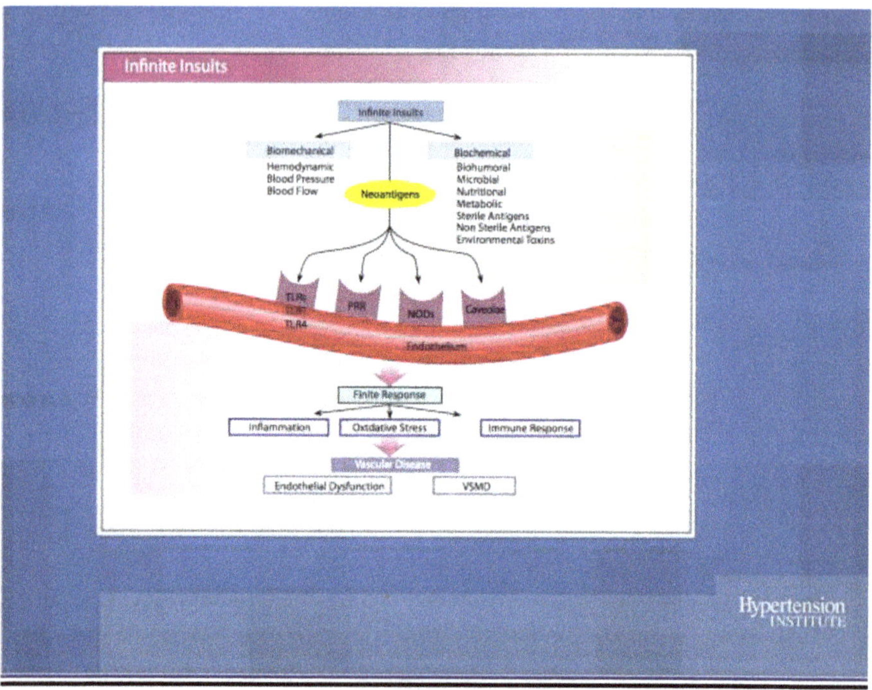

FIGURE 2 The infinite insults are divided into two major groups. These include the blood pressure and blood flow in the arteries and a variety of other causes such as infections, bad nutrition, and low levels of nutrients, high blood sugar, high blood lipids, toxins, and hormone problems. The three finite vascular responses of inflammation, oxidative stress, and vascular immune dysfunction lead to damage to the lining of the arteries, the endothelium, and this is called "endothelial dysfunction". In addition, there is damage to the heart and the wall of the arteries. This can make the heart enlarge (heart failure) or cause a heart attack and can make the arteries stiff, like a "rusty lead pipe," which will narrow the arteries, increasing blood pressure even more leading to rupture of the artery or form a blood clot inside the artery.

endothelium is the size of 6.5 tennis courts or about 14,000 ft.^{2}. (2–5, 11–14) If the endothelium becomes damaged and does not make nitric oxide but instead produces other compounds that damage the arteries and cause them to constrict then the blood pressure will increase. (2–5, 11–14) This "*endothelial dysfunction*" may precede the development of hypertension by decades. (2–5, 11–14) We will define and talk more about these finite responses, nitric oxide, the endothelium, endothelial dysfunction, and your genetics in greater detail later in this book.

Hypertension is a consequence of abnormal blood vessel health, both structure and function (this is called "**vascular biology**"), **inflammation, oxidative stress** and **immune disorders** of the artery, low levels of **nitric oxide**, **endothelial dysfunction**, and low levels of **micronutrients** (vitamins, minerals, and antioxidants) and **macronutrients** (organic high-quality protein, good fats (fish oil and olive oil), beneficial complex carbohydrates, vegetables, and fruits). (2–5, 11–14) Macronutrients and micronutrients are crucial in the regulation of blood pressure and subsequent cardiovascular disease. (2–5, 11–14) The appropriate measurement, interpretation, and treatment of these micronutrient and macronutrient levels and deficiencies, reducing inflammation, oxidative stress and immune vascular problems, increasing nitric oxide levels, and improving endothelial dysfunction may effectively lower blood pressure and decrease cardiovascular disease. (2–5, 11–14)

There are volumes of scientific information and clinical research on exercise, the nutritional inclusion of foods such as beets, pomegranate, garlic, olive oil, dark chocolate, green tea, the low "inflammation diet", the low-sodium diet, high-potassium and high-magnesium diets, fruits, and vegetables. In addition, clinical research is abundant on nutritional supplements including minerals, vitamins, and antioxidants such a coenzyme Q-10, magnesium, potassium, omega-3 fatty acids, vitamin C, various B vitamins, vitamin D, taurine, lycopene, carnitine, grape seed, and beet extract, Bonita fish extract and many more lower blood pressure very effectively without side effects.

This book will review the up to the minute information that you should know about hypertension that could save your life and prevent a deadly heart attack, heart failure, stroke, or kidney failure. What causes hypertension? How do you diagnose and measure blood pressure correctly? What are the complications of hypertension? How do you treat hypertension using the **Hypertension Institute Integrative Program** with nutrition, nutraceutical supplements, antioxidants, minerals, vitamins, anti-inflammatory agents, exercise, weight and body fat management, stress reduction, and other life style changes and drugs? The Hypertension Institute Integrative Program is designed to be a personalized, precision-based, and integrative program using the best that medicine can offer you. In a clinical trial at the Hypertension Institute, **62% of hypertensive patients evaluated over 1 year were able to stop or reduce their blood pressure medications!** (20) This is the reason we wrote this book. We want you to have all the knowledge that you can to keep you safe from the ravages of hypertension and be able to apply that knowledge to your heart and blood vessel health. Remember, "A wise healer uses that which works." You will learn and apply what works now in your life!

SUMMARY AND KEY TAKEAWAY POINTS

1. Hypertension is one of the most common reasons that patients see physicians.
2. Hypertension is a major cause of heart attack, heart failure, stroke, and kidney failure and a leading cause of death in the United States.
3. A normal blood pressure is 120/80 mm Hg, but it varies over 24 hours.
4. A large number of patients do NOT know they have hypertension, and many of those who are treated do not have their blood pressure controlled to normal recommended levels.
5. Hypertension occurs due to your genetics and family history as well as many nongenetic causes. These are termed primary (essential or genetic) and secondary causes.
6. Low levels of micronutrients and macronutrients are common in hypertension.

7. Hypertension occurs due to inflammation, oxidative stress, and immune dysfunction of the artery.
8. Nitric oxide improves blood pressure and decreases cardiovascular disease.
9. Endothelial dysfunction predicts future hypertension and cardiovascular events.
10. An integrative, personalized, and precision-based treatment using optimal nutrition, targeted supplements, vitamins, minerals, antioxidants, appropriate exercise, weight management, and stress reduction is the best approach to blood pressure control and reduction in cardiovascular events.

REFERENCES

1. Whelton PK, et al. ACC/AHA/AAPA/ABC/ACPM/AGS/APhA/ASH/ASPC/NMA/PCNA Guideline for the prevention, detection, evaluation, and management of high blood pressure in adults: a report of the American College of Cardiology/American Heart Association Task Force on Clinical Practice Guidelines. Hypertension. 2018 Jun;71(6):e13–e115.
2. Houston M. The role of nutrition and nutraceutical supplements in the treatment of hypertension. World J Cardiol. 2014;6(2):38–66.
3. Houston M. Nutrition and nutraceutical supplements for the treatment of hypertension: Part 1. J Clin Hypertens. 2013;15:752–757.
4. Houston M. Nutrition and nutraceutical supplements for the treatment of hypertension: Part II. J Clin Hypertens. 2013;15:845–851.
5. Houston M. Nutrition and nutraceutical supplements for the treatment of hypertension: Part III. J Clin Hypertens. 2013;15:931–937.
6. Borghi C, Cicero AF. Nutraceuticals with a clinically detectable blood pressure-lowering effect: a review of available randomized clinical trials and their meta-analyses. Br J Clin Pharmacol. 2017;83(1):163–171.
7. Sirtori CR, Arnoldi A, Cicero AF. Nutraceuticals for blood pressure control. Rev Ann Med. 2015;47(6):447–456.
8. Cicero AF, Colletti A. Nutraceuticals and blood pressure control: results from clinical trials and meta-analyses. High Blood Press Cardiovasc Prev. 2015;22(3):203–213.
9. Turner JM, Spatz ES. Nutritional supplements for the treatment of hypertension: a practical guide for clinicians. Curr Cardiol Rep. 2016;18(12):126.
10. Caligiuri SP, Pierce GN. A review of the relative efficacy of dietary, nutritional supplements, lifestyle and drug therapies in the management of hypertension. Crit Rev Food Sci Nutr. 2016;57(16):3508–3527.
11. Houston MC, Fox B, Taylor N. What Your Doctor May Not Tell You About Hypertension. The Revolutionary Nutrition and Lifestyle Program to Help Fight High Blood Pressure. AOL Time Warner, Warner Books, New York, NY, 2003.
12. Houston M. Treatment of hypertension with nutrition and nutraceutical supplement: Part 1. Altern Complement Med. 2019;24:260–275.
13. Houston M. Treatment of hypertension with nutrition and nutraceutical supplement: Part 2. Altern Complement Med. 2019;25:23–36.
14. Sinatra S, Houston M, Editors. Nutrition and Integrative Strategies in Cardiovascular Medicine. CRC Press, 2015.
15. The Seventh Report of the Joint National Committee on Prevention, Detection, Evaluation, and Treatment of High Blood Pressure (JNC-7). *JAMA*. 2003;289:2560–2572.

16. Thomopoulos C, Parati G, Zanchetti A. Effects of blood pressure lowering on outcome incidence in hypertension: 7. Effects of more vs. less intensive blood pressure lowering and different achieved blood pressure levels - updated overview and meta-analyses of randomized trials. J Hypertens. 2016;34(4):613–622.
17. Ettehad D, Emdin CA, Kiran A, Anderson SG, Callender T, Emberson J, Chalmers J, Rodgers A, Rahimi K. Blood pressure lowering for prevention of cardiovascular disease and death: a systematic review and meta-analysis. Lancet. 2016;387(10022):957–967.
18. ESH/ESC Task Force for the Management of Arterial Hypertension. 2013 Practice guidelines for the management of arterial hypertension of the European Society of Hypertension (ESH) and the European Society of Cardiology (ESC): ESH/ESC Task Force for the Management of Arterial Hypertension. J Hypertens. 2013;31:1925–1938.
19. Flack JM, Calhoun D, Schiffrin EL. The new ACC/AHA hypertension guidelines for the prevention, detection, evaluation, and management of high blood pressure in adults. Am J Hypertens. 2018;31(2):133–135.
20. Houston MC. The role of cellular micronutrient analysis and minerals in the prevention and treatment of hypertension and cardiovascular disease. Ther Adv Cardiovasc Dis. 2010;4:165–183.

1 Prevention of High Blood Pressure. Do Not Let This Happen to You. Actual Patient Cases of High Blood Pressure from the Hypertension Institute

Joe was a 43-year-old black male contractor who was diagnosed with hypertension at the age of 21. Joe was married and had two children in high school. He stopped taking all of his blood pressure medicines over 10 years ago due to side effects of fatigue, depression, and impotence. He loved his coffee and drank six large cups a day and then wound down after work with three to four ice cold beers. He went to work early one Monday morning, but about 2 hours later he started to have a severe headache followed by weakness in his right arm and leg and inability to speak. He was rushed to the hospital where he was diagnosed with severe hypertension and a stroke. Later that day, he went into a coma and died 24 hours later.

Maria is a 46-year-old married Hispanic female and a mother of four children. She has had hypertension for over 20 years. She has a lot of stress in her life taking her kids to school and various sporting activities. She says that she does not have any time for herself. She takes all three of her blood pressure medications almost every day but is overweight, does not exercise, and eats fast food with lots of sodium, high calories and she loves her sweets. She went to her doctor last week complaining of shortness of breath and some left-sided chest pain. He did an electrocardiogram and examined her and said everything looked good except her blood pressure was elevated. He added a fourth blood pressure medication and told her that she was just stressed. He then gave her another prescription for her stress and told her to get some rest and not to worry so much.

The next morning, she woke up with severe chest pain, shortness of breath, and heavy sweating. She called an ambulance. When the ambulance arrived at her home, she had a cardiac arrest and her heart stopped beating. She had CPR (cardiopulmonary resuscitation) by the ambulance team. At the hospital, she was revived and diagnosed with a massive heart attack.

Robert is a 62-year-old married white male who is relaxing in his big easy chair at the kidney dialysis unit. He has had kidney failure for 10 years due to uncontrolled hypertension and is on the dialysis machine 3–4 days a week. He had to go on disability and does not work now. He was the owner of a small grocery store. He can no longer play golf with his buddies which he loved so much. He misses most of his grandchildren's school and sporting events because he is too tired or has to be on the kidney dialysis machine.

Betty is a 58-year-old divorced white female who lives alone. She has one daughter who takes care of her. She has had hypertension since the age of 26 but refused to take her blood pressure medications because they made her "feel bad." She stays at home most of the time since she was diagnosed with end-stage congestive heart failure. She cannot walk more than 5 minutes without getting very short of breath. Her legs are swollen. She is on oxygen 24 hours a day. Her doctor has her on six medications and a very strict low-sodium diet. At night she has to sleep in a recliner since she cannot lie flat in her own bed because she cannot breathe. She is on the heart transplant list.

Mike was a healthy 42-year-old white male attorney, married, and father of three children. His mother and father both had hypertension, and they died when he was very young. He played football and basketball in high school and college and had a very good law practice. He ran every day, was not overweight, and felt great. He has not been to a physician for a physical exam since he was 22. On Saturday, he went out for his daily run. He was found dead in the park. His autopsy showed that he died from a ruptured thoracic aneurysm (the large artery that comes out of the heart in his chest burst). The pathologist noted that all of his arteries were severely damaged from chronic uncontrolled severe hypertension.

All of these people had one thing in common – hypertension. None of them should have died or had any of the complications. Many patients have no idea that something is not right until the damage is done. Even small increases in blood pressure will increase your risk for a cardiovascular event. For every mm Hg increase in your blood pressure, your risk for a heart attack, a stroke, or kidney disease increases. Even a small increase in blood pressure to 140/90 mm Hg will decrease your life by 10 years! Joe should have avoided the stroke and death. Maria should not have had a heart attack, Robert could have saved his kidneys, Betty would not be on the cardiac transplant list, and Mike would not have died from an artery that burst in his chest. If each of them had gone to their doctor for regular blood pressure checks and started the program to lower their blood pressure that we will describe in this book, they would not have suffered these cardiovascular events or died.

There are many things that you can start doing immediately to prevent high blood pressure, delay its onset, or reduce its severity. These will be discussed in detail in this book, but here is the list:

1. Maintain an ideal body weight, body fat, and visceral or belly fat for your gender and age.
2. Exercise at least 4 days per week for 1 hour each day with both aerobic and resistance training.
3. Get at least 8 hours of restful sleep per night.
4. Reduce dietary sodium chloride (table salt or NaCl) to less than 2000 mg (2 g) per day.
5. Increase potassium in your diet to at least 5000 mg/day (5 g).

6. Increase magnesium in your diet to at least 1000 mg/day (1 g).
7. Consume at least six servings of vegetables and six servings of fruit per day.
8. Reduce stress, meditate, and lower anxiety and relax.
9. Stop all tobacco products.
10. Reduce or stop alcohol.
11. Stop all sources of caffeine if you metabolize it slowly.
12. Consume specific types of foods and nutritional supplements that can prevent high blood pressure.

In the next chapter, we will start your journey on how to control your blood pressure, reduce all of these cardiovascular and kidney diseases, improve your life, and how long you live. We will start with a summary of the **Hypertension Institute program to lower your blood pressure.**

2 The Hypertension Institute Program to Lower Your Blood Pressure

Summary

Maintaining control of your blood pressure is a lifetime commitment. It requires that you follow all of the suggestions in this book to achieve the optimal goals for blood pressure levels and cardiovascular disease reduction. Some patients are tempted to only do part of the program or only do it for only a short period of time. You must make this commitment to keep yourself healthy and have a normal life expectancy. The goals are as follows: (1–5)

1. Lower the blood pressure to normal (120/80 mm Hg).
2. Improve both the function and structure of the arteries. This means improvement in endothelial function, increase in nitric oxide levels, increased elasticity of the arteries, dilation of the arteries, decrease thickness of the arteries and heart muscle, and reduction in inflammation, oxidative stress, and vascular immune dysfunction.
3. Reduce all cardiovascular events such as coronary heart disease, heart attack, heart failure, kidney disease, and large arterial disease.

It has been well established in numerous clinical blood pressure trials that certain blood pressure medications may lower the blood pressure, but they are not effective in improving the function and structure of the arteries or the heart, and they do not optimally reduce cardiovascular events compared to other blood pressure medications, especially coronary heart disease and heart attack. Specially, the diuretic, hydrochlorothiazide, and many older beta blockers such as atenolol are inferior to other drugs called angiotensin-converting enzyme inhibitors, angiotensin receptor blockers, and calcium channel blockers. (1–4) We will discuss these concepts and the blood pressure medications later in the book.

2.1 HERE IS A SUMMARY OF THE HYPERTENSION INSTITUTE PROGRAM

1. Determine the blood pressure level and other important measurements using a 24-hour ambulatory blood pressure monitor (24-hour ABPM) in conjunction with regular office blood pressures and home blood pressure readings.

2. Measure your blood micronutrient and macronutrient status and optimally replace all of those deficiencies with proper nutrition and supplements, antioxidants, and minerals.
3. Measure blood tests that determine the type of hypertension that is present. The two forms are called high-renin hypertension and low-renin hypertension. The blood tests include a plasma renin activity or PRA (a hormone that controls blood pressure and aldosterone), a hormone that controls blood pressure and blood volume. This will be discussed in detail later in this book.
4. Measure the genetics that determine your blood pressure and risk for coronary heart disease, heart attack, blood pressure, diabetes mellitus, cholesterol, and other blood fats.
5. Assess the presence and severity of the artery damage, artery elasticity and stiffness, endothelial function, nitric oxide levels, heart function and stiffness, heart size (enlargement), risk for coronary heart disease, coronary artery calcification, rest and exercise blood pressure, heart rate and its variability, the function of your nervous system and how it relates to blood pressure, and your overall cardiovascular risk with various noninvasive cardiovascular testing.
6. Exclude all of the secondary causes of hypertension.
7. Assess all of the new and emerging blood and urine tests that are called cardiovascular risk factors in addition to the usual measured risk factors such as blood fats and cholesterol, blood sugar (diabetes mellitus), homocysteine, and inflammation markers.
8. Properly measure obesity, total and regional body fat with a special machine called body impedance analysis. Maintain your ideal body weight, BMI, and body fat.
9. Determine the need for early and aggressive control of blood pressure based on the information listed above.
10. Start the Hypertension Institute blood pressure nutrition program.
11. Use specific blood pressure–lowering nutritional supplements.
12. Exercise regularly with both resistance and aerobic exercises using guidelines that are recommended in this book and by your physician.
13. De-stress your life with meditation, relaxation, and breathing exercises.
14. Stop all tobacco products.
15. Reduce or stop alcohol.
16. Stop caffeine if your genetics show that you cannot break down caffeine rapidly (slow metabolizer).
17. Stop or reduce all medications, if possible, that may increase your blood pressure.
18. Use the best medications to lower blood pressure, improve arterial function and structure, and decrease cardiovascular events.

In the next chapter, we will discuss more about what blood pressure is, how it is measured, and some of the complications associated with high blood pressure.

REFERENCES

1. Whelton PK, et al. ACC/AHA/AAPA/ABC/ACPM/AGS/APhA/ASH/ASPC/NMA/PCNA Guideline for the prevention, detection, evaluation, and management of high blood pressure in adults: a report of the American College of Cardiology/American Heart Association Task Force on Clinical Practice Guidelines. Hypertension. 2018;71(6):e13–e115.
2. Houston MC, Fox B, Taylor N. What Your Doctor May Not Tell You About Hypertension. The Revolutionary Nutrition and Lifestyle Program to Help Fight High Blood Pressure. AOL Time Warner, Warner Books, New York, NY, 2003.
3. Thomopoulos C, Parati G, Zanchetti A. Effects of blood pressure lowering on outcome incidence in hypertension: 7. Effects of more vs. less intensive blood pressure lowering and different achieved blood pressure levels – updated overview and meta-analyses of randomized trials. J Hypertens. 2016;34(4):613–622
4. Ettehad D, Emdin CA, Kiran A, Anderson SG, Callender T, Emberson J, Chalmers J, Rodgers A, Rahimi K. Blood pressure lowering for prevention of cardiovascular disease and death: a systematic review and meta-analysis. Lancet. 2016;387(10022):957–967.
5. Houston, MC. Handbook of Hypertension. Wiley Blackwell, 2009.

3 What Is Hypertension and How Is It Measured?

A Symptomless Disease

3.1 DEFINITION OF HYPERTENSION AND THE CARDIOVASCULAR SYSTEM

Your heart beats 60–80 times per minute or about 100,000 times per day depending on your exercise level, sleep, or stress level. During your lifetime, your heart pumps 3 billion beats and over 1 million barrels of blood. The heart and the blood vessels (arteries and veins) compose the cardiovascular system. The heart has four chambers (right and left atriums and right and left ventricles) enclosed by heart muscle (Figure 3.1). (2–5, 11–14)

Blood pressure is the force inside the artery that determines the flow of blood, oxygen, and nutrients throughout the body after it leaves the heart. (2–5, 11–14) The arteries carry blood away from the heart, while the veins carry blood back to the heart. The capillaries are the small vessels that lie between the arteries and the veins where oxygen and nutrients are given up to the cells and tissues. The veins are thin walled and do not have a high blood pressure force inside them, so they are not involved in these cardiovascular complications. We are primarily concerned with the arteries and the heart related to hypertension (Figure 3.1). The blood pressure force is also inside the heart. As the heart contracts, the systolic blood pressure (SBP) is produced. That is the top number of your blood pressure measurement. As the heart relaxes, the diastolic blood pressure (DBP) occurs that is the bottom number of your blood pressure. For example, 120/80 mm Hg is a normal blood pressure. The blood pressure number of 160/100 mm Hg is hypertension. If only the SBP is elevated (i.e., 160/80 mm Hg), it is termed systolic hypertension, while if only the DBP is elevated (i.e., 120/100 mm Hg) it is called diastolic hypertension. If both the systolic and diastolic numbers are elevated, it is called combined hypertension.

Perhaps, one the best ways to understand blood pressure is to look at the following formula that I learned in medical school (11, 20):

BP = CO × SVR

Blood pressure = cardiac output × systemic vascular resistance

OR

Pressure = force × resistance

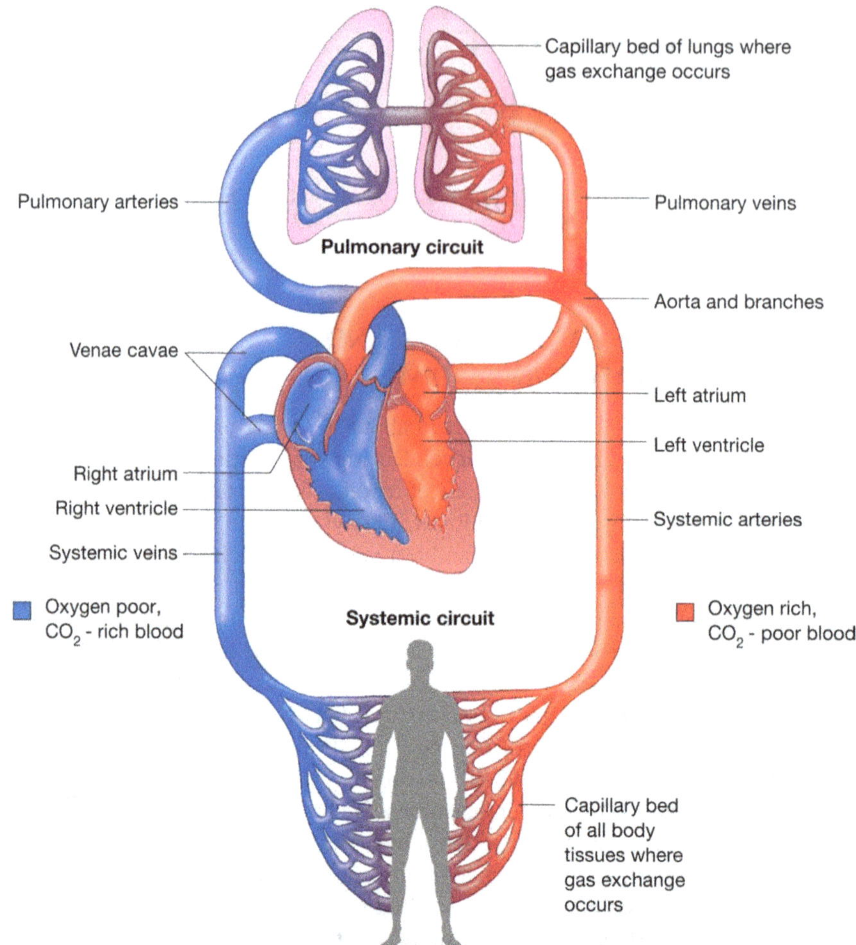

FIGURE 3.1 The circulatory system.

A simple analogy is a garden hose. If you turn the faucet on just a small amount, there is not much force available to propel the water out, so it just trickles out of the end of the hose. On the other hand, if you turn the faucet to full force, then you will have a lot of water coming out of the hose. This would be like the cardiac output or the amount of blood and force pumped out of the heart. The cardiac output is related to both your heart rate and the amount of blood pumped out of the heart with each beat (called the stroke volume). This is the force part of the equation. Let us look at the resistance side of this equation. Now, if you kink the hose or block the end of the same partially or completely, then the pressure inside the hose will build up faster and to high levels. If the hose is new and elastic, it can expand and the pressure does not increase as much. In contrast, if the hose is old or stiff, the pressure can build up quickly and to very high levels or the hose may spring a leak and burst. Your arteries can be just like the hose, that is, elastic or stiff. The consequences of the stiff artery with high resistance are higher blood pressure, possible rupture of the artery, or a clot in the artery.

There exists a continued risk of arterial damage and cardiovascular disease (CVD) for each 1 mm Hg increase in blood pressure. Normal BP is 120/80 mm Hg but the risk for cardiovascular events starts at 110/70 mm Hg for both SBP and DBP. For example, an increase in blood pressure of 20/10 mm Hg doubles the risk for heart attack, heart failure, and stroke. (2–5, 11–14) Remember that both the SBP and the DBP predict the risk for stroke, coronary heart disease, heart failure, heart attack, and kidney disease. The DBP is more predictive prior to age 55 years, while the SBP is more predictive after the age of 55 years of these cardiovascular events. As one ages, the SBP usually increases due to the loss of arterial elasticity, that is, the arteries are stiff.

If the blood pressure is too high, it will cause damage to the important lining of the artery, called the endothelium and also to the arterial wall, called the media or muscle of the artery which becomes thick and stiff (**see** Figure 3.2). (1–20) As the endothelium is damaged, it loses its ability to make nitric oxide and many other substances that allow the artery to dilate and help keep the blood pressure lower. This is called endothelial dysfunction. In addition, the loss of nitric oxide increases the risk of heart attack, heart failure, stroke, and generalized atherosclerosis with plaque build-up as well as hardening (stiffness or arteriosclerosis) of the arteries.

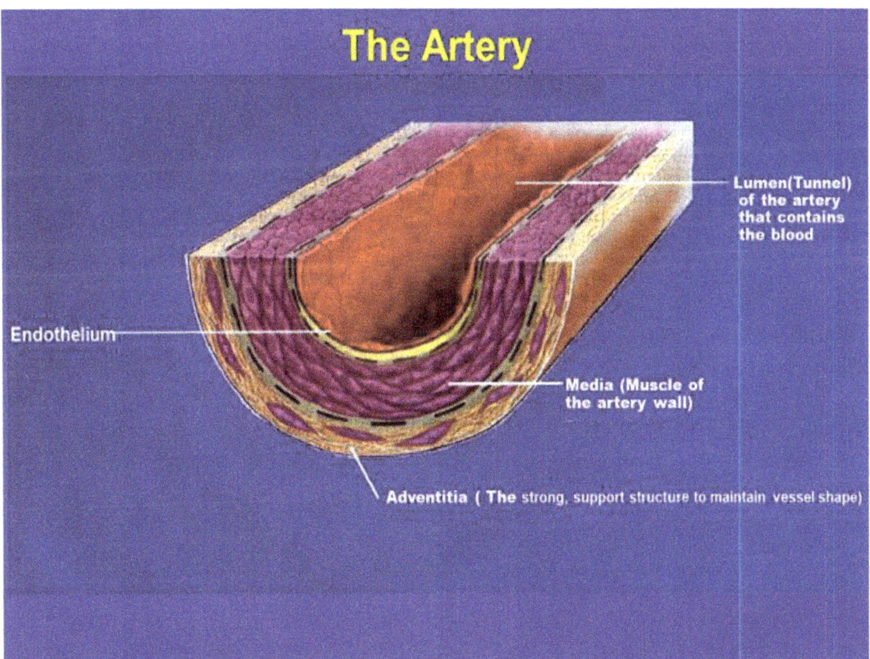

FIGURE 3.2 A the artery structure.

As the artery becomes stiff and loses its elastic stretch, the blood pressure goes higher and the artery can leak, burst, or form a clot. This results in a heart attack or a stroke. (1–20) The finite responses in the artery increase the blood pressure, as discussed in the introduction. These include inflammation, oxidative stress, and vascular immune dysfunction. (2–5, 11–14)

The left ventricle pumps blood into the aorta, then to the systemic arteries, then to the capillaries and to the veins that return the blood to the right atrium, then to the right ventricle, then to the lungs for oxygenation, then back to the left atrium, and finally to the left ventricle. The arteries are oxygen and nutrient rich, while the veins are oxygen and nutrient poor, with more carbon dioxide.

The artery is composed of **the innermost "tunnel like" part of the artery (lumen)** that has all the blood elements such as red blood cells, white blood cells and platelets, the lining of the blood artery called the **endothelium**, the muscle of the artery wall (**media**), and the structural outer support of the artery (**adventitia**). Between the endothelium and the lumen is the **glycocalyx** that is a "sugar coating or fur coat" layer or shield of cells with hair-like projections that serves as a protective role for the endothelium.

3.2 THE BLOOD PRESSURE COMPONENTS

3.2.1 Systolic and Diastolic Blood Pressure

SBP and DBP are the most commonly reported BP measures in clinical practice and clinical research studies because they are well-established CVD risk factors and can be indirectly measured. When considered separately, higher SBP and DBP are associated with increased cardiovascular risk. SBP is associated with cardiovascular events independently of DBP. In contrast, in some studies, as mentioned previously, the DBP is more predictive of cardiovascular events before the age of 50–55 years, while the SBP is more predictive of CVD after the same age. (1, 19, 20)

3.2.2 Pulse Pressure

The pulse pressure (PP) = the systolic pressure–the DBP (1, 19, 20). It is a marker of arterial stiffness, loss of artery elasticity and is a very strong predictor of CVD and death. For example, if the blood pressure is 120/80 mm Hg then the PP is 40 mm Hg that is normal, while in case the blood pressure is 160/60 mm Hg the PP is100 mm Hg that is very high. Higher levels of PP have been associated with increased risk for cardiovascular events, especially stroke, heart attack, and heart failure, independently of other blood pressure components.

3.2.3 The Central Blood Pressure

The central blood pressure (CBP) (21) is the pressure in the largest artery in the body, called the aorta, that takes all of the blood pumped from the heart (the left ventricle) during its contraction. As the heart has to pump against a higher CBP if you have hypertension, it will, over time, develop stiffness of the heart muscle, enlargement of the heart, then weakness of the heart muscle and result in heart failure. (21) The two types of heart failure are **diastolic heart failure** due to stiffness of the left ventricle, and **systolic heart failure** due a decrease of the pumping action of the left ventricle. The CBP is a more accurate predictor of CVD such as stroke, heart attack, and heart failure than the blood pressure that we measure in the upper arm, the brachial blood pressure. (21) New noninvasive blood pressure machines can now measure both the central and brachial blood pressure to see if they are the same. If they are not the same, the CBP measurement is preferred to predict future risk of cardiovascular events. Also, as we will discuss next in this book, some blood pressure medications may reduce the brachial blood pressure but will not decrease the CBP as much. This will result in a false sense of security about your blood pressure if the brachial artery blood pressure is normal but the CBP is elevated, which would mean that you are still at risk for cardiovascular events.

3.2.4 Exercise Effects on Blood Pressure

It is very important to know what happens to your blood pressure during various levels of exercise. You may have very high blood pressure during exercise and may not know it. This puts you at risk for a stroke or heart attack during exercise. A hypertensive response to exercise is an SBP over 200 mm Hg and any increase in the DBP in men or women. However, in men, an SBP over 165 mm Hg and graded upward to 180 and 200 mm Hg at moderate exercise increases the future risk for both cardiovascular events and for chronic hypertension. Ask your doctor to perform an exercise stress test and measure your blood pressure and heart rate and different levels of exercise. This could save you from a serious cardiovascular event or sudden death.

3.3 PREDICTORS OF NEW ONSET HYPERTENSION: THE 31 TOP CLUES

If you do not yet have hypertension but are concerned that you may be at risk, there are 31 TOP clinical clues and lab tests that will help predict that risk:

- Genetics: If one of your parents had high blood pressure, you have a 25% chance of developing high blood pressure yourself. If both parents had high blood pressure, then the risk is 50% that you will have high blood pressure. If your parents or a sibling developed high blood pressure before the age of 50 years, then your risk to develop hypertension is not only higher but also at an earlier age. Numerous genes that cause hypertension can be specific for drug, supplement, and diet treatment. The CardiaX genetic profile from Vibrant Labs in San Francisco measures 25 genes related to CVD and hypertension.
- Race: African-Americans are more likely to have hypertension (one in three) compared to Caucasians (one in four). It also occurs earlier, is more severe, and causes more cardiovascular damage and disease and a higher death rate.

- Gender: Men have more hypertension than women until about age 60 years, then women take the lead especially with systolic hypertension. However, women tend to fair better than their male counterparts with fewer cardiovascular complications.
- Age: As you age, your blood pressure, systolic especially, increases.
- Resting heart rate: Higher heart rates over 80 beats per minute at rest.
- Abnormal heart rate variability (the beat-to-beat pattern is abnormal).
- Stiff and nonelastic arteries (especially the small arteries) can be measured with noninvasive tests such as pulse wave velocity, augmentation index, and type of pulse wave curve. We will discuss these next in the book.
- Measures of glucose in your blood such as serum glucose fasting and post meal glucose, hemoglobin A1c, and fasting serum insulin.
- Increased leptin and decreased adiponectin are hormones that are related to fat tissue and risk for diabetes mellitus.
- Inflammation and increased high sensitivity C reactive protein.
- Oxidative stress.
- Low oxidative defense.
- Vascular immune dysregulation and dysfunction.
- Plasma renin activity is elevated. (A hormone made in the kidney that increases blood pressure and constriction of the arteries.)
- Plasma aldosterone and cortisol and urine aldosterone and cortisol are elevated. (Hormones made in the adrenal gland.)
- Renal disease and loss of protein and albumin in the urine (microalbuminuria).
- Overweight or obese. Percentages of total body fat and visceral fat are increased.
- Hyperuricemia (high uric acid) >6.0 mg/dl.
- Homocysteinemia (elevation of a blood compound homocysteine that damages the arteries and is related to low levels of B vitamins and genetics) >8.
- Dyslipidemia (cholesterol and other fats): LDL > 115 mg/dl and high levels of an abnormal LDL called oxidized LDL.
- Hypertensive response to exercise. An SBP over 200 mm Hg and any increase in DBP in men or women is abnormal. However, in men an SBP over 165 mm Hg and graded upward to 180 and 200 mm Hg at moderate exercise increases cardiovascular risk and events as well as hypertension risk in the future.
- Endothelial dysfunction with low nitric oxide levels.
- White coat hypertension (WCH): Your blood pressure is elevated in the doctor's office but is normal at home, out of the doctor's office.
- Masked hypertension (MH): Your blood pressure is elevated at home out of the doctor's office but is normal in the doctor's office.
- Alcohol abuse: Excessive alcohol consumption will increase blood pressure. Consumption should be limited to less than 20 g of alcohol per day for men and less than 10 g per day for women. That 20 g of pure alcohol would be about 7 oz of wine and 18 oz of beer.
- Medications and drug abuse: See Table 3.1 for a list of these.
- Tobacco use of any kind and smoking.

TABLE 3.1
Causes of Secondary Hypertension (1, 11, 19, 20)

A number of conditions can cause secondary hypertension and should be excluded with proper testing by your physician.

- **Diabetes mellitus damage to the kidneys (diabetic nephropathy).** Diabetes can damage your kidneys' filtering system, which can lead to hypertension.
- **Polycystic kidney disease.** This is a genetic condition where cysts in your kidneys prevent them from working normally, leading to kidney failure and hypertension.
- **Glomerular disease.** Your kidneys filter waste, sodium, and other compounds using microscopic-sized filters called glomeruli that may become damaged or leak leading to hypertension.
- **Renovascular hypertension.** The arteries to the kidneys become narrowed or blocked. Renovascular hypertension is often caused fatty plaques (atherosclerosis) or due to the muscle and fibrous tissues of the renal artery wall that thickens and forms rings (fibromuscular dysplasia).
- **Cushing syndrome.** Overuse of corticosteroid medications or excess production of the hormone ACTH (adrenocorticotropic hormone) from a pituitary tumor or overproduction of cortisol from the adrenal glands increases blood volume and causes hypertension.
- **Aldosteronism.** A growth (tumor) in one or both of the adrenal glands, increased growth of normal cells (hyperplasia) in one or both of the adrenal glands cause the adrenal glands to release an excessive amount of the hormone aldosterone. This makes your kidneys retain salt and water and lose potassium, which causes hypertension.
- **Pheochromocytoma.** This is a rare tumor that is usually found in an adrenal gland which increases the production of the hormones adrenaline and noradrenaline leading to severe and labile (blood pressure spikes) hypertension. Symptoms may include headache, fast heart rate, skipped heart beats, and sweating.
- **Thyroid problems.** If the thyroid gland (located in your neck) does not make enough thyroid hormone (hypothyroidism) or produces too much thyroid hormone (hyperthyroidism), then hypertension may occur.
- **Acromegaly (gigantism):** This occurs due to overproduction of growth hormone by the pituitary gland in the brain.
- **Hyperparathyroidism.** The parathyroid glands are positioned in your neck behind the thyroid gland and they regulate levels of calcium and phosphorus in your blood and tissues. If the glands secrete too much parathyroid hormone, the amount of calcium in your blood rises and phosphorus falls and the blood pressure increases.
- **Coarctation of the aorta.** This is a disease usually present at birth where the body's main artery (aorta) is narrowed (coarctation). This forces the heart to pump harder to get blood through the narrowing and to the rest of your body. The leg blood pressures are lower than they should be compared to the arm blood pressure.
- **Sleep apnea (OSA or obstructive sleep apnea)** is associated with severe snoring, breathing repeatedly stops and starts during sleep, causing you to not get enough oxygen and increasing carbon dioxide. Sleep apnea causes the nervous system to be overactive and release adrenaline and noradrenaline as well as cortisol that increases blood pressure and causes arterial damage.
- **Obesity increases blood pressure due to many factors.** Fat tissue (adipose tissue) especially around the abdomen makes over 45 "adipokines" that are types of hormones and other compounds that cause inflammation, oxidative stress, salt and water retention, hypertension, and cardiovascular disease.
- **Pregnancy.** Pregnancy can make existing high blood pressure worse or may cause high blood pressure to develop during pregnancy such as pregnancy-induced hypertension, preeclampsia, or eclampsia.

(*Continued*)

TABLE 3.1 ***(Continued)***
Causes of Secondary Hypertension (1, 11, 19, 20)

- **Stress, anxiety, and depression.**
- **Alcohol.**
- **Caffeine** in patients that metabolize it slowly due to their genetics.
- **Smoking and other tobacco products.**
- **Nicotine** in smokers or in other compounds.
- **Heavy metals** such as lead, mercury, arsenic, and cadmium.
- **Pollution** of any type (air, water, soil).
- **Sodas** of any type. (Regular and those with artificial sweeteners.)
- **Plastic containers** and bottles, especially bottled water (BPA-bisphenol A).
- **Fructose** (high fructose corn syrup).
- **Artificial sweeteners.**
- **Proton pump inhibitors (PPI) and H2 blockers** that reduce stomach acid.
- **Medications and supplements.** A variety of prescription medications and ever the counter medications may increase blood pressure.

- Poor diet with high sodium, low potassium, low magnesium, not enough fruits and vegetables, not enough quality protein, too much trans fats and certain saturated fat, too much sugar and refined carbohydrates and starches, and possibly caffeine. We will discuss this in detail in the nutrition chapters in this book.
- Too much emotional stress, anxiety, hostility, or depression.
- Low income is associated with higher blood pressure for unknown reasons.
- Less education is associated with higher blood pressure for unknown reasons.

3.4 PROPER MEASUREMENT OF BLOOD PRESSURE: THE AMERICAN HEART ASSOCIATION (AHA) CRITERIA AND KOROTKOFF SOUNDS

A proper and accurate measurement of blood pressure in your physician's office is the first and most important step to determine if you have hypertension using the American Heart Association (AHA) criteria. These will be listed next. Office blood pressure on your first visit should be measured in both arms, in three positions, lying, sitting, and standing, and in your legs with a heart rate for each blood pressure reading. (1, 19, 20) Normally, the arm pressures are the same, but some arterial problems can cause a significant difference between the two arms. This is called "**interarm variation of blood pressure**" and if it is over 10 mm Hg SBP, then an underlying problem may be present 80% of the time and should be identified. (1, 19, 20) Some of these causes include increased arterial stiffness, atherosclerosis, muscular beading of the arm artery, vasculitis (artery inflammation), radiation arteritis, a blockage in the artery from an outside structural problems with pressure on the artery (thoracic outlet syndrome,) subclavian artery stenosis (the big artery in the chest that goes into the arm to form the brachial artery), dissecting aortic aneurysm (weakness in the artery muscle that causes tears in the aorta and risk for dilation and rupture), and finally various types of congenital abnormalities.

The leg SBP should be at least 10 mm Hg higher than the arm SBP. If the leg pressure is less than 10 mm Hg systolic, it suggests an arterial disease or blockage between the heart and the leg. (1, 19, 20) Supine leg pressure is higher by 17 mm in ankle and 10 mm Hg in the calf versus the arm. There are several sounds that your doctor will listen for with their stethoscope to determine your systolic and DBP. These called the **Korotkoff sounds and have five phases**. (1, 19, 20)

Phase I: Marked by the first appearance of faint, clear tapping sounds that gradually increase in intensity. Phase I should be used as the SBP.

Phase II: Period during which a murmur or swishing sound is heard.

Phase III: Period during which sounds are crisper and increase in intensity.

Phase IV: Period marked by the distinct, abrupt muffling of sound (soft, blowing quality is heard).

Phase V: The point at which sounds disappear. Phase V should be used as the DBP (except on rare occasions, e.g., aortic valve insufficiency, which is a leaky valve).

3.4.1 BP Measurement in the Office

In your physician's office, the blood pressure is measured noninvasively with a blood pressure cuff called a sphygmomanometer with two methods (1, 19, 20). The traditional method involves placing a stethoscope over the brachial artery by your doctor to detect the appearance and muffling or disappearance of the blood pressure sounds called **Korotkoff sounds** that determine the systolic and the DBP. Over the past 30 years, other automated techniques, also using an arm cuff to listen to the brachial artery, have been developed for office and home use. The accuracy of the blood pressure readings relies on standardized techniques and appropriate observer training. You must purchase a validated and good home blood pressure machine and be instructed in their proper use by your doctor to avoid inaccurate blood pressure readings. *Automated wrist cuffs and finger cuffs are not recommended for either office or home use as they are not accurate or reliable*.

The proper measurement of the arm blood pressure is published by the **American Heart Association and the American College of Cardiology (see next)**. (1, 19) You should observe if the suggestions are followed in the doctor's office to be sure that you have an accurate blood pressure reading.

1. The patient should be seated in a chair with their back supported and feet on the floor for 5 minutes in a quiet, comfortable environment. The arm should be free of restrictive clothing (bare arm) or other materials and supported at heart level. The patient should avoid exertion, temperature extremes, eating, caffeine, alcohol, or smoking for 1 hour before measuring blood pressure. They should have an empty bladder and should not talk or move during the blood pressure measurement.

2. The observer (clinician) should be at eye level of the meniscus of the mercury column of the blood pressure equipment or centered in front of the blood pressure gauge to avoid a strained posture. The arm of the patient should be supported and held at the level of their heart.
3. The appropriate cuff size should be selected (standard, large, or pediatric). The cuff bladder should be 20% wider than the diameter of the extremity. The bladder length should be approximately twice the recommended width. There are white lines on the cuff to assist in this technique.
4. The deflated cuff should be placed at least 2.5 cm (1 in.) above the antecubital space (the area opposite the elbow). The cuff should fit smoothly and snugly around the arm, with the bladder centered directly over the brachial artery.
5. Palpate for the brachial pulse. To estimate the SBP, rapidly inflate the cuff until the brachial pulse can no longer be felt.
6. Place the bell of the stethoscope over the previously palpated brachial artery. Rapidly inflate the cuff to 30 mm Hg above the point at which the brachial pulse disappears; deflate the cuff at the rate of 2–3 mm Hg/s.
7. Record the SBP as the first Korotkoff sound and DBP as the fifth Korotkoff sound.
8. Allow 1–2 minutes between BP determinations.
9. The blood pressure should then be determined in the upright posture after the patient has been standing for 2 minutes with pulse rate. The arm should be positioned at heart level, with the forearm at the horizontal level of the fourth intercostal space (the rib cage space on the front of the chest).
10. On the initial visit, blood pressure readings should be performed in both arms and in the thigh. Subsequent BP determinations should be performed in the arm with the higher reading, if there is more than a 10 mm Hg discrepancy in BP reading.
11. Automated wrist cuffs and finger cuffs are not recommended for either office or home use as they are not accurate or reliable!

3.5 COMMON MISTAKES IN BLOOD PRESSURE MEASUREMENT (1, 19, 20)

1. Failure to keep the person in the supine position for 5 minutes before measuring the supine blood pressure.
2. Failure to keep the arm at the level of the heart and supported. If the arm is lower than the heart level, the blood pressure is falsely high. If the arm is elevated above the heart level, the blood pressure is falsely low.
3. If the Korotkoff sounds cannot be heard, failure to completely deflate the cuff before determining blood pressure and failure to wait 1–2 minutes before doing further determinations.
4. Observer error, because of hearing impairment, bias (preferring some digits over others), or unconscious bias toward underreading or over-reading blood pressure depending on dividing line of normal.

5. Failure to keep the eyes at the level of the mercury manometer or the gauge.
6. Deflating the cuff too rapidly. The cuff should be deflated at a rate of 2–3 mm Hg/s.
7. Failure to use appropriate cuff size. Use of a regular adult cuff for obese patients or those with a large arm leads to a high blood pressure reading, while using a large cuff on a normal-size arm will underestimate the blood pressure. So, it is recommended to use a large adult cuff or thigh cuff for obese persons and a child's cuff for children. The cuff should cover two-thirds of the arm above the antecubital space.
8. Failure to position the cuff correctly. The cuff should be placed 2–3 cm above the antecubital space.
9. Failure to provide a conducive environment: Comfortable room temperature and quiet surroundings free of noises and distracting stimuli.
10. Missing the heartbeat during auscultation in patients with excessive bradycardia.
11. Patient has consumed alcohol, caffeine, smoked recently, is under stress, has a full bladder, or is talking.
12. Using noncalibrated or nonvalidated blood pressure devices.

3.6 CLASSIFICATION OF HYPERTENSION: AHA/ASH/ACC

Blood pressure categories (1, 19) in the new guideline are as follows:

- **Normal**: Less than 120/80 mm Hg.
- **Elevated**: Systolic between 120 and 129 *and* diastolic less than 80.
- **Stage 1**: Systolic between 130 and 139 *or* diastolic between 80 and 89.
- **Stage 2**: Systolic at least 140 *or* diastolic at least 90 mm Hg.
- **Hypertensive crisis**: Systolic over 180 and/or diastolic over 120, with patients needing prompt changes in medication if there are no other indications of problems, or immediate hospitalization if there are signs of organ damage.

The guidelines eliminated the category of prehypertension, categorizing patients as having either elevated (120–129 and less than 80) or stage 1 hypertension (130–139 or 80–89).

3.6.1 Twenty-Four-Hour Ambulatory Blood Pressure Monitoring (24-hour ABPM)

The 24-hour ABPM (twenty-four-hour ambulatory blood pressure monitoring) is the "gold standard" for the measurement of blood pressure, to predict cardiovascular events, for the proper selection of both supplement and drug therapies and to avoid either over or under treatment of hypertension (1, 11, 19, 20, 22). This test is simple to perform, very accurate and provides essential and valuable information to your doctor. A blood pressure cuff is attached to the arm which is connected to a small hand size computer that attaches to your waist and measures the blood pressure and heart rate at preset intervals for 24 hours. This allows numerous blood pressure and heart rate readings during the day, at night, during rest, during exercise, and other times of the day. You can determine the time of day for each reading, what you are doing at the time and many other important measurements as noted next. It is my opinion that this is a mandatory test for hypertension patients for all the next reasons.

3.6.2 Dipping Pattern

Normal dipping. At night, the average blood pressure should fall 10% below the average daytime blood pressure. Failure to do this increases the nighttime blood pressure force in the arteries and increases the risk of cardiovascular events. The arteries never get to "relax."

Excessive dipping at night is a drop in the nighttime blood pressure more than 10% of the average daytime blood pressure. This increases the risk for strokes related to blood clots, called ischemic strokes and heart attack.

Reverse dipping at night is an actual increase in the average nighttime blood pressure of less than 10% compared to the average daytime blood pressure. This increases the risk of bleed into the brain known as a hemorrhagic stroke or intracranial hemorrhage.

The nighttime blood pressure drives the risk for heart attack, stroke, and heart failure more than any other blood pressure measurement. It is important to know this and the dipping pattern to determine what time your doctor gives your medications (morning or night) as well as the type and dose of the medications.

Morning blood pressure surges increase the risk for stroke and heart attack, as well as heart enlargement, called left ventricular hypertrophy. An increase in the SBP over 35 mm Hg from the ideal of SBP of 121. 5 mm Hg is the definition of elevated morning blood pressure surges.

The blood pressure load is the number of blood pressure readings that are over 140/90 mm Hg. The normal blood pressure load should be less than 15%. Any blood pressure readings that are over this percentage increase the risk for cardiovascular events.

Blood pressure variability with wide swings of more than 20 mm Hg for SBP and more than 10 mm Hg for DBP increases cardiovascular events and kidney disease. Recent studies suggest that the even swings of SBP over 13 mm Hg will increase by four times the risk for coronary heart disease and heart attack.

White coat hypertension means that your blood pressure is elevated in the office but not at home. Recent studies suggest that WCH increases cardiovascular events. This occurs in about 20–25% of patients with hypertension. We will discuss this in more detail later in the book.

Masked hypertension means that your blood pressure is higher at home than in the office when your doctor measures it. MH is also associated with higher cardiovascular events, higher blood glucose levels, and loss of protein through the kidneys. MH has in incidence of about 10% in patients with hypertension. We will discuss this in more detail later in the book.

3.7 PRIMARY (ESSENTIAL OR GENETIC) AND SECONDARY HYPERTENSION

Hypertension is divided into two major groups. Primary hypertension, which means hypertension that runs in families, is also called **essential or genetic hypertension**, (1, 11, 19, 20) is the most common, and accounts for about 90–95% of all adult cases of hypertension.

Primary hypertension is diagnosed in the absence of a **secondary** or identifiable cause. **Secondary hypertension** – the other major group – accounts for around 5–10% of the cases of adult hypertension for which an underlying cause can be identified. Secondary hypertension can be caused by conditions that affect your kidneys, arteries, heart, or endocrine system (Table 3.1). Secondary hypertension can also occur during pregnancy. Importantly, secondary forms of hypertension, such as primary hyperaldosteronism (overproduction of the hormone aldosterone from the adrenal gland), account for 20% of resistant hypertension (hypertension in which BP is >140/90 mm Hg despite the use of medications from three or more drug classes, one of which is a diuretic).

3.8 SUMMARY AND KEY TAKEAWAY POINTS

1. Blood pressure = systemic vascular resistance × cardiac output.
2. A normal blood pressure is 120/80 mm Hg. The SBP is the top number when the heart pumps and the DBP is the bottom number when the heart is relaxed. Both predict cardiovascular events. SBP predicts cardiovascular events best in patients over the age of 55 years, while the DBP predicts the risk of cardiovascular events best in patients under the age of 55 years.
3. You can predict your risk of developing hypertension with the **31 CLUES** of clinical evaluations and lab testing.
4. Endothelial dysfunction, low nitric oxide, and damaged, enlarged, and stiff arteries walls (muscle or media) lead to cardiovascular events.
5. The blood vessel has only three finite responses to the infinite number of insults that can damage it. These include inflammation, oxidative stress, and vascular immune dysfunction or dysregulation.
6. The blood pressure must be properly and accurately measured in your doctor's office of the first and all subsequent visits using the AHA criteria. During the first office visit, the blood pressure is measured in both arms, the legs, and in three positions (lying, sitting, and standing).
7. The CBP predicts cardiovascular events better than the arm (brachial) blood pressure.
8. The exercise blood pressure must be measured. The SBP should not go over 180 mm Hg and the DBP should stay the same or decrease from the baseline resting levels.
9. The blood pressure measured by your doctor or nurse in the office may be measured by auscultation or by an oscillometric blood pressure machine.

10. Home blood pressure monitoring is important but you must obtain a reliable and validated blood pressure machine and be instructed in its proper use.
11. The 24-hour ABPM is the gold standard for the diagnosis and treatment of hypertension. It provides essential and valuable information such as dipping status, nighttime blood pressures, morning surges, liability and variability, blood pressure load, heart rate, WCH, and MH.
12. Your doctor should evaluate you for secondary causes of hypertension and measure your genetics for hypertension and CVD.

Pain relievers and arthritis medications such as aspirin and acetaminophen (Tylenol) and all of the **nonsteroidal anti-inflammatory drugs and cyclooxygenase inhibitors (COX-2 inhibitors)**:

1. Celecoxib (Celebrex).
2. Diclofenac (Cambia, Cataflam, Voltaren-XR, Zipsor, Zorvolex).
3. Ibuprofen (Motrin, Advil).
4. Indomethacin (Indocin).
5. Ketoprofen (Active-Ketoprofen [Orudis – discontinued brand]).
6. Naproxen (Aleve, Anaprox, Naprelan, Naprosyn).
7. Oxaprozin (Daypro).
8. Piroxicam (Feldene).

- **Birth control pills.**
- **Antidepressants** especially tricyclic antidepressants and MAO inhibitors.
- **Drugs used after organ transplants** such as cyclosporin.
- **Miscellaneous drugs and supplements**

1. Ginseng.
2. Licorice.
3. Ephedra (ma-Huang).
4. Diet pills.
5. Cocaine.
6. Amphetamines and methamphetamine.
7. Adderall, Ritalin, Concerta.
8. Decongestants and antihistamines, especially those containing pseudoephedrine.
9. Erythropoietin that is used for anemia in kidney disease.
10. Anabolic steroids.
11. Lithium.
12. Thallium.
13. Ergotamine.
14. Bromocriptine.
15. Metoclopramide.
16. Digitalis.
17. Disulfiram.
18. Migraine headache medications.

REFERENCES

1. Whelton PK, et al. ACC/AHA/AAPA/ABC/ACPM/AGS/APhA/ASH/ASPC/NMA/PCNA Guideline for the prevention, detection, evaluation, and management of high blood pressure in adults: a report of the American College of Cardiology/American Heart Association Task Force on Clinical Practice Guidelines. Hypertension. 2018 Jun;71(6):e13–e115.
2. Houston M. The role of nutrition and nutraceutical supplements in the treatment of hypertension. World J Cardiol. 2014;6(2):38–66.
3. Houston M. Nutrition and nutraceutical supplements for the treatment of hypertension: Part 1. J Clin Hypertens. 2013;15:752–757.
4. Houston M. Nutrition and nutraceutical supplements for the treatment of hypertension: Part II. J Clin Hypertens. 2013;15:845–851.
5. Houston M. Nutrition and nutraceutical supplements for the treatment of hypertension: Part III. J Clin Hypertens. 2013;15:931–937.
6. Borghi C, Cicero AF. Nutraceuticals with a clinically detectable blood pressure-lowering effect: a review of available randomized clinical trials and their meta-analyses. Br J Clin Pharmacol. 2017;83(1):163–171.
7. Sirtori CR, Arnoldi A, Cicero AF. Nutraceuticals for blood pressure control. Rev Ann Med. 2015;47(6):447–456.
8. Cicero AF, Colletti A. Nutraceuticals and blood pressure control: results from clinical trials and meta-analyses. High Blood Press Cardiovasc Prev. 2015;22(3):203–213.
9. Turner JM, Spatz ES. Nutritional supplements for the treatment of hypertension: a practical guide for clinicians. Curr Cardiol Rep. 2016;18(12):126. Review.
10. Caligiuri SP, Pierce GN. A review of the relative efficacy of dietary, nutritional supplements, lifestyle and drug therapies in the management of hypertension. Crit Rev Food Sci Nutr. 2016 Aug 5:0. [Epub ahead of print].
11. Houston MC, Fox B, Taylor N. What Your Doctor May Not Tell You About Hypertension. The Revolutionary Nutrition and Lifestyle Program to Help Fight High Blood Pressure. AOL Time Warner, Warner Books, New York, NY, 2003.
12. Houston M. Treatment of hypertension with nutrition and nutraceutical supplement: Part 1. Altern Complement Med. 2019;24:260–275.
13. Houston M. Treatment of hypertension with nutrition and nutraceutical supplement: Part 2. Altern Complement Med. 2019;25:23–36.
14. Sinatra S, Houston M, Editors. Nutrition and Integrative Strategies in Cardiovascular Medicine. CRC Press, 2015.
15. The seventh report of the Joint National Committee on prevention, detection, evaluation, and treatment of high blood pressure (JNC-7). JAMA. 2003;289:2560–2572.
16. Thomopoulos C, Parati G, Zanchetti A. Effects of blood pressure lowering on outcome incidence in hypertension: 7. Effects of more vs. less intensive blood pressure lowering and different achieved blood pressure levels – updated overview and meta-analyses of randomized trials. J Hypertens. 2016;34(4):613–622.
17. Ettehad D, Emdin CA, Kiran A, Anderson SG, Callender T, Emberson J, Chalmers J, Rodgers A, Rahimi K. Blood pressure lowering for prevention of cardiovascular disease and death: a systematic review and meta-analysis. Lancet. 2016;387(10022):957–967.
18. ESH/ESC Task Force for the Management of Arterial Hypertension. 2013 Practice guidelines for the management of arterial hypertension of the European Society of Hypertension (ESH) and the European Society of Cardiology (ESC): ESH/ESC Task Force for the Management of Arterial Hypertension. J Hypertens. 2013;31:1925–1938.

19. Flack JM, Calhoun D, Schiffrin EL. The new ACC/AHA Hypertension Guidelines for the prevention, detection, evaluation, and management of high blood pressure in adults. Am J Hypertens. 2018;31(2):133–135.
20. Houston MC. Handbook of Hypertension. Wiley Blackwell, 2009.
21. Park CM, Korolkova O, Davies JE, et al. Arterial pressure: agreement between a brachial cuff-based device and radial tonometry. J Hypertens. 2014 Apr;32(4):865–872.
22. Yang WY, Melgarejo JD Thijs L. Association of office and ambulatory blood pressure with mortality and cardiovascular outcomes. JAMA. 2019;322(5):409–420.

4 The Arteries, the Endothelium, Endothelial Dysfunction, Nitric Oxide, and Hypertension

The arteries are the vessels that carry blood from the heart to all the cells and tissues throughout the body. All of the arteries in the body have basically the same structure that consists of the following four parts (Figure 4.1) (1–13):

1. *The lumen (Figure 4.2).*
2. *The endothelium (Figures 4.3 and 4.4).*
3. *The artery muscle (media) (Figure 4.1).*
4. *The adventitia (Figure 4.1).*

The **lumen** is the inside of the artery (Figure 4.2) which would be similar to the inside of a water hose. Inside the lumen is the blood that contains red blood cells, white blood cells, platelets, plasma with various types of proteins like albumin, clotting factors, nutrients, and other blood components. The red blood cells carry oxygen to the cells and tissues throughout the body. If the red blood cell count is low, this is anemia and can result in poor oxygen delivery to vital organs such as the heart, brain, and kidneys. The white blood cells are involved in protecting us from infections, help to repair injuries, and provide an immune response to outside invaders. The white blood cells are involved in inflammation as well as immune function. The platelets and the coagulation factors help to form clots in the artery lumen if we bleed. The proteins, such as the globulins, are involved in immune function, and the plasma albumin helps to maintain the blood volume and blood flow. Lastly, all of the nutrients that are absorbed from our diet following digestion in the gastrointestinal tract are delivered into the blood for delivery to all of the cells and tissues. Many of the immune white blood cells, under certain conditions, are involved in hypertension as they may cause damage to the endothelium and artery muscle which will constrict and increase the blood pressure. Remember, inflammation is one of the three finite responses of the artery that induces high blood pressure. (1–13)

The endothelium is one of the most important parts of the artery and its role in protecting us from hypertension and cardiovascular disease is crucial. It is like the air traffic control tower that communicates to the blood cells and to the arterial muscle. (1–13) The **endothelium** is a thin layer of cells (Figure 4.3) that separates the blood from the muscle of the artery, called the **media** (Figure 4.1). The left side of the panel in Figure 4.3 is a normal endothelium, but the right side of the panel in the

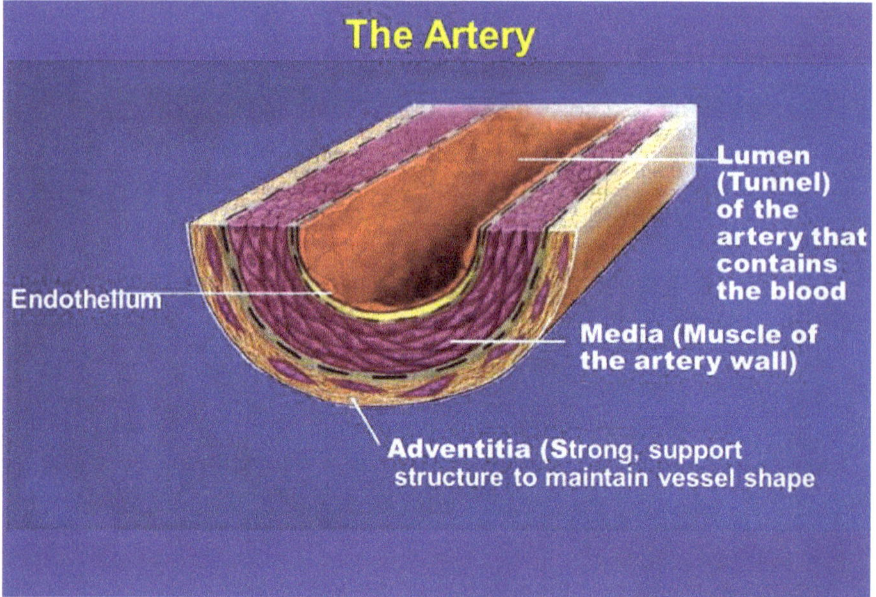

FIGURE 4.1 The artery.

figure is a damaged endothelium. There are many things that can damage the endothelium such as hypertension, high cholesterol, high blood sugar, and more. Both the structure and function of the endothelium are changed in the right panel. These changes are abnormal and are causes of the endothelium not to function in its usual

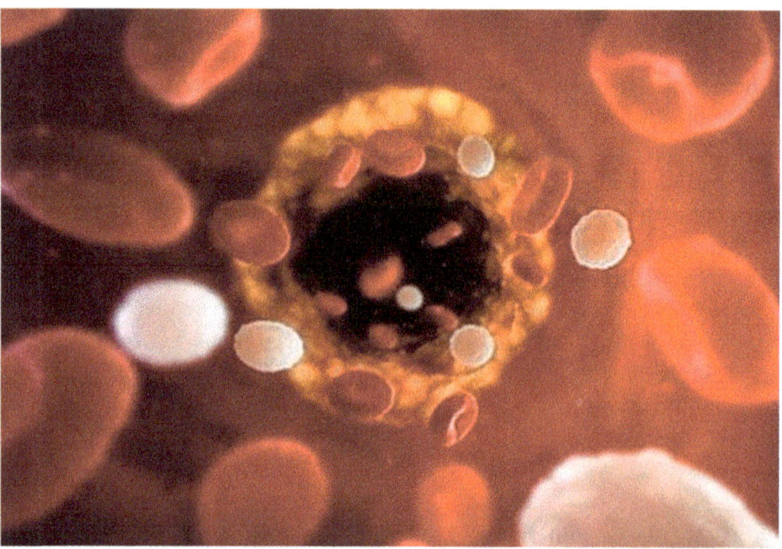

FIGURE 4.2 The lumen.

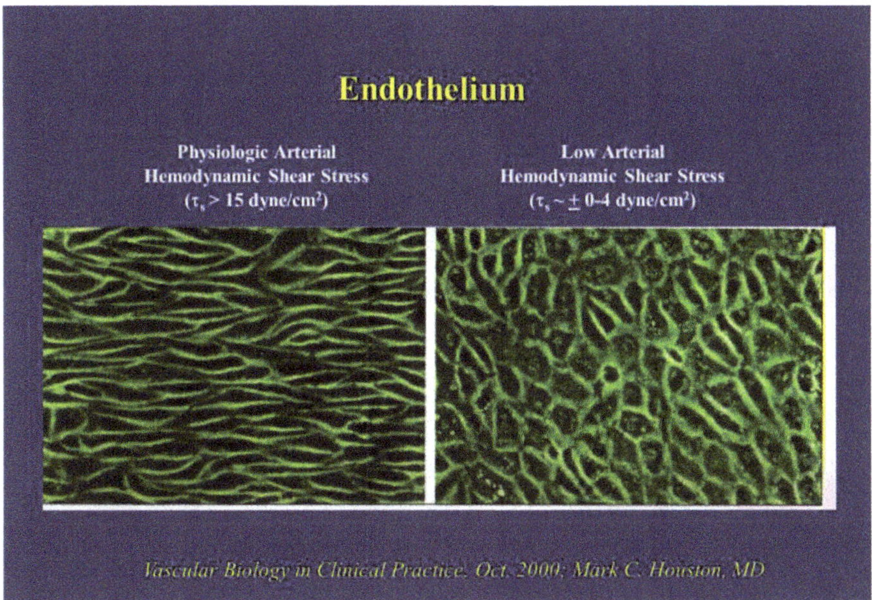

FIGURE 4.3 The endothelium.

fashion. The medical term for this is **endothelial dysfunction**. The endothelium serves a barrier (like a solid plank fence) to prevent things in the blood from crossing over into the arterial muscle. (1–13) However, just like the planks in the fence can be damaged and you can cross to the other side of the fence, the endothelium may be damaged, some of the endothelial cells get separated, it will start to leak (**see the right side of the panel in** Figure 4.3).

The endothelium lies in a very key area and determines what can happen in the blood and in the artery muscle (Figure 4.4). (1–13) The alterations in the blood will make the platelets stick together and form blood clots, make the white blood cells attach to the endothelial lining and cause inflammation, oxidative stress, immune dysfunction of the artery, and start the process of total arterial damage with accumulation of cholesterol, fats, and other substance leading to a blockage in the artery (a plaque or **atherosclerosis**) which can cause a heart attack or a stroke. If the blood pressure is high, then this process of forming a plaque will progress faster and be more severe.

The alterations to the arterial muscle include leaking of the blood vessel with the loss of proteins into the cells and organs. If this happens in the kidney, then the proteins spill into the urine, which is very abnormal, and predict future kidney disease. Another alteration is the constriction or narrowing of the artery with reduced blood flow and hypertension. Finally, there may be abnormal growth, thickening, and stiffness of the artery which leads the medical disease called **arteriosclerosis**.

The endothelium acts like an endocrine organ that makes a lot of compounds that regulate the blood pressure and overall arterial health. One of these compounds is **nitric oxide** that helps to dilate the artery and lower the blood pressure. Nitric oxide

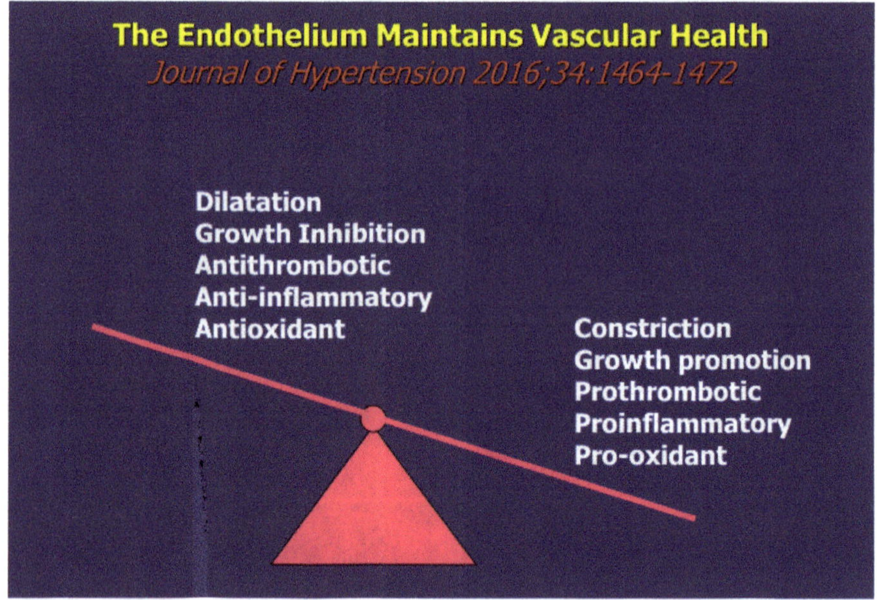

FIGURE 4.4 The vascular endothelium.

is a short-live gas that also provides numerous other health benefits to the artery and to reduce cardiovascular disease. The endothelium must function normally to prevent hypertension. (1–13) The endothelium is the largest organ in the body. (2–5, 11–13) Its size is of 6.5 tennis courts or about 14,000 square feet. (2–5, 11–13)

If the endothelium becomes damaged and does not make as much nitric oxide but rather produces other compounds that damage the arteries, it causes them to constrict increase the blood pressure. (2–5, 11–13) This "*endothelial dysfunction*" may precede the development of hypertension by decades. (2–5, 11–13)

As the endothelium is damaged, in addition to losing its ability to make *nitric oxide* and many other substances that allow the artery to dilate and help keep the blood pressure lower, inflammation, oxidative stress, and immune artery dysfunction occur. All of these consequences increase the risk of heart attack, heart failure, stroke, and generalized *atherosclerosis* with plaque build-up as well as hardening (stiffness or *arteriosclerosis*) of the arteries. As the artery becomes stiff and losses its elastic stretch, the blood pressure goes higher and the artery can leak, burst, or form a clot. This results in a heart attack or a stroke. (1–13)

4.1 THE ARTERY MUSCLE OR MEDIA

The media is the muscle of the artery (Figure 4.1). This would be similar to an actual outside of a water hose. The muscle of the artery can dilate or constrict which will change the flow in the artery and the blood pressure. Depending on the size of the artery, there may more or less muscle. For example, the aorta is the largest artery in the body and has a significant amount of muscle. However, the smaller arteries in the coronary heart arteries and the brain have less muscle and more endothelium. If the blood pressure is elevated, it will cause all of the arteries to become thicker and stiffer, which may seriously reduce the blood flow in the smaller arteries to the heart, brain, and kidney resulting in disease. Also, the arteries could primarily become stiff and thick due to other reasons such as high blood sugar, high cholesterol, smoking, and genetics which lead to hypertension.

4.2 THE ADVENTITIA

The adventitia (Figure 4.1) is the outermost layer of the artery that surrounds the muscle and provides support to the artery and also supplies blood to the artery through small arteries called the vasa vasorum.

4.3 WHAT COMES FIRST, BAD ARTERIES OR HYPERTENSION?

Recent scientific studies suggest that the abnormalities of the arterial muscle, heart muscle, and endothelial dysfunction occur decades before the blood pressure increases. However, once the blood pressure increases, there is more damage to the endothelium and the arteries. In other words, the blood pressure and artery have a "bidirectional" effect on one another, that is, it goes both ways. The abnormal artery increases the blood pressure and then the blood pressure causes more damage to the artery. It is a continuous back-and-forth process that causes cardiovascular disease. This is important because we have endothelial, artery, and heart tests that can be measured noninvasively to determine the presence of abnormalities and start treatments before the blood pressure starts to increase. If you have a family history of hypertension, it is likely that your arteries and your heart start to develop functional and structural abnormalities that your doctor can find before your blood pressure starts to increase. Hypertension may then initially be a disease of the artery and one of the ways that arterial disease will show up in you is hypertension!

4.4 SUMMARY AND KEY TAKEAWAY POINTS

1. The arteries have four parts: lumen, endothelium, muscle, and adventitia.
2. The endothelium is like the air traffic control system of the artery and determines what happens in the blood and the artery muscle such as clotting, leakage or contraction of the muscle, growth, inflammation, oxidative stress or immune dysfunction of the artery, atherosclerosis, arteriosclerosis, and hypertension.
3. The endothelium makes nitric oxide that helps one to reduce blood pressure and cardiovascular disease.
4. Endothelial dysfunction and artery and heart abnormalities may precede the development of hypertension by decades.
5. Hypertension is a disease of the artery function and structure which occurs first and is genetic.
6. The effects of the blood pressure on the artery are bidirectional.

REFERENCES

1. Whelton PK et al. ACC/AHA/AAPA/ABC/ACPM/AGS/APhA/ASH/ASPC/NMA/PCNA Guideline for the prevention, detection, evaluation, and management of high blood pressure in adults: a report of the American College of Cardiology/American Heart Association Task Force on Clinical Practice Guidelines. Hypertension. Jun 2018;71(6):e13–e115.
2. Houston M. The role of nutrition and nutraceutical supplements in the treatment of hypertension. World J Cardiol. 2014;6(2):38–66.
3. Houston M. Nutrition and nutraceutical supplements for the treatment of hypertension: Part 1. J Clin Hypertens. 2013;15:752–757.
4. Houston M. Nutrition and nutraceutical supplements for the treatment of hypertension: Part II. J Clin Hypertens. 2013;15:845–851.
5. Houston M. Nutrition and nutraceutical supplements for the treatment of hypertension: Part III. J Clin Hypertens. 2013;15:931–937.
6. Borghi C, Cicero AF. Nutraceuticals with a clinically detectable blood pressure-lowering effect: a review of available randomized clinical trials and their meta-analyses. Br J Clin Pharmacol. 2017;83(1):163–171.
7. Sirtori CR, Arnoldi A, Cicero AF. Nutraceuticals for blood pressure control. Rev Ann Med. 2015;47(6):447–456.
8. Cicero AF, Colletti A. Nutraceuticals and blood pressure control: results from clinical trials and meta-analyses. High Blood Press Cardiovasc Prev. 2015;22(3):203–213.
9. Turner JM, Spatz ES. Nutritional supplements for the treatment of hypertension: a practical guide for clinicians. Curr Cardiol Rep. 2016;18(12):126. Review.
10. Caligiuri SP, Pierce GN. A review of the relative efficacy of dietary, nutritional supplements, lifestyle and drug therapies in the management of hypertension. Crit Rev Food Sci Nutr. 2017;57:3508–3527.
11. Houston MC, Fox B, Taylor N. What Your Doctor May Not Tell You About Hypertension. The Revolutionary Nutrition and Lifestyle Program to Help Fight High Blood Pressure. AOL Time Warner, Warner Books, New York, NY, 2003.
12. Houston M. Treatment of hypertension with nutrition and nutraceutical supplement: Part 1. Altern Complement Med. 2019;24:260–275.
13. Houston M. Treatment of hypertension with nutrition and nutraceutical supplement: Part 2. Altern Complement Med. 2019;25:23–36.

5 The Three Finite Vascular Responses That Cause Hypertension

Inflammation, Oxidative stress, and Vascular Immune Dysfunction

Hypertension is one of the insults, "**biomechanical**," that will damage the arteries and the heart. (1–12) Changes in the blood pressure and the blood flow will stimulate **receptors** on the artery that have long fancy names as shown in Figure 5.1 that result in one or all of the three finite responses of inflammation, oxidative stress, and immune artery dysfunction (Figures 5.1 and 5.2). (1–12) The receptors in the artery are like a "**lock and key system**." The insults are the keys and the arterial receptors are the locks. However, we have discussed in the previous chapter, the relationship between the blood pressure and the function and structure of the artery is "**bidirectional**," that is it goes both ways. (1–12) The abnormal artery increases the blood pressure and then the blood pressure causes more damage to the artery. It is a continuous back-and-forth process that causes cardiovascular disease.

There are other insults called "**biochemical**" that include high cholesterol, high blood sugar, diabetes mellitus, toxins, metabolic issues, and infections that can also stimulate the same receptors and exacerbate the hypertension or cause cardiovascular disease. (1–12) If you start to add more and more insults, then there will be more cardiovascular disease. For example, hypertension with high cholesterol or diabetes mellitus is much worse than any of these by itself to cause cardiovascular disease. Some of the insults are considered to be like a "foreign invader" and are called **antigens or neoantigens** (new antigen or like an antigen). This simply means that the body does not recognize them as friendly and will send out the troops and military to fight. The finite processes are designed to protect the artery from damage in the acute setting. However, if they become chronic, then the blood pressure starts to increase and the artery is damaged.

As we will discuss, it is important to find the cause of the finite responses and treat them in order to manage and control the blood pressure better and thus reduce cardiovascular disease. (1–12)

Oxidative stress is an imbalance of radical oxygen species **(ROS)** (the bad guys) with a decrease in antioxidant defenses (the good guys) that contributes to

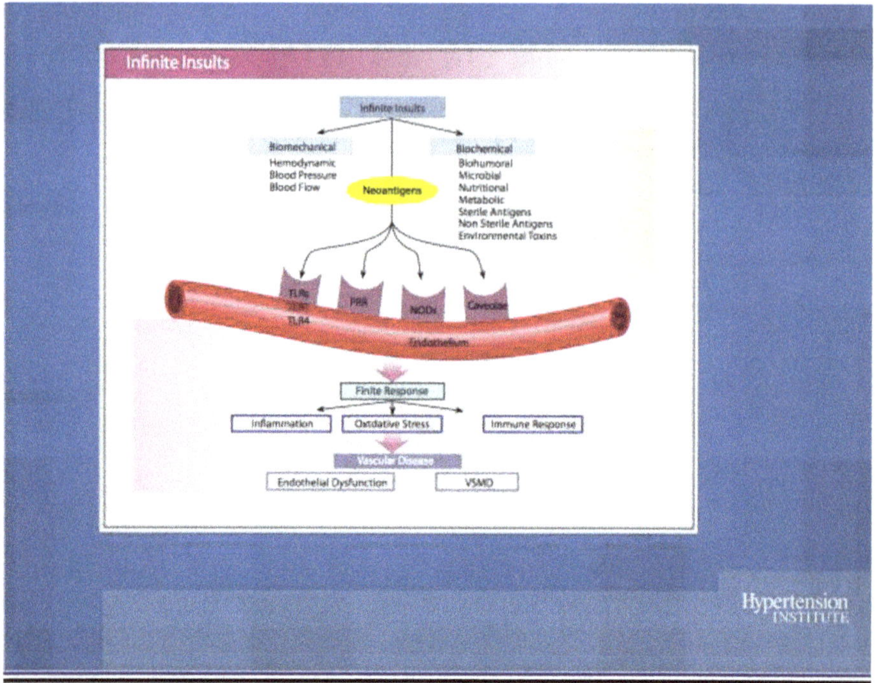

FIGURE 5.1 Infinite insults (biomechanical and biochemical groups noted in "*blue*") to the blood vessel (noted in "*red*") result in only three finite responses of inflammation, oxidative stress, and vascular immune dysfunction. The biomechanical insults are the blood pressure and blood flow. These insults attach to receptors (in purple) sitting on the artery to induce the arterial and heart disease. The receptors have various names like **pattern recognition receptors (PRR), toll-like receptors (TLR)**, noted in "*purple*" and others that control what happens in the endothelium and the artery called vascular smooth muscle dysfunction or **VSMD** as noted.

hypertension in humans on the basis of genetics and environment. (2–5, 11–14, 23–37). Oxidative stress is like having too much fire, i.e., too much ROS, and no fire extinguishers to put out the fire, i.e., not having enough antioxidants. The oxidative stress will damage cells to the point that they do not function or they die. If this happens in the arteries, then you get hypertension, arteriosclerosis, or atherosclerosis (defined in previous chapters). If it happens in the heart, you get coronary heart disease, a heart attack, or heart failure. If this happens in the brain, then you get a stroke. If it happens in the kidney, you get kidney failure. It is important that we balance the oxidative stress and the oxidative defense. The predominant ROS produced by cells is called **superoxide anion** and is part of our normal metabolism or break down of our food to make energy. In addition, the **superoxide anion reduces nitric oxide** that leads to endothelial dysfunction and hypertension. (24, 27) Our antioxidant defense is supplied by various compounds called enzymes that will break down the ROS and also by the intake of vitamins, minerals, and antioxidants in our diet or in

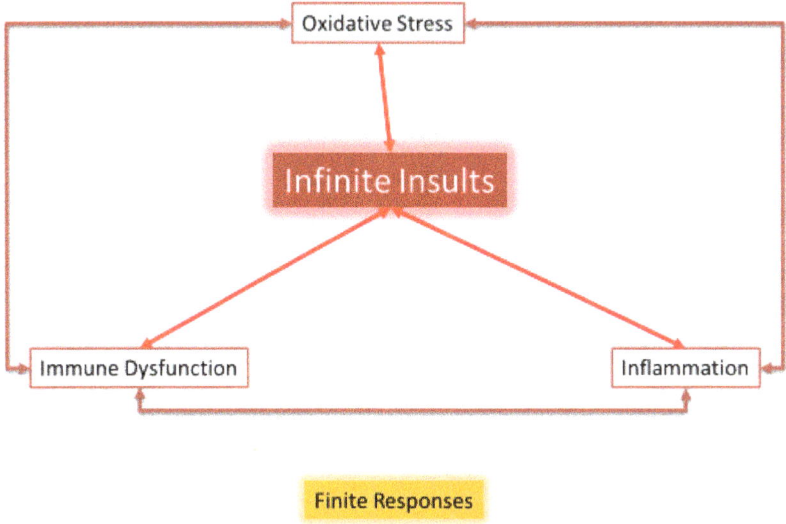

FIGURE 5.2 Infinite insults, such as hypertension, start the process of the three finite vascular responses of inflammation, oxidative stress, and vascular immune dysfunction leading to endothelial dysfunction, cardiac and vascular dysfunction.

supplements. Antioxidant deficiency with an excess of ROS has been implicated in human hypertension in many clinical studies. (29–31)

Inflammation is due to white blood cells and called T cells and B cells that attack invaders such as bacteria, viruses, and other insults to contain, remove, and kill them. The redness, swelling, and pain that you would see on your skin after a burn or an infection with bacteria is inflammation. This same response occurs in the arteries and causes hypertension and artery damage. Acute and chronic inflammation with abnormal vascular immune responses and the involvement of **pattern recognition receptors** and **toll-like receptors** are definitely involved in hypertension on the basis of recent research and clinical studies (2–5, 11–14, 33–50) There are numerous inflammatory compounds that can be measured in the blood and that are excellent markers for hypertension and cardiovascular disease. (2–5, 11–14, 33–50) For example, an elevated high sensitivity C reactive protein (hs-CRP) is both a risk marker and a risk factor for hypertension and cardiovascular disease. (2, 38, 39) Increases in hs-CRP of over 3 μg/ml in the blood may increase blood pressure rapidly that is proportional to the blood hs-CRP level. (38–39) Nitric oxide is also inhibited by hs-CRP and this can directly increase blood pressure by attaching to receptors on the artery causing constriction and narrowing of the artery. (38, 39, 44, 49)

The **immune system** is closely involved with inflammation with the same T cells and B cells and other immune and inflammation cells. The immune system is like a continuous "security system" that is monitoring your blood for invaders such as bacteria, other infections, and toxins. (2–4, 35–36, 40–50) The immune system is there to protect you and your arteries from harm. However, if those immune responses become chronic or imbalanced then the artery, heart, and kidney will be damaged and result in hypertension, cardiovascular disease, and kidney disease. (2–4, 35–36, 40–50) Monocytes, which are a type of white blood cell, sneak across the damaged endothelial cell lining and form new and larger cells called **macrophages** that cause atherosclerosis and increase blood pressure. (41, 44, 49–50) Many of these cells may play a major role in starting hypertension and keeping it going. (41)

In conclusion, oxidative stress, inflammation, and immune artery dysfunction cause hypertension. Controlling and treating all three of these finite artery responses will help one to lower the blood pressure. In other words, we have to rethink the older concepts of hypertension. It is now proven that your genetics interact with your environment to cause the three finite responses, hypertension and cardiovascular disease. Hypertension is an inflammatory, oxidative stress and immunologic disease and process!

5.1 SUMMARY AND KEY TAKEAWAY POINTS

1. The artery has only three finite artery responses to an infinite number of insults. If they become chronic, the blood pressure increases.
2. The insults are divided into two major groups: biomechanical and biochemical. Some of these insults are called "antigens" or "neoantigens" (a new antigen or like an antigen).
3. The insults attach to artery receptors (lock and key system) to produce oxidative stress, inflammation, and immune artery dysfunction.
4. Hypertension is a bidirectional (back-and-forth) process where arterial damage increases the blood pressure and hypertension damages the artery.
5. The finite responses can be measured with blood tests.
6. The finite response if treated correctly will reduce the blood pressure and reduce cardiovascular disease.

REFERENCES

1. Whelton PK, et al. ACC/AHA/AAPA/ABC/ACPM/AGS/APhA/ASH/ASPC/NMA/PCNA Guideline for the prevention, detection, evaluation, and management of high blood pressure in adults: a report of the American College of Cardiology/American Heart Association Task Force on Clinical Practice Guidelines. Hypertension. Jun 2018;71(6):e13–e115.
2. Houston M. The role of nutrition and nutraceutical supplements in the treatment of hypertension. World J Cardiol. 2014;6(2):38–66.
3. Houston M. Nutrition and nutraceutical supplements for the treatment of hypertension: Part 1. J Clin Hypertens. 2013;15:752–757.
4. Houston M. Nutrition and nutraceutical supplements for the treatment of hypertension: Part II. J Clin Hypertens. 2013;15:845–851.
5. Houston M. Nutrition and nutraceutical supplements for the treatment of hypertension: Part III. J Clin Hypertens. 2013;15:931–937.
6. Borghi C, Cicero AF. Nutraceuticals with a clinically detectable blood pressure-lowering effect: a review of available randomized clinical trials and their meta-analyses. Br J Clin Pharmacol. 2017;83(1):163–171.
7. Sirtori CR, Arnoldi A, Cicero AF. Nutraceuticals for blood pressure control. Rev Ann Med. 2015;47(6):447–456.

8. Cicero AF, Colletti A. Nutraceuticals and blood pressure control: results from clinical trials and meta-analyses. High Blood Press Cardiovasc Prev. 2015;22(3):203–213.
9. Turner JM, Spatz ES. Nutritional supplements for the treatment of hypertension: a practical guide for clinicians. Curr Cardiol Rep. 2016;18(12):126. Review.
10. Caligiuri SP, Pierce GN. A review of the relative efficacy of dietary, nutritional supplements, lifestyle and drug therapies in the management of hypertension. Crit Rev Food Sci Nutr. 2017;57:3508–3527.
11. Houston MC, Fox B, Taylor N. What Your Doctor May Not Tell You About Hypertension. The Revolutionary Nutrition and Lifestyle Program to Help Fight High Blood Pressure. AOL Time Warner, Warner Books, New York, NY, 2003.
12. Houston M. Treatment of hypertension with nutrition and nutraceutical supplement: Part 1. Altern Complement Med. 2019;24:260–275.
13. Houston M. Treatment of hypertension with nutrition and nutraceutical supplement: Part 2. Altern Complement Med. 2019;25:23–36.
14. Sinatra S, Houston M, Editors. Nutrition and Integrative Strategies in Cardiovascular Medicine. CRC Press, 2015.
15. The seventh report of the Joint National Committee on prevention, detection, evaluation, and treatment of high blood pressure (JNC-7). JAMA. 2003;289:2560–2572.
16. Thomopoulos C, Parati G, Zanchetti A. Effects of blood pressure lowering on outcome incidence in hypertension: 7. Effects of more vs. less intensive blood pressure lowering and different achieved blood pressure levels – updated overview and meta-analyses of randomized trials. J Hypertens. 2016;34(4):613–622.
17. Ettehad D, Emdin CA, Kiran A, Anderson SG, Callender T, Emberson J, Chalmers J, Rodgers A, Rahimi K. Blood pressure lowering for prevention of cardiovascular disease and death: a systematic review and meta-analysis. Lancet. 2016;387(10022):957–967.
18. ESH/ESC Task Force for the Management of Arterial Hypertension. 2013 Practice guidelines for the management of arterial hypertension of the European Society of Hypertension (ESH) and the European Society of Cardiology (ESC): ESH/ESC Task Force for the Management of Arterial Hypertension. J Hypertens. 2013;31:1925–1938.
19. Flack JM, Calhoun D, Schiffrin EL. The new ACC/AHA Hypertension Guidelines for the prevention, detection, evaluation, and management of high blood pressure in adults. Am J Hypertens. 2018;31(2):133–135.
20. Appel LJ; American Society of Hypertension Writing Group. ASH position paper: dietary approaches to lower blood pressure. J Am Soc Hypertens. 2009;3:321–331.
21. Eaton SB, Eaton SB III, Konner MJ. Paleolithic nutrition revisited: a twelve-year retrospective on its nature and implications. Eur J Clin Nutr. 1997;51:207–216.
22. Layne J, Majkova Z, Smart EJ, Toborek M, Hennig B. Caveolae: a regulatory platform for nutritional modulation of inflammatory diseases. J Nutr Biochem. 2011;22:807–811.
23. Dandona P, Ghanim H, Chaudhuri A, Dhindsa S, Kim SS. Macronutrient intake induces oxidative and inflammatory stress: potential relevance to atherosclerosis and insulin resistance. Exp Mol Med. 2010;42(4):245–253.
24. Kizhakekuttu TJ, Widlansky ME. Natural antioxidants and hypertension: promise and challenges. Cardiovasc Ther. 2010;28(4):e20–e32.
25. Houston MC. New insights and approaches to reduce end organ damage in the treatment of hypertension: subsets of hypertension approach. Am Heart J. 1992;123:1337–1367.
26. Nayak DU, Karmen C, Frishman WH, Vakili BA. Antioxidant vitamins and enzymatic and synthetic oxygen-derived free radical scavengers in the prevention and treatment of cardiovascular disease. Heart Dis. 2001;3:28–45.
27. Ritchie RH, Drummond GR, Sobey CG, De Silva TM, Kemp-Harper BK. The opposing roles of NO and oxidative stress in cardiovascular disease. Pharmacol Res. 2017;116:57–69.

28. Russo C, Olivieri O, Girelli D, Faccini G, Zenari ML, Lombardi S, Corrocher R. Antioxidant status and lipid peroxidation in patients with essential hypertension. J Hypertens. 1998;16:1267–1271.
29. Tse WY, Maxwell SR, Thomason H, Blann A, Thorpe GH, Waite M, Holder R. Antioxidant status in controlled and uncontrolled hypertension and its relationship to endothelial damage. J Hum Hypertens. 1994;8:843–849.
30. Galley HF, Thornton J, Howdle PD, Walker BE, Webster NR. Combination oral antioxidant supplementation reduces blood pressure. Clin Sci. 1997;92:361–365.
31. Dhalla NS, Temsah RM, Netticadam T. The role of oxidative stress in cardiovascular diseases. J Hypertens. 2000;18:655–673.
32. Loperena R, Harrison DG. Oxidative stress and hypertensive diseases. Med Clin North Am. 2017;101(1):169–193.
33. Pietri P, Vlachopoulos C, Tousoulis D. Inflammation and arterial hypertension: from pathophysiological links to risk prediction. Curr Med Chem. 2015;22(23):2754–2761.
34. Amer MS, Elawam AE, Khater MS, Omar OH, Mabrouk RA, Taha HM. Association of high-sensitivity C reactive protein with carotid artery intima media thickness in hypertensive older adults. J Am Soc Hypertens. 2011;5(5):395–400.
35. Kvakan H, Luft FC, Muller DN. Role of the immune system in hypertensive target organ damage. Trends Cardiovasc Med. 2009;19(7):242–246.
36. Rodriquez-Iturbe B, Franco M, Tapia E, Quiroz Y, Johnson RJ. Renal inflammation, autoimmunity and salt-sensitive hypertension. Clin Exp Pharmacol Physiol. 2012;39(1):96–103.
37. Mansego ML, Solar Gde M, Alonso MP, Martinez F, Saez GT, Escudero JC, Redon J, Chaves FJ. Polymorphisms of antioxidant enzymes, blood pressure and risk of hypertension. J Hypertens. 2011;29(3):492–500.
38. Vongpatanasin W, Thomas GD, Schwartz R, Cassis LA, Osborne-Lawrence S, Hahner L, Gibson LL, Black S, Samois D, Shaul PW. C-Reactive protein causes downregulation of vascular angiotensin subtype 2 receptors and systolic hypertension in mice. Circulation. 2007;115(8):1020–1028.
39. Razzouk L, Munter P, Bansilal S, Kini AS, Aneja A, Mozes J, Ivan O, Jakkula M, Sharma S, Farkouh ME. C reactive protein predicts long-term mortality independently of low-density lipoprotein cholesterol in patients undergoing percutaneous coronary intervention. Am Heart J. 2009;158(2):277–283.
40. Tian N, Penman AD, Mawson AR, Manning RD Jr, Flessner MF. Association between circulating specific leukocyte types and blood pressure. The atherosclerosis risk in communities(ARIC) study. J Am Soc Hypertens. 2010;4(6):272–283.
41. Muller DN, Kvakan H, Luft FC. Immune-related effects in hypertension and target-organ damage. Curr Opin Nephrol Hypertens. 2011;20(2):113–117.
42. Leibowitz A, Schiffin EL. Immune mechanisms in hypertension. Curr Hypertens Rep. 2011;13(6):465–472.
43. Xiong S, Li Q, Liu D, Zhu Z. Gastrointestinal tract: a promising target for the management of hypertension. Curr Hypertens Rep. 2017;19:(4):31.
44. Caillon A, Mian MO, Fraulob-Aquino JC, Huo KG, Barhoumi T, Ouerd S, Sinnaeve PR, Paradis P, Schiffrin EL. Gamma delta T cells mediate angiotensin II-induced hypertension and vascular injury. Circulation. 2017;135(22):2155–2162. pii: CIRCULATIONAHA.116.027058. doi: 10.1161/CIRCULATIONAHA.116.027058.
45. Rudemiller NP, Crowley SD The role of chemokines in hypertension and consequent target organ damage. Pharmacol Res. 2017;119:404–411.
46. De Ciuceis C, Agabiti-Rosei C, Rossini C, Airò P, Scarsi M, Tincani A, Tiberio GA, Piantoni S, Porteri E, Solaini L, Duse S, Semeraro F, Petroboni B, Mori L, Castellano M, Gavazzi A, Agabiti-Rosei E, Rizzoni D. Relationship between different subpopulations of circulating CD4+ T lymphocytes and microvascular or systemic oxidative stress in humans. Blood Press. 2017;26(4):237–245.

47. Caillon A, Schiffrin EL. Role of inflammation and immunity in hypertension: recent epidemiological, laboratory, and clinical evidence. Curr Hypertens Rep. Mar 2016;18(3):21.
48. Abais-Battad JM, Dasinger JH, Fehrenbach DJ, Mattson DL. Novel adaptive and innate immunity targets in hypertension. Pharmacol Res. 2017;120:109–115. pii: S1043-6618(16)30860-X. doi: 10.1016/j.phrs.2017.03.015.
49. Biancardi VC, Bomfim GF, Reis WL, Al-Gassimi S, Nunes KP. The interplay between angiotensin II, TLR4 and hypertension. Pharmacol Res. 2017;120:88–96. pii: S1043-6618(16)30910-0. doi: 10.1016/j.phrs.2017.03.017.
50. Justin Rucker A, Crowley SD. The role of macrophages in hypertension and its complications. Pflugers Arch. 2017;469(3–4):419–430.

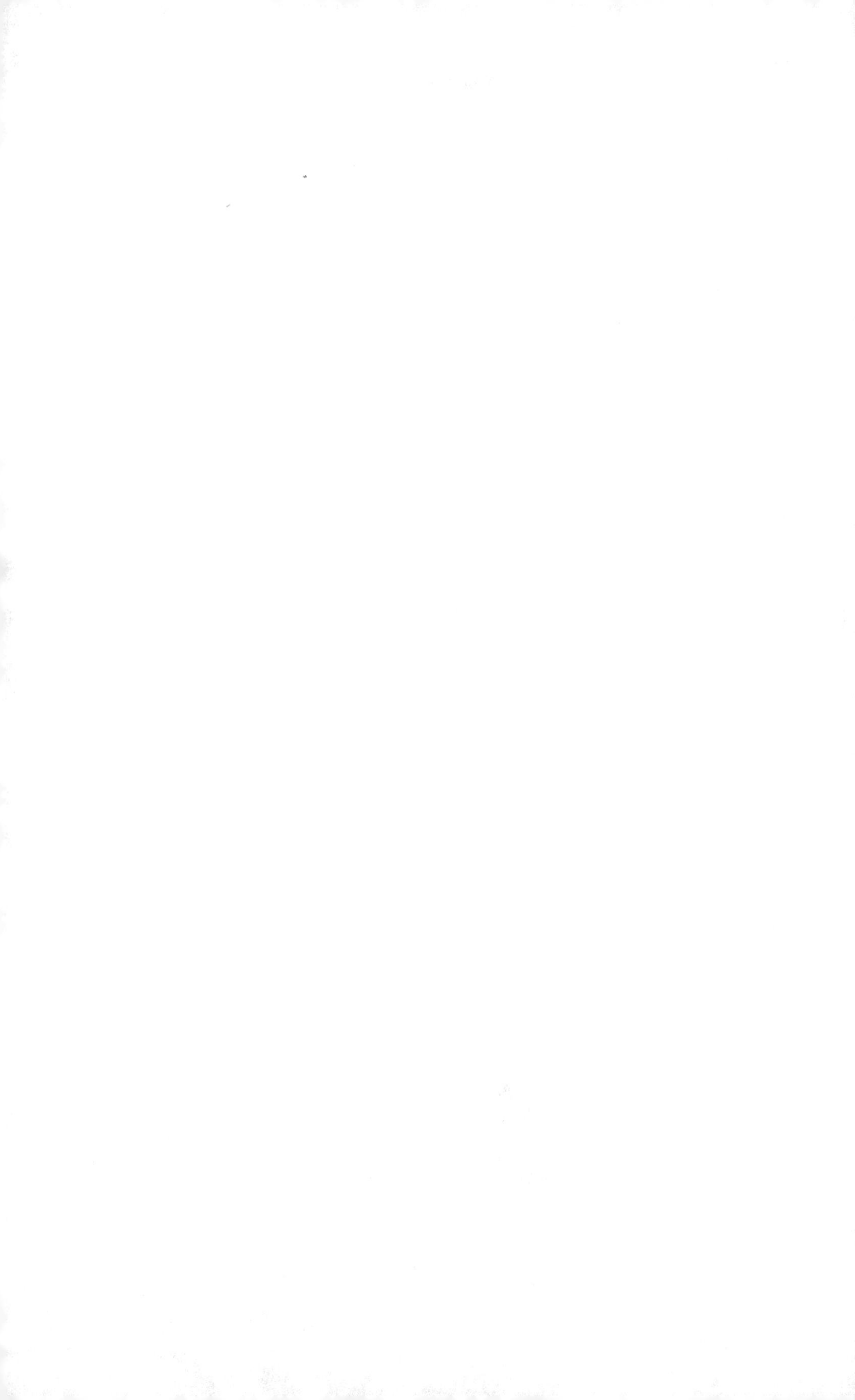

6 The Balance of Hypertension: Injury and Repair

Hypertension is a balance of **vascular damage and repair** (Figure 6.1). The **vascular damage** is caused by the three finite responses: angiotensin II, endothelin, and aldosterone. (1–9) Angiotensin II is a potent hormone that is made from several hormones that are first made in the liver. Angiotensin II produces inflammation, oxidative stress, and immune arterial dysfunction and causes the arteries to constrict, and the muscle of the artery becomes stiff, grown, and thickened, and it also remodels (change in structure of the artery), which increases blood pressure and atherosclerosis. (1–9) This "**remodeling**" means that the artery muscle not only grows and becomes thicker and stiffer, but also the lumen is smaller, which reduces the blood flow and oxygen delivery to the organs such as brain, heart, and kidney (Figure 6.2). (1–9) Endothelin is another potent hormone that increases blood pressure by causing marked constriction of the arteries, growth, stiffness, thickening, and "remodeling". Endothelin is also a cause of heart attack (Figure 6.2). (1–9) Aldosterone is a hormone that is made in the adrenal gland that sits on top of the kidney. Aldosterone also causes the arteries to grow, become stiff, and thicken, which increases blood pressure (Figure 6.2). It produces inflammation, oxidative stress, and immune arterial dysfunction. Aldosterone increases the reabsorption of sodium and water, which causes an increase in blood volume that may make the legs swell. Aldosterone will cause loss of potassium from the kidney, which may cause palpitations of the heart, fatigue, and leg cramps. The growth, thickening, and stiffness of the artery means that under times of stress or anxiety when you produce more adrenalin or the stress hormone cortisol, the artery is more likely to constrict to a greater degree which accounts for more labile and severe hypertension. (1–9) *The **vascular protection and repair*** is nitric oxide and bone marrow–derived endothelial progenitor cells (**EPCs**) (Figure 6.1). (1–9) The EPCs are young cells that are made in the bone marrow, migrate to the lining of the artery, the endothelium, deposit there, and mature into healthy normal endothelial cells. These new endothelial cells are able to make more nitric oxide, lower blood pressure, and keep the artery healthy to prevent damage to the arteries and heart disease. The endothelium maintains communication between the circulating blood cells and the arterial muscle. The EPCs are one of the most predictive of all known cardiovascular risk factors. If the EPCs are in low number or they are not healthy then you will have a higher risk of hypertension, diabetes, high cholesterol, and cardiovascular disease such as heart attack, angina, and stroke. (1–9)

It is very important to maintain a normal balance between the hormones that damage the artery and the EPCs that repair the artery. If our scale in Figure 6.1

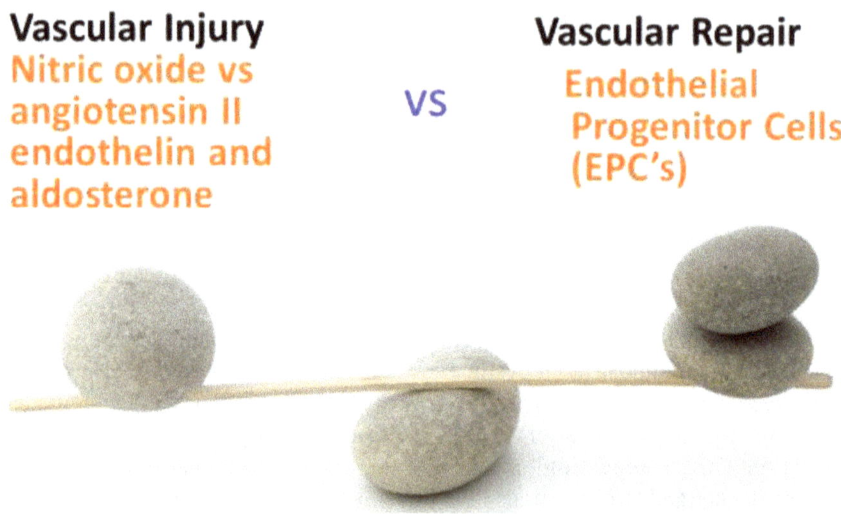

FIGURE 6.1 Cardiovascular disease is a balance of vascular injury and vascular repair.

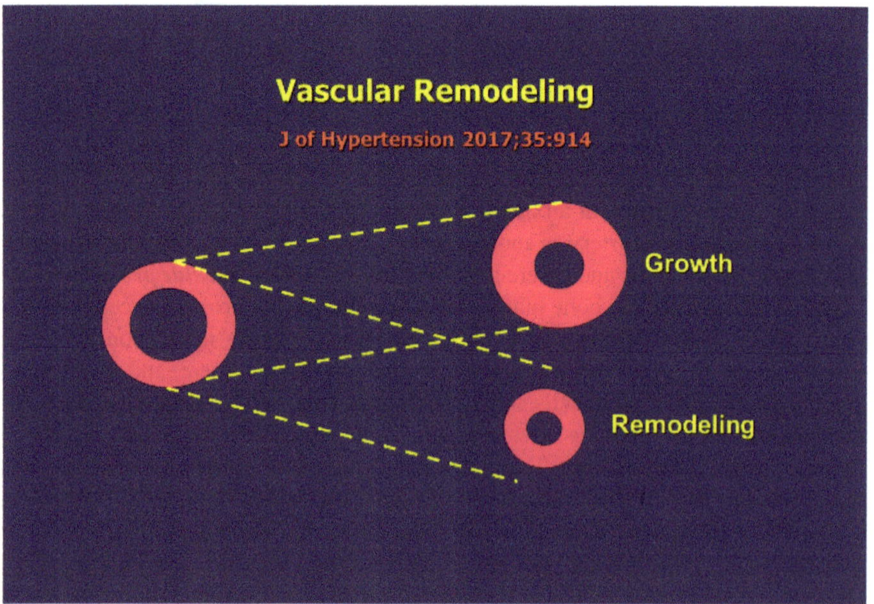

FIGURE 6.2 Artery thickness, growth, stiffness, and remodeling. Notice the thick arterial wall and the smaller lumen.

is overbalanced with angiotensin II, endothelin, or aldosterone, there will be an increase in the blood pressure acutely and chronically. (2–9) There are many treatments such as blood pressure–lowering drugs and some supplements that will be discussed later in the book, which can block or lower the levels of these hormones. The EPCs decrease with aging, smoking, high levels of angiotensin II, inflammation, oxidative stress, and arterial immune dysfunction. (2–9) The EPCs can be stimulated and increased by exercise, nitric oxide, certain blood pressure medications, statins (drugs used to lower cholesterol), and a supplement called resveratrol that comes from grapes, beets, and dark green leafy vegetables such as kale and spinach. (2–9)

6.1 SUMMARY AND KEY TAKEAWAY POINTS

1. The artery health is a balance between artery damage and repair.
2. The arterial damage is caused by many factors but especially due to inflammation, oxidative stress, and the hormones: angiotensin II, endothelin, aldosterone, adrenalin, and cortisol.
3. The arterial damage induces endothelial dysfunction and the artery becomes stiff, thick, grown, and remodeled, causing more arterial constriction and higher blood pressure.
4. The arterial repair is by nitric oxide and endothelial progenitor cells.
5. Many factors and treatments can improve the hormone levels and may impair or improve the production of endothelial progenitor cells.

REFERENCES

1. Whelton PK, et al. ACC/AHA/AAPA/ABC/ACPM/AGS/APhA/ASH/ASPC/NMA/PCNA guideline for the prevention, detection, evaluation, and management of high blood pressure in adults: a report of the American College of Cardiology/American Heart Association Task Force on Clinical Practice Guidelines. Hypertension. 2018;71(6): e13–e115.
2. Houston M. The role of nutrition and nutraceutical supplements in the treatment of hypertension. World J Cardiol. 2014;6(2):38–66.
3. Houston M. Nutrition and nutraceutical supplements for the treatment of hypertension: Part 1. J Clin Hypertens. 2013;15:752–757.
4. Houston M. Nutrition and nutraceutical supplements for the treatment of hypertension: Part II. J Clin Hypertens. 2013;15:845–851.
5. Houston M. Nutrition and nutraceutical supplements for the treatment of hypertension: Part III. J Clin Hypertens. 2013;15:931–937.
6. Houston MC, Fox B, Taylor N. What Your Doctor May Not Tell You About Hypertension. The Revolutionary Nutrition and Lifestyle Program to Help Fight High Blood Pressure. AOL Time Warner, Warner Books, New York, NY, 2003.
7. Houston M. Treatment of hypertension with nutrition and nutraceutical supplement: Part 1. Altern Compliment Med. 2019;24:260–275
8. Houston M. Treatment of hypertension with nutrition and nutraceutical supplement: Part 2. Altern Compliment Med. 2019;25:23–36
9. Sinatra S, Houston M, Editors. Nutrition and Integrative Strategies in Cardiovascular Medicine. CRC Press, 2015.

7 The Hypertension Syndrome: The Hypertension Partners and Special Forms of Hypertension: White Coat Hypertension and Masked Hypertension and Gender Differences in Hypertension

Hypertension does not usually occur by itself. Frequently, hypertension is associated with a variety of other medical problems or diseases. This is called the **Hypertension Syndrome** (Figure 7.1). (1–10) In fact, about 70% of the time one or more of the following is associated with hypertension: decreased arterial compliance (stiff, non-elastic arteries), endothelial dysfunction, abnormal blood glucose (blood sugar), or diabetes mellitus, neurohormonal dysfunction (imbalance of the nervous system and the hormones) that we discussed in the previous chapter, such as angiotensin II, endothelin, aldosterone, adrenalin, and cortisol (stress hormones made in the adrenal gland). In addition, there are changes in the kidney (renal function with loss of protein in the urine and poor kidney function), blood clots, insulin resistance (insulin does not work well to maintain a normal blood sugar), enlarged heart (left ventricular hypertrophy and dysfunction), atherosclerosis arteriosclerosis and atherogenesis, abnormal lipids (fats and cholesterol in the blood), and obesity.

7.1 WHY IS IT IMPORTANT THAT YOU KNOW ABOUT THE HYPERTENSION SYNDROME?

If you have hypertension, you must have the other parts of the Hypertension Syndrome evaluated by your doctor. There are several important reasons to do this.

SIDE BAR ON INSULIN RESISTANCE

Insulin resistance *means that the insulin that is released from the pancreas to the rest of the body does not work like it is supposed to because the organs have a "block" on its ability to enter the cells and reduces its effects inside the cell. In other words, those organs are partly or completely resistant to the effects of insulin to move glucose (blood sugar) into those cells for metabolism and energy production. This usually occurs in fat tissue (adipose tissue) especially the belly fat (called visceral fat) and the skeletal muscle. When this happens, the blood insulin level increases, the glucose increases, and these organs or tissues become "starved" of glucose that would normally provide energy. However, the kidney remains insulin sensitive, and the insulin works well. When insulin attaches to receptors in the kidney, it will cause an increase in the reabsorption of sodium and water to increase the blood volume and elevate the blood pressure. The insulin also causes inflammation of the arteries and makes them constrict which further elevates blood pressure and causes cardiovascular disease. Patients who are obese and have a large amount of belly or visceral fat are particularly likely to be insulin resistant.*

1. Each additional abnormality or disease that you have will increase your risk for cardiovascular disease (CVD). The more that you have, the greater the risk. For example, if you have hypertension and diabetes mellitus, depending on the severity and duration of each, your risk for a cardiovascular event could be two to five times greater.
2. Treatment of your hypertension not only can change the blood pressure level but also can either improve or worsen the other parts of the Hypertension Syndrome. For example, a good nutrition or supplement program usually improves blood pressure and other parts of the syndrome. However, some blood pressure lowering medications can have either a good or a bad effect on the other parts of the syndrome. For example, the blood pressure classes called ACEI (angiotensin-converting enzyme inhibitors) and ARBs (angiotensin receptor blockers) improve most of the other parts of the Hypertension Syndrome. However, other blood pressure lowering drugs such as beta blockers and many diuretics (water pills) may increase blood sugar, the blood cholesterol, and fats as well as worsen other parts of the Hypertension Syndrome. We will discuss all the blood pressure lowering medications later in the book. Your physician should check for all the parts of the syndrome with blood tests, urine tests, and noninvasive vascular tests at the beginning of your treatment and then they should be followed to be sure that all of the parts of the Hypertension Syndrome are improved.
3. Additional treatments may be needed in addition to your blood pressure lowering medications to improve the other parts of the Hypertension Syndrome such as your cholesterol, blood sugar, or kidney function.

7.2 WHITE COAT HYPERTENSION

The term "white coat hypertension" (WCH) means that your blood pressure is elevated in the doctor's office (i.e., the white coat designation), but it is normal at home when you are out of the doctor's office. (11–14) It used to be thought that WCH was benign and not associated with CVD compared to a person who has normal blood pressure. However, recent clinical studies suggest otherwise. (11–14) It has been shown that the cardiovascular risk for coronary heart disease, heart attack, stroke, heart failure, and kidney disease is somewhere in between the risk of a patient with chronic hypertension and a patient with normal blood pressure. (11–12)

- In untreated patients, WCH was associated with a 38% increased risk of CVD and a 20% increase in total mortality (death) compared with patients with normal blood pressure.
- In the mixed population of patients, both on blood pressure lowering medications and those not on medications, WCH was associated with a 19% increased risk of CVD and a 50% increases in total mortality.
- In the patients treated with blood pressure lowering drugs to a normal blood pressure, neither the risk of CVD nor total mortality was increased in WCH.

In addition, a recent study showed that alterations in heart structure and function (called left ventricular hypertrophy with heart enlargement and muscle thickness), in WCH patients, as defined by ambulatory blood pressure monitoring, are intermediate between chronic hypertensive patients and patients with normal blood pressure. (13)

In another large study, untreated WCH, but not treated WCH, was associated with an increased risk for cardiovascular events by 36%, cardiovascular mortality (death) by 209%, and an increase in overall total deaths by 33%. (14)

7.3 MASKED HYPERTENSION

Masked hypertension (MH) means that your blood pressure is normal in your doctor's office but is elevated at home, out of the doctor's office. This MH increases the risk for future hypertension, causes heart enlargement and dysfunction, aortic artery stiffness, thickening of the carotid artery (artery in the neck that supplies blood to the brain), and increases cardiovascular events, cardiovascular death, and overall death. (15–18)

7.4 THE RISK FOR FUTURE HYPERTENSION IS INCREASED IN BOTH WCH AND MH

In a study conducted over 11 years (18), the rate of progression to chronic hypertension was increased in both MH and WCH.

- Normal blood pressure was an 18% risk of progression to hypertension.
- WCH was a 52% risk of progression to hypertension.
- MH was a 73% risk of progression to hypertension.
- Thus, there is a three- to fourfold greater risk with WCH and MH to develop hypertension in the future.

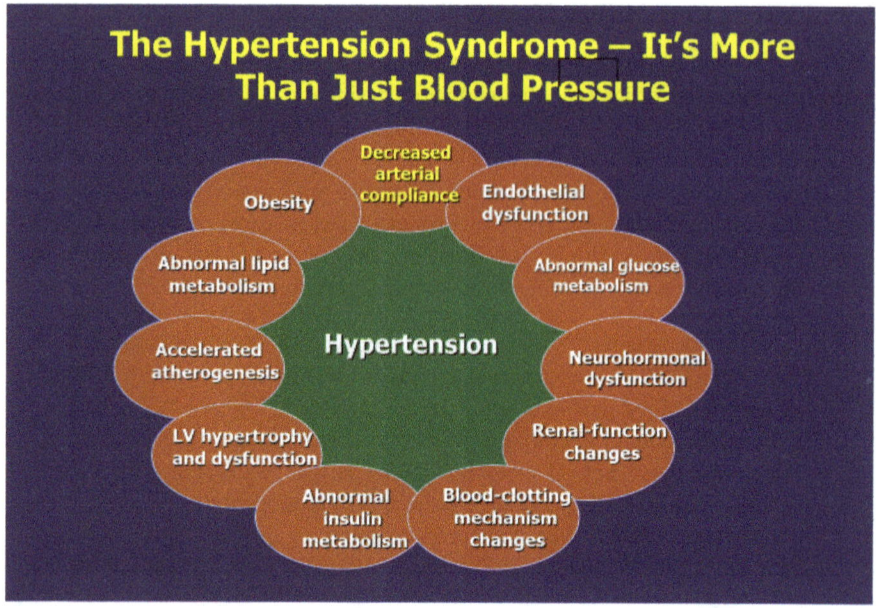

FIGURE 7.1 Hypertension Syndrome.

All of the studies support the view that WCH and MH should not be further considered benign medical problems. WCH and MH increase the risk of future hypertension, cause heart enlargement and dysfunction, arterial and aortic artery stiffness, thickness of the carotid artery, and increase cardiovascular events, cardiovascular death, and overall death. (11–18) Out-of-office BP monitoring with a 24-hour ambulatory blood pressure monitor or accurate home monitoring is critical in the diagnosis and management of hypertension.

7.5 GENDER DIFFERENCES IN HYPERTENSION

Several hypertension studies using office, home, and 24-hour ambulatory blood pressure monitoring compared the outcome between men and women of the same age group. Men are at greater risk for cardiovascular and renal disease than are age-matched, premenopausal women. After menopause, however, blood pressure increases in women to levels even higher than in men. Increasing hypertension and incident ischemic stroke was almost 2× more prevalent in women compared with men. (19–21) The leading cause of death in the United States is heart disease, and the primary modifiable risk factor for heart disease is hypertension. Although a larger percentage of men (24.4%) die from heart disease than women (22.3%), women are more likely to develop adverse consequences as a result of their hypertension. For each 10 mm Hg increase in SBP in women, there is a 25% increased risk of developing CVD. In men, the risk is only increased by 15%. (19–21) Women also have a greater incidence of WCH.

A study that analyzed blood pressure control rates among hypertensive women with coronary artery disease showed that women who had a prior myocardial infarction (MI) or revascularization procedure were at a higher risk for stroke, MI, and death (Sava et al. 2019). These women were also women with elevated blood pressures and also more likely to develop left ventricular hypertrophy, diastolic dysfunction, increased arterial stiffness, diabetes, stroke, and chronic kidney disease. (19–21)

Observed gender differences in hypertension, which exist in human and animal populations, are due to both biological and behavioral differences. The biological factors include sex hormones, chromosomal differences, and other biological sex differences that are protective against hypertension in women. These biological factors become evident during adolescence and persist through adulthood until women reach menopause, at which point gender differences in hypertension become correspondingly smaller or nonexistent. While a female is premenopausal, she is benefiting from estrogen's protective effects. Estrogen has been found to activate nitric oxide, leading to inhibition of the sympathetic system, thus causing vasodilation and other vascular beneficial effects. Women have more arterial estrogen receptors than men, and a premenopausal woman, who has the highest level of estrogen production, is able to most benefit from the vascular effect. There also may be a greater anti-inflammatory immune profile in women with hypertension which may be a compensatory mechanism to limit increases in blood pressure. Evidence shows that ovarian hormones can reduce plasma renin levels and ACE activity, thus leading to decreased angiotensin II levels and stimulation of the angiotensin I receptor that induces vasoconstriction and increases blood pressure. In addition, angiotensin type II receptors, which promote an anti-inflammatory profile, vasodilation, and lower blood pressure, have greater activity in women. (19–21)

The side effect profile of antihypertensive drugs varies between sexes. Women are 1.5–1.7 times more likely to develop side effects than men. With diuretic use, women are more likely to develop hyponatremia, hypokalemia, and arrhythmias. Women also more commonly develop ACEI-related cough and calcium-channel blocker-related peripheral edema. (19–21)

7.6 SUMMARY AND KEY TAKEAWAY POINTS

1. The Hypertension Syndrome is a group of medical problems and diseases frequently associated with hypertension that increase your risk for CVD, are improved by nutrition and nutritional supplements, but may be favorably or unfavorably affected by blood pressure medications. You may require additional medications to control the associated problems or diseases.
2. WCH and MH increase the risk of future hypertension, cause heart enlargement and dysfunction, arterial and aortic artery stiffness, thickening of the carotid artery, increase cardiovascular events, cardiovascular death, and overall death.

3. The 24-hour ambulatory blood pressure monitor or accurate home monitoring is essential to determine if you have white coat or MH.
4. There are important gender differences in hypertension that impact risk and treatment.

REFERENCES

1. Whelton PK, et al. ACC/AHA/AAPA/ABC/ACPM/AGS/APhA/ASH/ASPC/NMA/PCNA Guideline for the prevention, detection, evaluation, and management of high blood pressure in adults: a report of the American College of Cardiology/American Heart Association Task Force on Clinical Practice Guidelines. Hypertension. Jun 2018;71(6):e13–e115.
2. Houston M. The role of nutrition and nutraceutical supplements in the treatment of hypertension. World J Cardiol. 2014;6(2):38–66.
3. Houston M. Nutrition and nutraceutical supplements for the treatment of hypertension: Part 1. J. Clin Hypertens. 2013;15:752–757.
4. Houston M. Nutrition and nutraceutical supplements for the treatment of hypertension: Part II. J. Clin Hypertens. 2013;15:845–851.
5. Houston M. Nutrition and nutraceutical supplements for the treatment of hypertension: Part III. J Clin Hypertens. 2013;15:931–937.
6. Houston MC, Fox B, Taylor N. What Your Doctor May Not Tell You About Hypertension. The Revolutionary Nutrition and Lifestyle Program to Help Fight High Blood Pressure. AOL Time Warner, Warner Books, New York, NY, 2003.
7. Houston M. Treatment of hypertension with nutrition and nutraceutical supplement: Part 1. Altern Complement Med. 2019;24:260–275.
8. Houston M. Treatment of hypertension with nutrition and nutraceutical supplement: Part 2. Altern Complement Med. 2019; 25: 23–36.
9. Sinatra S, Houston M, Editors. Nutrition and Integrative Strategies in Cardiovascular Medicine. CRC Press, 2015.
10. Houston MC. Handbook of Hypertension. Wiley-Blackwell, Oxford, UK, 2009.
11. Briasoulis A, Androulakis E, Palla M, Papageorgiou N, Tousoulis D. White-coat hypertension and cardiovascular events: a meta-analysis. J Hypertens. Apr 2016;34(4):593–599.
12. Huang Y, Huang W, Mai W, Cai X, An D, Liu Z, Huang H, Zeng J, Hu Y, Xu D. White-coat hypertension is a risk factor for cardiovascular diseases and total mortality. J Hypertens. Apr 2017;35(4):677–688.
13. Cuspidi C, Rescaldani M, Tadic M, Sala C, Grassi G, Mancia G. White-coat hypertension, as defined by ambulatory blood pressure monitoring, and subclinical cardiac organ damage: a meta-analysis. J Hypertens. Jan 2015;33(1):24–32.
14. Cohen JB, Lotito MJ, Trivedi UK, Denker MG, Cohen DL, Townsend RR. Ann cardiovascular events and mortality in white coat hypertension: a systematic review and meta-analysis. Intern Med. Jun 18, 2019;170(12):853–862.
15. Koletsos N, Dipla K, Triantafyllou A, Gkaliagkousi E, Sachpekidis V, Zafeiridis A, Douma S. A brief submaximal isometric exercise test 'unmasks' systolic and diastolic masked hypertension. J Hypertens. Apr 2019;37(4):710–719.
16. Hänninen MR, Niiranen TJ, Puukka PJ, Kesäniemi YA, Kähönen M, Jula AM. Target organ damage and masked hypertension in the general population: the Finn-Home study. J Hypertens. Jun 2013;31(6):1136–1143.
17. Tadic M, Cuspidi C, Vukomanovic V, Celic V, Tasic I, Stevanovic A, Kocijancic VJ. Does masked hypertension impact left ventricular deformation?. Am Soc Hypertens. Sep 2016;10(9):694–701.

18. Sivén SS, Niiranen TJ, Kantola IM, Jula AMJ. White-coat and masked hypertension as risk factors for progression to sustained hypertension: the Finn Home Study. Hypertens. Jan 2016;34(1):54–60.
19. Everett B, ZaJacova A. Gender differences in hypertension and hypertension awareness among young adults. Biodemography Soc Biol. 2015;61(1):1–17.
20. Reckelhoff JF. Sex differences in regulation of blood pressure. Adv Exp Med Biol. 2018;1065:139–151.
21. Tadic M, Cuspidi C, Grassi G, Ivanovic B. Gender-specific therapeutic approach in arterial hypertension – challenges ahead. Pharmacol Res. Mar 2019;141:181–188.

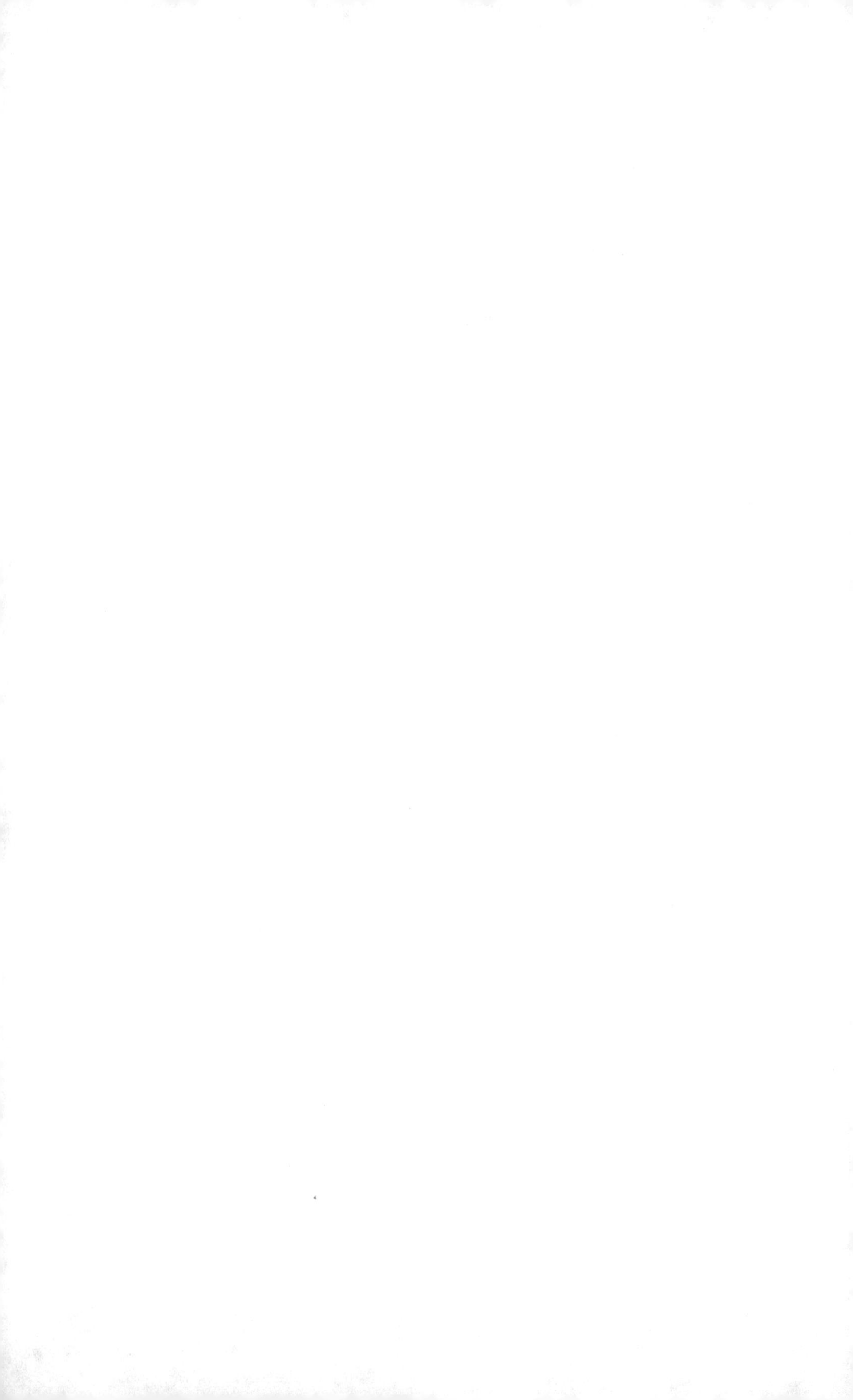

8 How Does Excess Blood Pressure Harm Us?

Cardiovascular Diseases and Hypertension

Why should we be so concerned and afraid of hypertension? All of the pressure inside of the arteries will damage the arteries and heart. The arteries are not able to withstand this high pressure inside without becoming thicker, stiffer, weaker, developing clots or atherosclerosis, or even rupturing. The heart has to pump against a high pressure, work harder and longer and will eventually enlarge, thicken, become stiff, weaken, dilate, and start to lose its pumping action resulting in congestive heart failure. Whether you are sleeping, resting, working, or exercising, your heart is working overtime. The longer you have hypertension and the higher the blood pressure level, the more like you are to have coronary heart disease, a heart attack, a stroke, enlarged heart, congestive heart failure, an aneurysm (a weak dilated artery that will burst), kidney failure, brain damage with vascular dementia and loss of memory, eye problems with visual loss, and an early death. If you have other diseases or problems related to the **Hypertension Syndrome** (Chapter 7), then your risk for any of these cardiovascular events is increased. Hypertension is associated with a wide variety of cardiovascular complications and diseases as well as increased death rate with a shortened life expectancy (Tables 8.1 and 8.2). (1–19)

Let us have a look at how untreated poorly controlled hypertension wreaks havoc on many of your vital organs

TABLE 8.1
Vital Organ Damage from Hypertension

1. **Coronary heart disease and heart attack.**
2. **Congestive heart failure.**
3. **Stroke.**
4. **Vascular dementia.**
5. **Kidney disease.**
6. **Aneurysms.**
7. **Eyes.**
8. **Endothelial dysfunction, arterial damage, and atherosclerosis.**

TABLE 8.2
Life Expectancy and Blood Pressure
If you are a 35-year-old man, this is the life expectancy according to the blood pressure levels:

Blood Pressure Level (mm Hg)	Life Expectancy (years)
120/80	76
130/90	67.5
140/90	66
140/95	62.5
150/100	55

8.1 CORONARY HEART DISEASE (ANGINA) AND HEART ATTACK (MYOCARDIAL INFARCTION)

As we discussed in Chapter 7, there are many other diseases, problems, and risk factors associated with hypertension in the Hypertension Syndrome. High cholesterol and other blood fats, high blood glucose, diabetes mellitus and obesity are three of the other top risk factors for coronary heart disease and heart attack along with smoking and hypertension. Coronary heart disease or coronary artery disease is a blockage in one or more of the arteries in the heart due to plaque formation and also constriction and endothelial dysfunction of the heart arteries (Figure 8.1). This leads to reduction delivery of blood, oxygen, and nutrients to the heart that results in angina (chest pain or pressure or shoulder or neck or arm paint with exertion and shortness of breath) or a heart attack or myocardial infarction. (1–19) You can imagine with all of the high pressure in the coronary arteries how it will force cholesterol fats and other blood components into the artery wall and form a blockage with a plaque. You are literally clogging up your coronary arteries!

8.2 CONGESTIVE HEART FAILURE

If you have hypertension, then the heart has to pump against an increased pressure in the **aorta** (largest artery in the body adjacent to the heart where all the blood is pumped), and it becomes overworked and will thicken, get stiff, enlarge, and dilate resulting in a decrease in the heart's pumping force with an eventual failure of the pump, especially the **left ventricle (see** Chapter 3, Figure 8.1). In addition, if the coronary arteries are blocked the heart muscle will not function optimally. (1–19) The amount of blood that the heart pumps out during 1-minute **(cardiac output – CO)** is directly related to the heart (pulse) rate **(HR)** and the amount of blood pumped during each beat **(ejection fraction)**.

This can be represented by the following formula:

$$\textbf{Cardiac Output (CO)} = \textbf{Ejection Fraction (EF)} \times \textbf{Heart Rate (HR)}$$

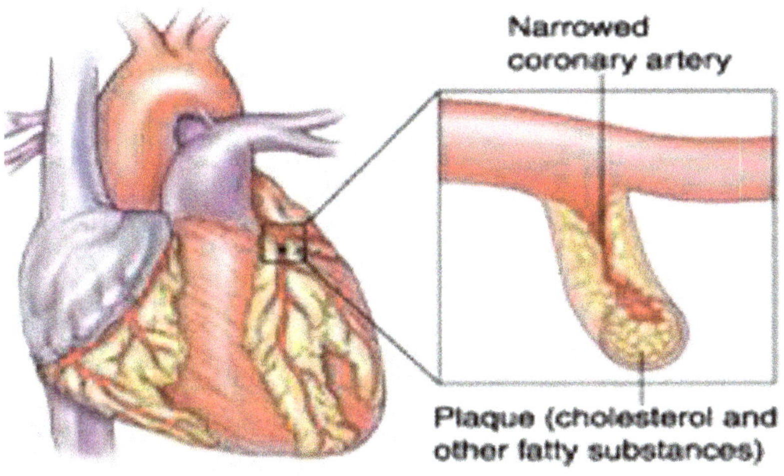

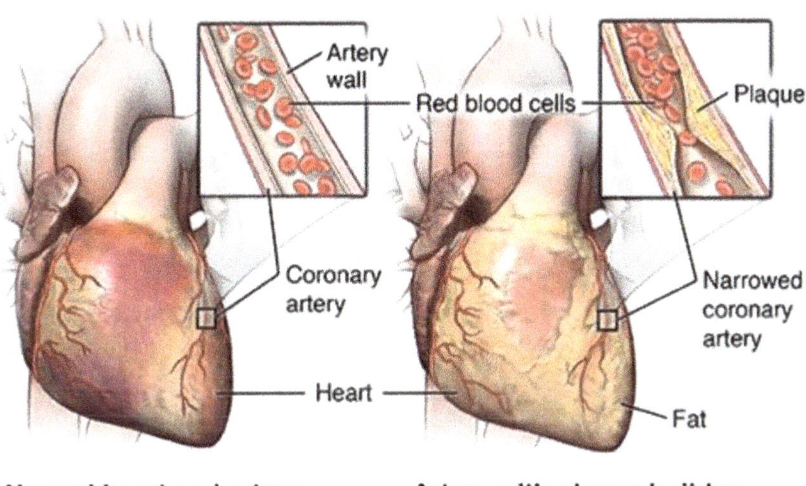

FIGURE 8.1 Coronary heart disease with plaque obstructing a coronary artery compared to a normal heart.

There are two types of heart failure, **diastolic heart failure and systolic heart failure** (Figure 8.2). (1–19) **Diastolic dysfunction or diastolic heart failure** is stiffening and thickening of the left ventricle in which the pumping action of the heart is initially normal (**ejection fraction**), but due to the stiffness and loss of elasticity of the left ventricle's heart muscle, the blood "backs up" into the lungs, legs, and abdomen to cause shortness of breath, fluid in the lungs (pulmonary edema) with leg and abdominal swelling (edema) (Figure 8.2). As the diastolic dysfunction or heart

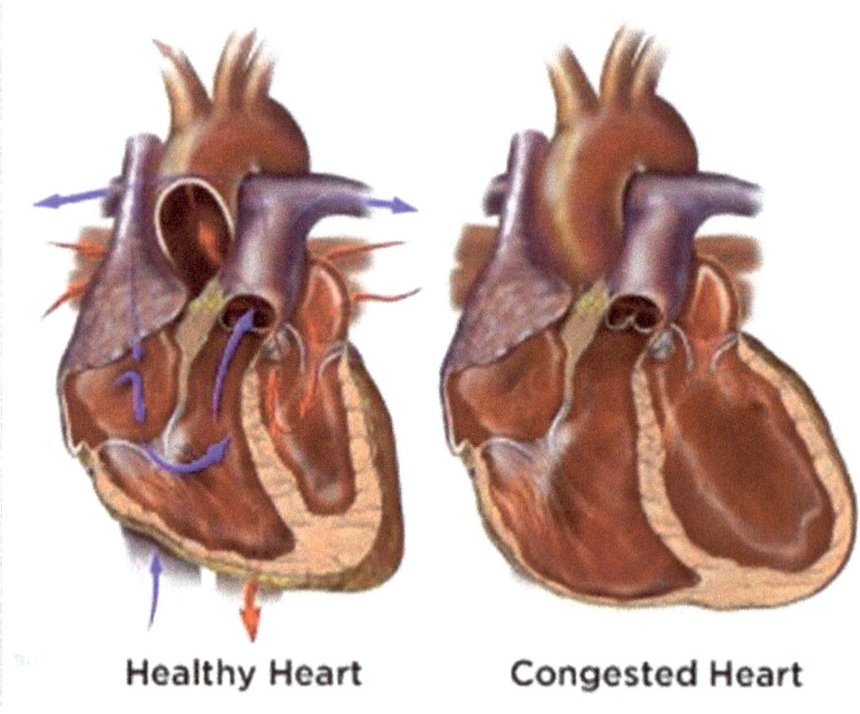

FIGURE 8.2 Normal heart and heart with congestive heart failure.

failure gets worse so will the clinical symptoms. The second type of heart failure is **systolic heart failure** commonly known as **congestive heart failure,** meaning that the lungs and other organs like the liver, abdomen, and legs become congested and are full of fluid. In this type of heart failure, the left ventricle starts to lose the ability or efficiency to pump blood out of the heart into the aorta, so the blood backs up in the heart increasing the pressure inside the heart due to the increased workload (Figure 8.2). The heart enlarges (**cardiomegaly**), dilates, becomes flabby, the ejection fraction falls, delivery of blood, oxygen, and nutrients to the body decreases, the heart cannot meet the body's demands, congestion of fluid occurs in the lungs, abdomen, liver, and legs, and you get bulging of your neck veins (**jugular venous distention**). As the left ventricle starts to fail, then the right ventricle will start to fail as well (**see** Chapter 3, Figure 8.1). (1–19) The clinical symptoms you experience include shortness of breath, chest pain, fatigue dizziness, passing out, inability to lie flat in bed due to shortness of breath and edema. (1–19)

8.3 STROKE OR CEREBROVASCULAR ACCIDENT (CVA)

Hypertension is the number one cause of stroke **(cerebrovascular accident – CVA)** and a major cause of disability. The pressure inside the brain arteries can cause a clot (thrombosis), become full of plaque or become obstructed, and reduce

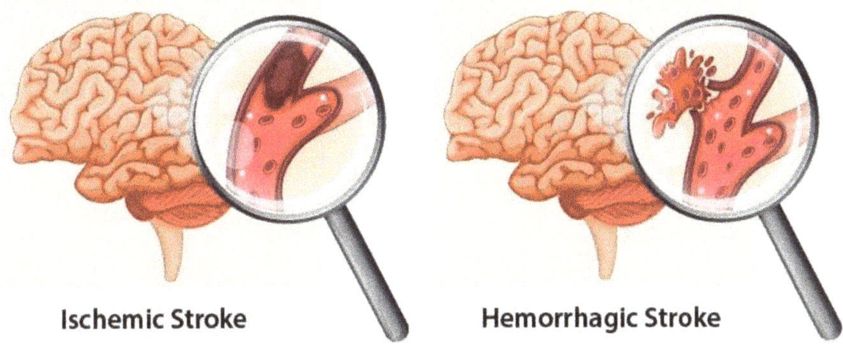

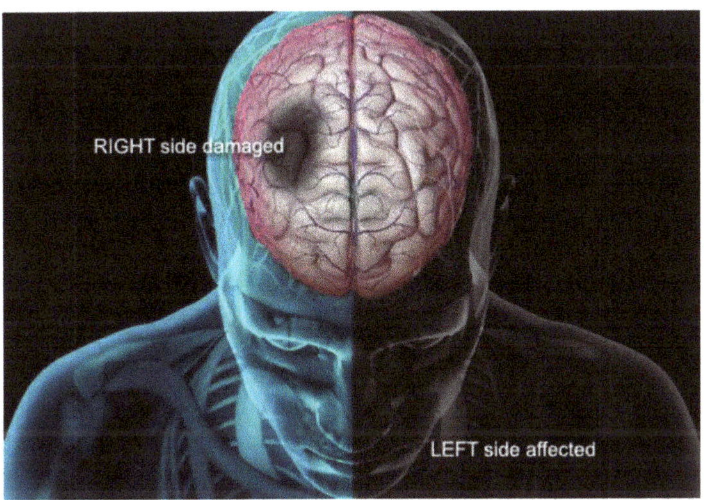

FIGURE 8.3 Two types of stroke: ischemic and hemorrhagic.

blood flow to the brain or the arteries can rupture (Figure 8.3). (1–19) The two most common types of strokes are **ischemic stroke** or a **thrombotic stroke** (a clot in the artery) and **hemorrhagic stroke** (a bleed into the brain from a leaking or ruptured artery) (Figure 8.3). Both are related to the duration and severity of the hypertension. (1–19) Thrombotic strokes are the most common of the two types. A less common third type is an embolic stroke where a free-floating clot breaks off from the heart, carotid artery, or other location, lodges in the brain, and obstructs a brain artery and blood flow. In either type of stroke, brain tissue is damaged and suffers from the lack of oxygen and nutrients. This results in weakness, paralysis, or numbness of an arm or leg, speech problems, eye problems, or death. One out of three strokes is fatal and it is the third leading cause of death in the United States. (1–19)

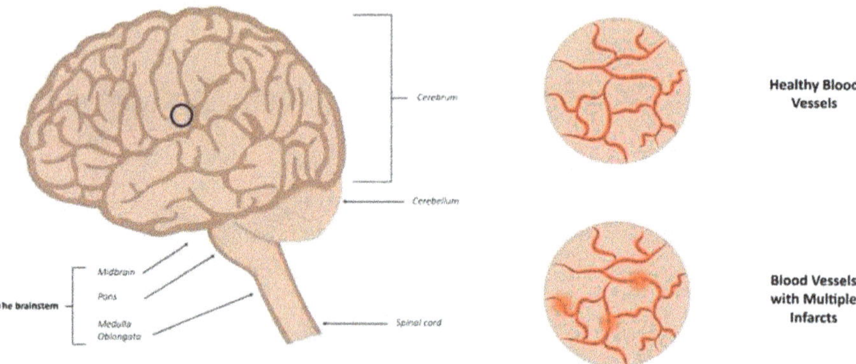

FIGURE 8.4 Vascular dementia with healthy brain arteries compared to multi-infarct dementia (top) and cerebral white matter disease (CWMD) (bottom).

8.4 VASCULAR DEMENTIA

Vascular dementia is a common type of memory loss and brain dysfunction due to hypertension that can look like Alzheimer's disease. (1–19) The hypertension causes a "mini stroke" in the very small arteries throughout the brain causing a syndrome known as **microinfarct-induced brain damage or cerebral (brain tissue) white matter disease** (Figure 8.4). (1–19) The cerebral white matter (CWM) can be seen on brain scans such as a computerized tomography (CT) or magnetic resonance imaging/arteriogram (MRI/MRA). This vascular dementia may actually be more common than Alzheimer's disease as a cause of loss of brain function and dementia in the United States. The symptoms include memory loss, cognitive, behavioral, and emotional abnormalities. The presence of high blood sugar, diabetes mellitus, high cholesterol, smoking high levels of homocysteine, and even obesity can also be to blamed. (1–19)

8.5 KIDNEY DISEASE OR CHRONIC KIDNEY DISEASE (CKD)

Hypertension is the second most common cause of kidney disease, kidney failure **(end-stage renal disease – ESRD**), and dialysis in the United States second only to diabetes mellitus (Table 8.3). (1–20)

Chronic kidney disease is a condition where the kidneys are damaged. Hypertension and kidney disease have a kind of reciprocal relationship such that hypertension causes kidney disease and kidney disease can cause hypertension.

The nephrons (the primary unit of filtration in the kidney) in the **kidneys** are supplied with a dense network of small blood vessels and capillaries (the glomerulus) and high volumes of blood flow through them. (20) Over time, in uncontrolled hypertension there is reduced oxygen and nutrients to the kidney that can cause arteries around the **kidneys** to narrow, weaken, or harden. These damaged arteries are not

TABLE 8.3
Causes of Kidney Disease and Failure in the United States Listed in Order of Frequency

1. High blood sugar (diabetes).
2. High blood pressure.
3. Chronic glomerulonephritis (kidney damage).
4. Autoimmune disease.
5. Polycystic kidney disease.
6. Blocked urinary tract.
7. Kidney infection.

able to deliver enough blood to the kidney tissue, and the kidney is unable to perform its function of filtering waste from the blood into collecting ducts into the urine for excretion. Toxins and waste products build up in the blood along with an increase in blood volume leading the clinical condition called **uremia** (Figure 8.5). The body literally starts to drown in its own waste. (1–20)

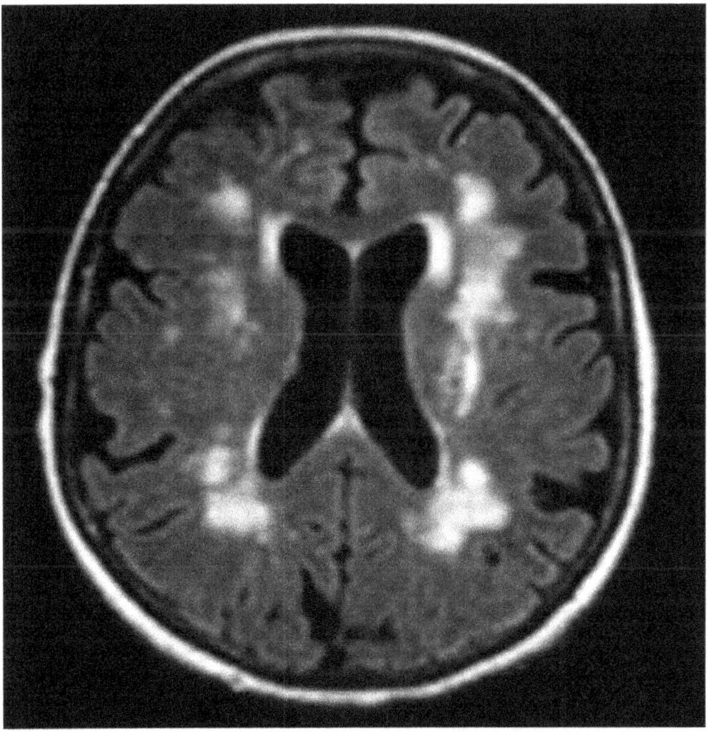

FIGURE 8.5 The white areas represent cerebral white matter disease with microinfarcts of small brain arteries.

Kidney damage can be estimated using the **serum creatinine**, persons' age, race, and gender. This calculation is known as the **eGFR**. Damage can also be proved by using markers such as the urinary protein or by documenting unusual findings on imaging studies such as the renal ultrasound. Kidney disease is divided into five stages, based upon the **eGFR levels** measured over at least a 3-month time frame. (1–20)

Stage 1 (≥90 ml/min)
Stage 2 (60 ml–89 ml/min)
Stage 3 (30 ml–59 ml/min)
Stage 4 (15 ml–29 ml/min)
Stage 5 (<15 ml/min)

8.6 ANEURYSMS

An aneurysm is an abnormal enlargement and bulging of an artery due to weakness in the muscle wall (Figure 8.6). (1–23) It may look like a "balloon" in the artery. These can occur in any size artery and in any location such as the aorta (thoracic and abdominal), legs, brain, heart, kidney, arteries in the abdomen, spleen, and other vital organs. (21–23) Aneurysms can develop slowly over many years and often have no symptoms.

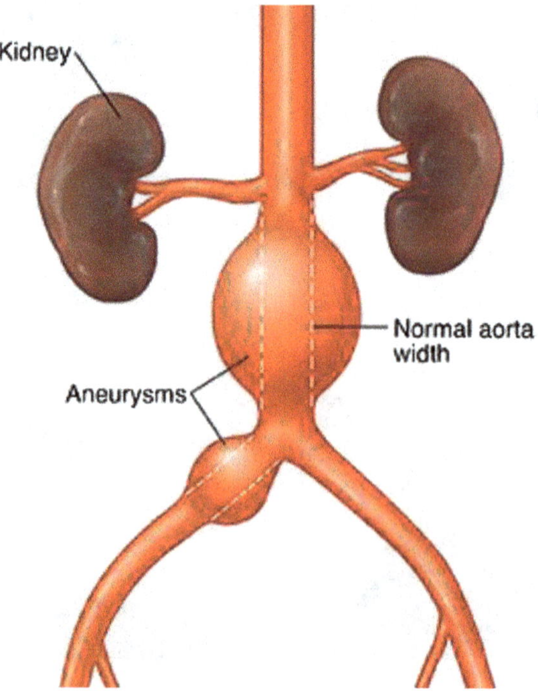

FIGURE 8.6 An aortic aneurysm in the abdomen and in the large iliac artery in the leg.

If an aneurysm expands quickly or ruptures, symptoms may develop suddenly and include the following:

- Pain.
- Clammy skin.
- Dizziness.
- Nausea and vomiting.
- Rapid HR.
- Shock.
- Low blood pressure.

They are prone to rupture with devastating effects and potentially life-threatening consequence depending on the location. The risk of rupture depends on the size of the aneurysm, the level of blood pressure, your cholesterol level, and whether you smoke. In some cases, aneurysms may be genetic. (21–23) An aortic aneurysm rupture if not treated within minutes will result in death. A brain aneurysm rupture produces a bleed into the brain, hemorrhagic stroke with paralysis, weakness, neurological symptoms, or death. There are several tests that can determine if you have an aneurysm such as an ultrasound, CT scans, MRI/MRA scans (MRI/angiogram), and arteriograms that require injections of a type of contrast dye into the artery in question. Control of the blood pressure is the most important treatment as this reduces the force and pressure in the artery that slows the growth of the aneurysm and the risk for rupture. Some aneurysms may require surgery to reinforce the artery wall with a stent, a coiling procedure, or other types of surgery.

8.7 EYES

Hypertension is a risk factor for a number of visual-threatening eye conditions that damage the eye, specifically the retina, a delicate membrane inside and at the back of the eye that receives the image by the lens and then sends it to the brains via the optic nerve (Figure 8.7). (24) This can be visualized by your doctor or an ophthalmologist with an ophthalmoscope. Narrowing of the arterioles, a stiffened artery compressing a vein (AV nicking), proteins from the damaged arteries, leak into the retina (exudates), hemorrhages, edema, retinal vascular occlusion, retinal microaneurysm, and anterior ischemic optic neuropathy can indicate the presence, chronicity, and severity of hypertension. (24) The type and severity of the retinal damage is defined by the Keith–Wagener–Barker classification in Table 8.4. In addition, hypertension may exacerbate the vision-threatening effects of diabetic retinopathy and has been implicated in the pathogenesis of age-related macular degeneration. The effects of sustained hypertension are directly visible in the eye as hypertensive retinopathy and choroidopathy, reflecting a pathological process occurring throughout the body (Figure 8.7). (24) The retinal visualization with an ophthalmoscope is one of the best ways to see what is going on the arteries in the rest of the body. It is like a "window" into the arteries of the brain. (24) These types of eye damage will result in poor vision or even blindness if the blood pressure is not controlled.

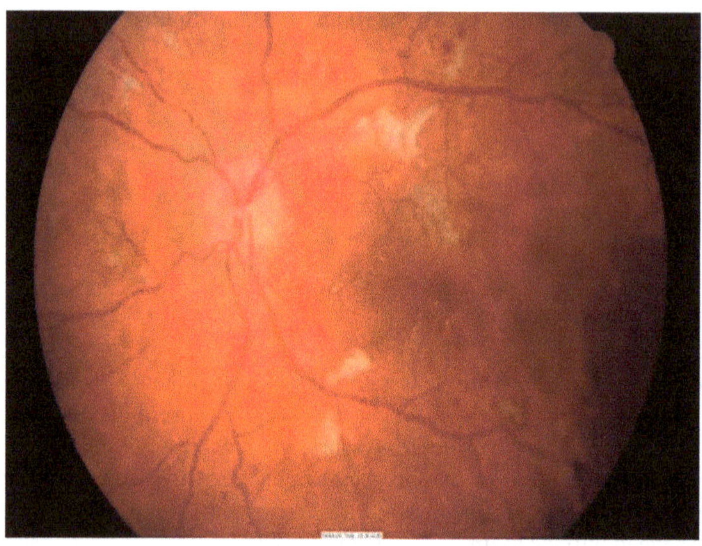

FIGURE 8.7 Hypertension retinopathy with AV nicking, hemorrhages, and exudates.

TABLE 8.4
Keith-Wagener-Barker Classification of Hypertensive Retinopathy

Classification

- **Keith-Wagener-Barker classification**

Grade	Description
Grade 1	Slight narrowing, sclerosis, and tortuosity of the retinal arterioles; mild, asymptomatic hypertension
Grade 2	Definite narrowing, focal constriction, sclerosis, and AV nicking; blood pressure is higher and sustained; few, if any, symptoms referable to blood pressure
Grade 3	Retinopathy (cotton-wool patches, arteriolosclerosis, hemorrhages); blood pressure is higher and more sustained; headaches, vertigo, and nervousness; mild impairment of cardiac, cerebral, and renal function
Grade 4	Neuroretinal edema, including papilledema; Siegrist streaks, Elschnig spots; blood pressure persistently elevated; headaches, asthenia, loss of weight, dyspnea, and visual disturbances; impairment of cardiac, cerebral, and renal function

8.8 ENDOTHELIAL DYSFUNCTION, GLYCOCALYX DAMAGE, ARTERIAL DAMAGE, ARTERIOSCLEROSIS, AND ATHEROSCLEROSIS

Hypertension attacks and damages the arteries by eroding their linings that include the **glycocalyx** (protective "fur coat") overlying the **endothelium**. The endothelium becomes stiff and thicker (**endothelial dysfunction**), (**arteriosclerosis**) then depositing plaque with cholesterol and inflammatory cells in the lumen that narrows the passageways and may completely block blood flow (**atherosclerosis**) (Figures 8.8–8.11). If the glycocalyx and/or the endothelium are damaged (**glycocalyx dysfunction and endothelial dysfunction**) and the single layer of endothelial cells becomes disorganized, then they are unable to perform all their biochemical chores such as producing nitric oxide and much more (Figures 8.8–8.11). The vessels constrict, the muscle gets thick and stiff, platelets clumps, clots form, inflammation, oxidative stress, and immune dysfunction of the arteries occur, and artery leaks. As the process develops, the artery becomes fibrotic, more diseased with more plaque, more obstruction, and calcified. Hypertension, high cholesterol and lipids, high blood sugar, diabetes mellitus, obesity and high body and belly fat, and smoking are the major risk factors for this process of atherosclerosis. The process of **atherosclerosis** is shown in Figure 8.11.

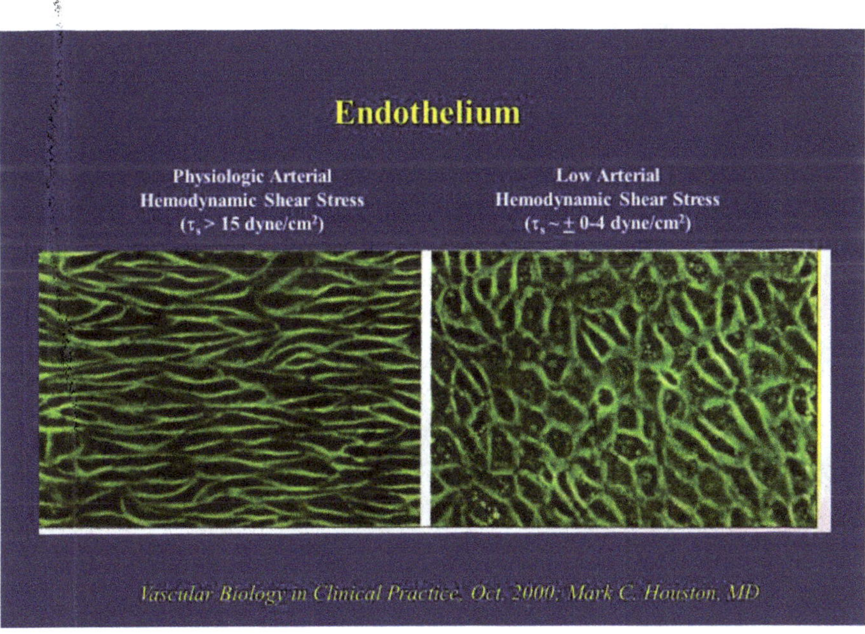

FIGURE 8.8 The endothelium and endothelial dysfunction. Normal endothelium is on the left and the abnormal endothelium is on the right.

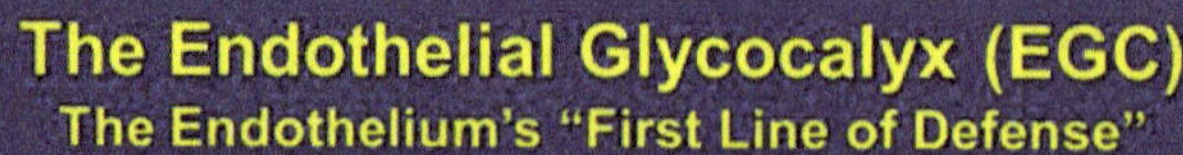

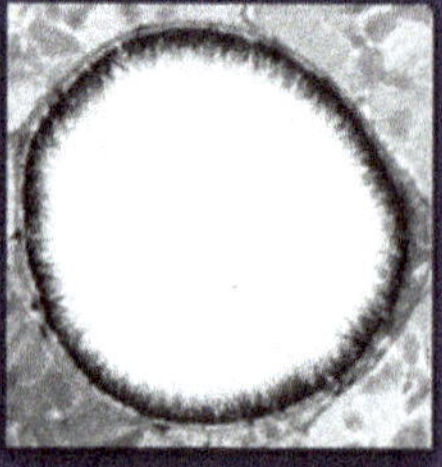

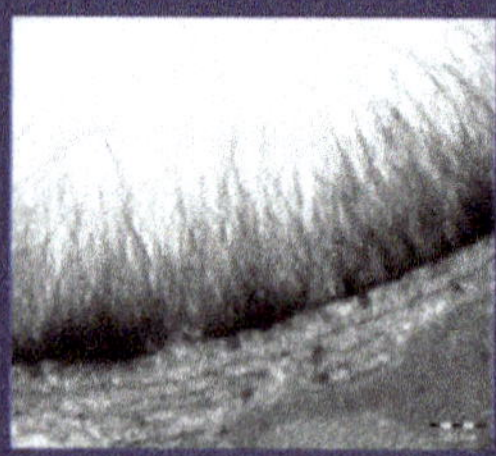

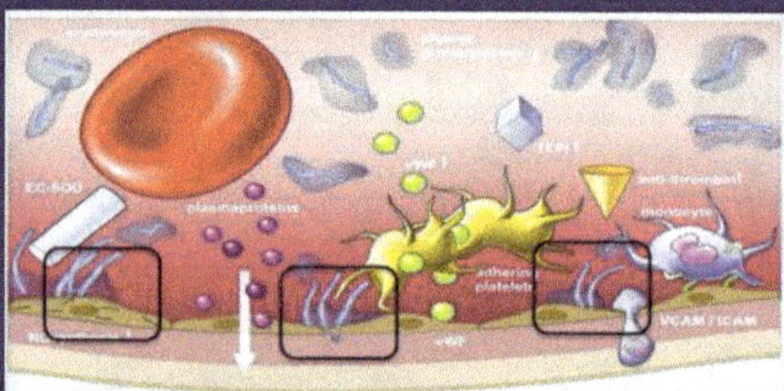

FIGURE 8.9 Endothelial glycocalyx.

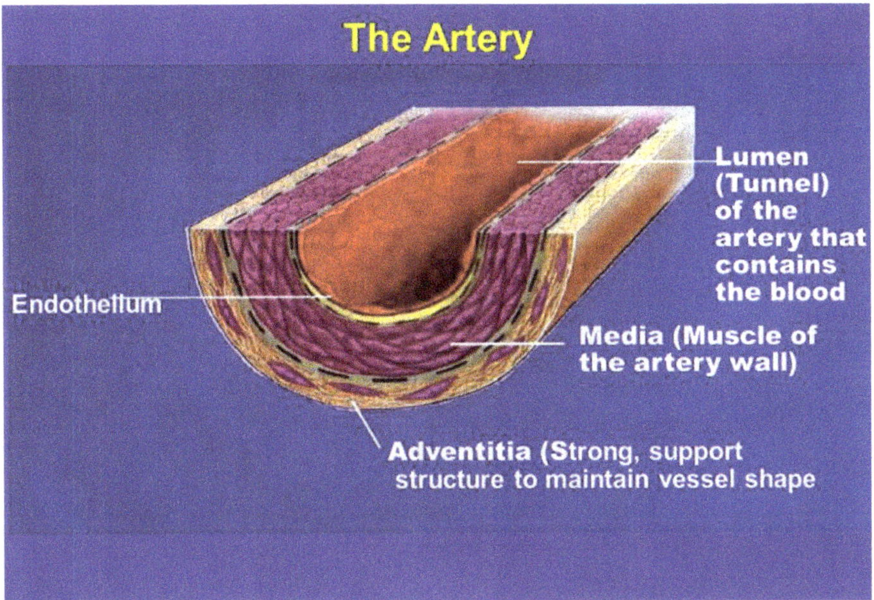

FIGURE 8.10 The artery components with the lumen endothelium, muscle or media, and adventitia.

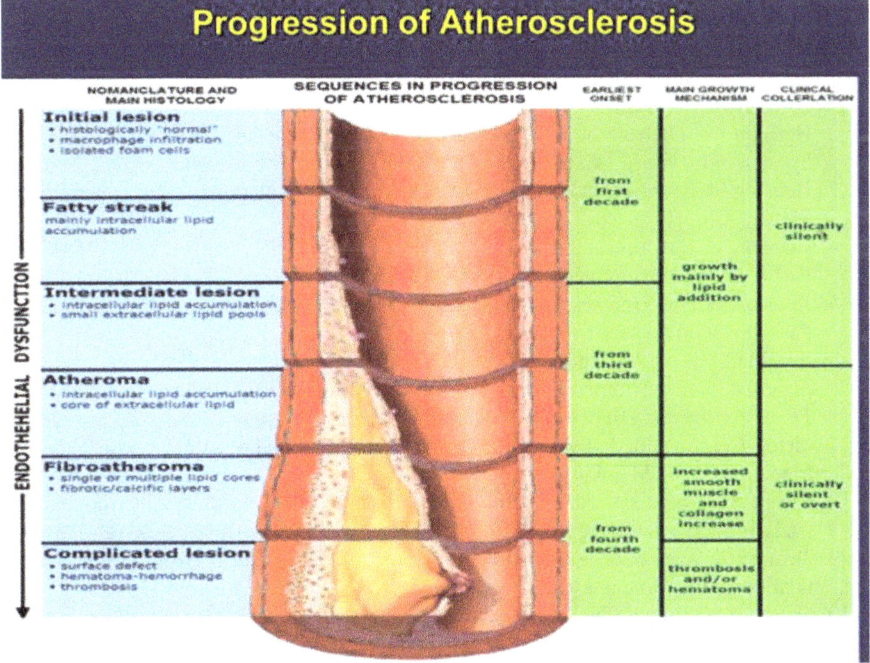

FIGURE 8.11 The progression of atherosclerosis.

8.9 SUMMARY AND KEY TAKEAWAY POINTS

1. Hypertension is one of the top five major risk factors for cardiovascular disease.
2. Even small increases in blood pressure will increase the risk for cardiovascular disease and early death.
3. Hypertension causes coronary heart disease, heart attack (myocardial infarction), congestive heart failure (diastolic and systolic heart failure), stroke (ischemic and hemorrhagic), kidney failure (ESRD), aneurysms, retinal damage to the eye, endothelial dysfunction, arterial damage (arteriosclerosis), and atherosclerosis.
4. The duration and severity of the hypertension are directly related to the cardiovascular damage.
5. The presence of other risk factors or diseases such as high cholesterol and fats, high blood sugar, diabetes mellitus, obesity with high body and belly (visceral) fat, and smoking will increase the risk of cardiovascular disease even more.
6. Lowering the blood pressure to normal and controlling other risk factors and diseases will reduce the risk for cardiovascular disease and increase life expectancy.

REFERENCES

1. Whelton PK, et al. ACC/AHA/AAPA/ABC/ACPM/AGS/APhA/ASH/ASPC/NMA/PCNA Guideline for the prevention, detection, evaluation, and management of high blood pressure in adults: a report of the American College of Cardiology/American Heart Association Task Force on Clinical Practice Guidelines. Hypertension. Jun 2018;71(6):e13–e115.
2. Houston M. The role of nutrition and nutraceutical supplements in the treatment of hypertension. World J Cardiol. 2014;6(2):38–66.
3. Houston M. Nutrition and nutraceutical supplements for the treatment of hypertension: Part 1. J Clin Hypertens. 2013;15:752–757.
4. Houston M. Nutrition and nutraceutical supplements for the treatment of hypertension: Part II. J Clin Hypertens. 2013;15:845–851.
5. Houston M. Nutrition and nutraceutical supplements for the treatment of hypertension: Part III. J Clin Hypertens. 2013;15:931–937.
6. Borghi C, Cicero AF. Nutraceuticals with a clinically detectable blood pressure-lowering effect: a review of available randomized clinical trials and their meta-analyses. Br J Clin Pharmacol. 2017;83(1):163–171.
7. Sirtori CR, Arnoldi A, Cicero AF. Nutraceuticals for blood pressure control. Rev Ann Med. 2015;47(6):447–456.
8. Cicero AF, Colletti A. Nutraceuticals and blood pressure control: results from clinical trials and meta-analyses. High Blood Press Cardiovasc Prev. 2015;22(3):203–213.
9. Turner JM, Spatz ES. Nutritional supplements for the treatment of hypertension: a practical guide for clinicians. Curr Cardiol Rep. 2016;18(12):126. Review.
10. Caligiuri SP, Pierce GN. A review of the relative efficacy of dietary, nutritional supplements, lifestyle and drug therapies in the management of hypertension. Crit Rev Food Sci Nutr. 2017;57:3508–3527.

11. Houston MC, Fox B, Taylor N. What Your Doctor May Not Tell You About Hypertension. The Revolutionary Nutrition and Lifestyle Program to Help Fight High Blood Pressure. AOL Time Warner, Warner Books, New York, NY, 2003.
12. Houston M. Treatment of hypertension with nutrition and nutraceutical supplement: Part 1. Altern Complement Med. 2019;24:260–275.
13. Houston M. Treatment of hypertension with nutrition and nutraceutical supplement: Part 2. Altern Complement Med. 2019;25:23–36.
14. Sinatra S, Houston M, Editors. Nutrition and Integrative Strategies in Cardiovascular Medicine. CRC Press, 2015.
15. The seventh report of the Joint National Committee on prevention, detection, evaluation, and treatment of high blood pressure (JNC-7). JAMA. 2003;289:2560–2572.
16. Thomopoulos C, Parati G, Zanchetti A. Effects of blood pressure lowering on outcome incidence in hypertension: 7. Effects of more vs. less intensive blood pressure lowering and different achieved blood pressure levels – updated overview and meta-analyses of randomized trials. J Hypertens. 2016;34(4):613–622.
17. Ettehad D, Emdin CA, Kiran A, Anderson SG, Callender T, Emberson J, Chalmers J, Rodgers A, Rahimi K. Blood pressure lowering for prevention of cardiovascular disease and death: a systematic review and meta-analysis. Lancet. 2016;387(10022):957–967.
18. ESH/ESC Task Force for the Management of Arterial Hypertension. 2013 Practice guidelines for the management of arterial hypertension of the European Society of Hypertension (ESH) and the European Society of Cardiology (ESC): ESH/ESC Task Force for the Management of Arterial Hypertension. J Hypertens. 2013;31:1925–1938.
19. Flack JM, Calhoun D, Schiffrin EL. The New ACC/AHA Hypertension Guidelines for the prevention, detection, evaluation, and management of high blood pressure in adults. Am J Hypertens. 2018;31(2):133–135.
20. Sun HJ. Current opinion for hypertension in renal fibrosis. Adv Exp Med Biol. 2019;1165:37–47.
21. Kokubo Y, Matsumoto C. Hypertension is a risk factor for several types of heart disease: review of prospective studies. Adv Exp Med Biol. 2017;956:419–426.
22. Fraga-Silva RA, Trachet B. Editorial: Novel insights on aortic aneurysm. Curr Pharm Des. 2015;21(28):3993–3995.
23. Ajiboye N, Chalouhi N, Starke RM, Zanaty M, Bell R. Unruptured cerebral aneurysms: evaluation and management. Sci World J. 2015;2015:954954.
24. Fraser-Bell S, Symes R, Vaze A. Hypertensive eye disease: a review. Clin Exp Ophthalmol. Jan 2017;45(1):45–53.

9 Clinical Symptoms, Signs, Blood Tests, and Noninvasive Vascular Testing for Hypertension and Cardiovascular Disease

9.1 CLINICAL SYMPTOMS OF HYPERTENSION

Hypertension is referred to as the "**silent killer**" for good reasons. Often, the first symptom or sign of hypertension is a tragic cardiovascular event such as a heart attack, stroke, ruptured aneurysm in the brain or the aorta, renal failure, or death. In fact, until the blood pressure gets very high, there may not be any symptoms at all. (1–19) It is the utter lack of pain or any other warning symptoms that makes hypertension so insidious. The level at which blood pressure may cause symptoms is variable depending on many factors such as age, gender, duration, the rapidity of the blood pressure changes, and other medical problems or diseases. However, most of the time if the blood pressure is over 180/110 mm Hg, the patient will have one or more of the symptoms listed next. Even though you may not have one of the tragic cardiovascular events, your arteries are being damaged by the high blood pressure that could result in kidney damage, vascular brain damage, coronary heart disease, heart attack, heart enlargement, asymptomatic enlargement of an aortic or brain aneurysm, congestive heart failure, valvular heart disease, retinal damage, arteriosclerosis, and atherosclerosis. If you wait too long, these chronic problems may be irreversible. The only way that you can avoid these severe cardiovascular events is to have your blood pressure checked by your doctor on a regular basis and make sure that it is controlled. If the blood pressure is high enough, you may experience some of the following symptoms. (1–19)

- **Severe headache** especially in the back of the head (occiput). Often the headache may occur on the temples or side of head and it is pulsating. The headache may get worse with exercise. High blood pressure can cause headaches because it affects the blood-brain barrier. Hypertension can result in excess pressure on the brain, which can cause blood to leak from the blood

vessels in the brain. This causes edema, or swelling, that is problematic because the brain sits within the skull and has no space to expand.
- Fatigue or overall weakness.
- Confusion.
- Memory problems and difficulty with focus.
- Seizures.
- Vision problems such as blurred vision and decreased visual acuity.
- Chest pain or chest heaviness.
- Shoulder, arm, and neck pain.
- Difficulty breathing (dyspnea).
- Irregular heartbeat or palpitations.
- Fast heart rate (tachycardia).
- Pounding in your chest, neck, or ears.
- Nausea or vomiting.
- Blood in the urine (hematuria).
- Excessive urination at night (nocturia).
- Ringing in the ears (tinnitus).
- Dizziness.
- Blackouts (syncope).
- Numbness or weakness on one side in the arms or legs.
- Water retention (edema) in the legs.
- Nosebleed (epistaxis).
- Flushing in the face.
- Sweating (diaphoresis).
- Anxiety.
- Insomnia.

Also, review the list of the 32 clues that predict your risk for hypertension in Chapter 3. This will help you to alert early in life that you may develop hypertension, encourage you to have regular medical examinations, and see if your blood pressure is elevated. If you have any of these symptoms, immediately seek medical advice to get your blood pressure checked and have a history and physical exam by your doctor.

9.2 CLINICAL SIGNS, BLOOD TESTS, AND NONINVASIVE VASCULAR TESTING FOR HYPERTENSION AND CARDIOVASCULAR DISEASE

There are many clinical signs, blood tests, and other noninvasive vascular tests that your doctor can order to determine if you have developed any damage to your arteries, endothelium, heart, brain, kidneys, eyes, or aorta. These tests will accurately define your present clinical cardiovascular damage that is related to hypertension and also predict your risk of future cardiovascular events such as a coronary heart disease, heart attack, stroke, heart failure, kidney failure, retinal damage, or aortic aneurysm. Let us take a look at each of these organs that can be damaged and what tests are available and discuss what they mean.

9.2.1 Arteries

The computerized arterial pulse wave analysis is a machine (**CV Profiler – see sources section on testing equipment**) that can measure the stiffness or elasticity of the large-, medium-, and small-size arteries throughout the body in a noninvasive manner that uses a computer analysis. (20–24) The results are standardized on the basis of your age and gender to give you a score called **"compliance of the arteries" that is a measure of their elasticity. The scores for compliance** for the big and medium arteries are called the C-1 compliance, while for the small resistance arteries it is called the C-2 compliance. The higher the compliance number, the more elastic the artery and the lower is your risk of a future cardiovascular event. The stiffer the artery, the lower the compliance score and the more likely you already had damage from hypertension. This gives you a point in time that estimates your vascular age very accurately and your future risk for a stroke, heart attack, and possibly kidney disease. In many cases, the smaller resistance arteries may be stiff before the blood pressure increases. This is an excellent clinical tool to detect and then treat you early before more arterial damage might occur. (20–24)

9.2.2 Endothelial Function and Dysfunction

One of the best validated early detection tests for functional abnormalities of the endothelium is the **EndoPAT (see sources section)** that determines endothelial

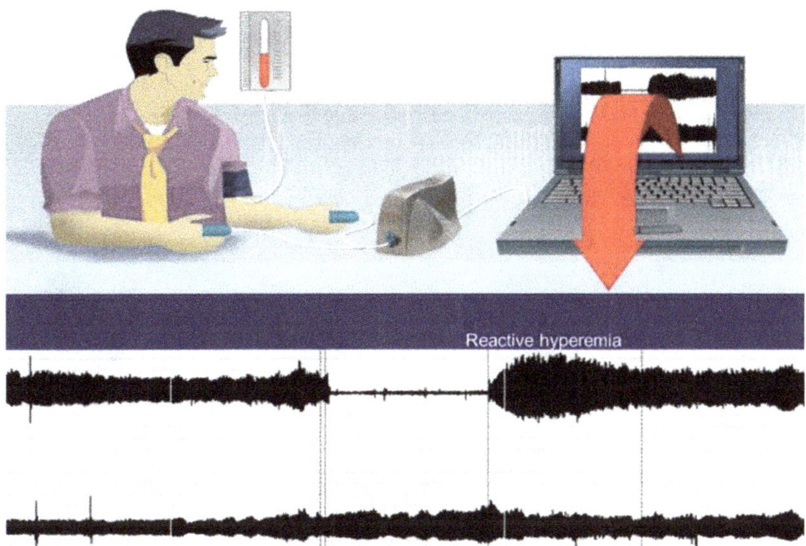

FIGURE 9.1 The measurement of endothelial function and dysfunction with the EndoPAT. The top curve below shows a normal artery with proper dilation after a brief occlusion of the brachial artery. Note the height of the black curve, called **reactive hyperemia**, that is increased compared to the other arm at the bottom. The ratio of the two curves determines the score for the EndoPAT.

function and dysfunction. (25–29) The EndoPAT measures the blood flow **(called reactive hyperemia)** in your arm after a 5-minute occlusion of the brachial (arm) artery which is an excellent indirect measure of nitric oxide (NO) bioavailability. Endothelial dysfunction in the arteries may predict future hypertension or be directly related to hypertension that now exists and is causing arterial damage (Figure 9.1). The EndoPAT that shows endothelial dysfunction not only predicts accurately the future risk for hypertension, coronary heart disease, angina, heart attack, congestive heart failure, cardiac death, hospitalization, coronary artery bypass graft, stent restenosis, but also the presence of plaque in the coronary arteries that are rupture prone, peripheral arterial disease (PAD) and stroke. (25–29) Endothelial dysfunction is defined as a score of less than 1.67. A really good score is over 2.1.

9.2.3 Carotid Artery Ultrasound

The carotid arteries are located on both sides of the neck and supply blood to the brain. They can become thick, stiff, or blocked with plaque that will reduce the blood supply to the brain, or a piece of the plaque could break off and go to the brain and cause a stroke (embolic stroke) (Figures 9.2 and 9.3). (28–30) Hypertension is a common cause of plaque and stroke, especially if there are other risk factors such as diabetes mellitus, high cholesterol, obesity, or smoking. The thickness of the endothelium and the muscle of the carotid artery is called the **carotid IMT or intimal**

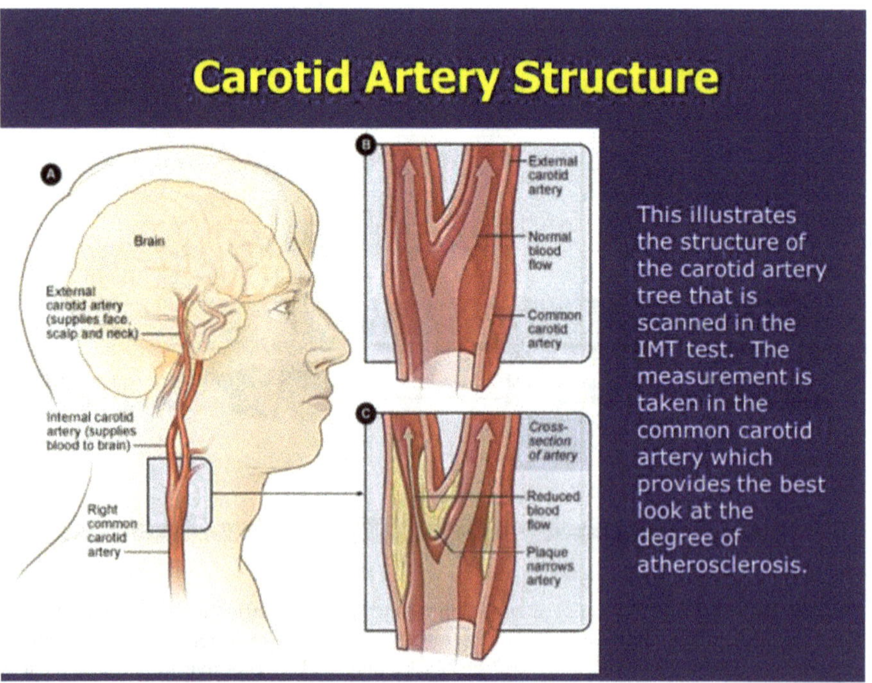

FIGURE 9.2 Carotid artery structure showing the IMT and plaque.

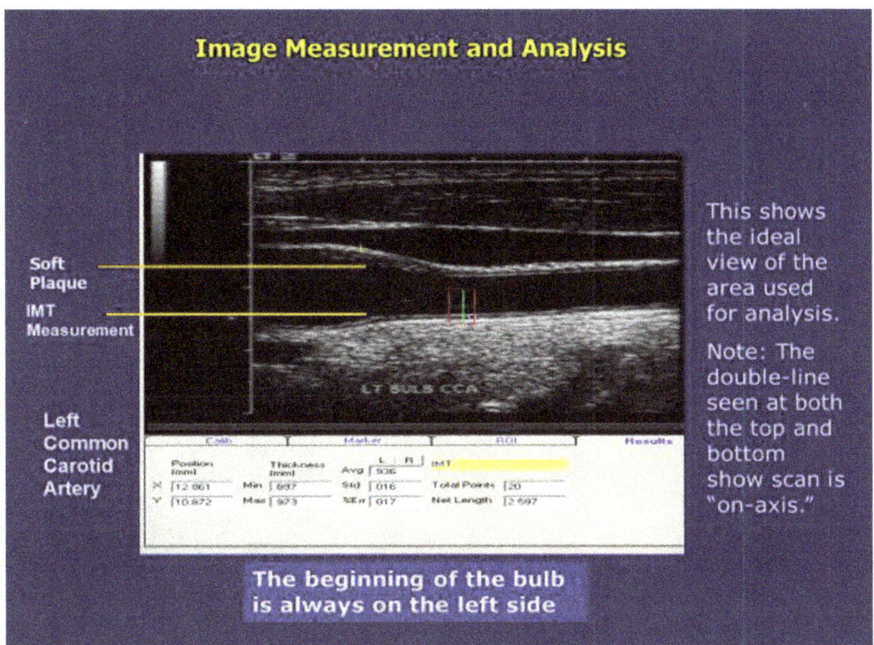

FIGURE 9.3 Actual carotid ultrasound with the IMT and plaque measurement.

media thickness. This **IMT** predicts future risk of both heart attack and stroke. (30–32) Normal values for the carotid IMT must be adjusted for age and gender. A carotid IMT of less than 0.6 mm is normal to low risk, 0.6–0.7 mm is moderate risk, and 0.7–0.95 mm is high risk for future heart attack or stroke. The normal carotid IMT growth rate is less than 0.016 mm/year. The risk for a heart attack is 26% greater per 0.10 mm growth of the carotid artery IMT difference over 5 years, while the risk for stroke is 32% higher. (30–32)

9.2.4. The Eye and the Retina

The retina or fundus examination (back of the eye) that contains the retinal arterioles is a window to the arteries in the brain and correlates highly with hypertension and with disease in the small arteries in other organs throughout the body. (33–36) Retinal damage indicates microvascular (small vessels) disease. Retinal microvascular endothelial dysfunction assessed with special eye testing shows that the retinal artery health and dilation is dependent on nitric oxide and predicts hypertension, stroke, and heart attack. (33–36) In addition hemorrhages, exudates, artery thickening, and damage may be seen (Figure 9.4).

9.2.5 Coronary Artery Calcification (CAC)

As the coronary arteries age, calcium can be deposited in the muscular wall of the artery or in a plaque inside the artery lumen that will obstruct the blood flow (Figure 9.5). (37–40)

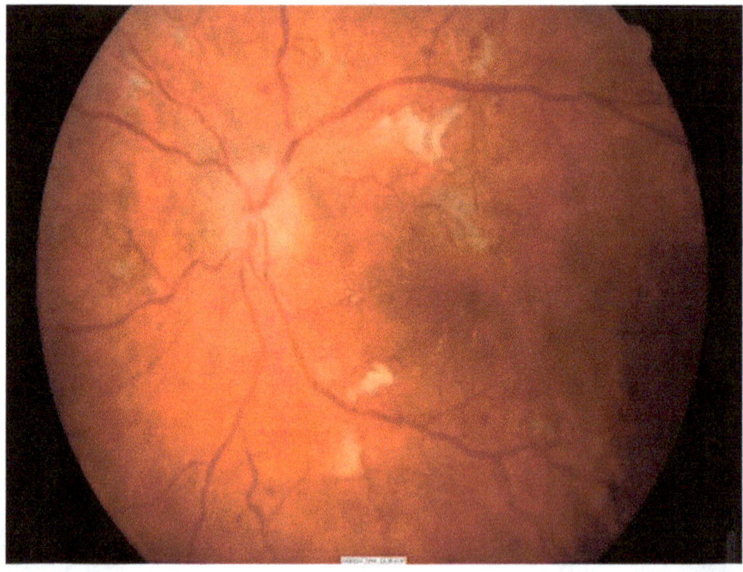

FIGURE 9.4 Hypertension retinopathy with AV nicking, hemorrhages, and exudates.

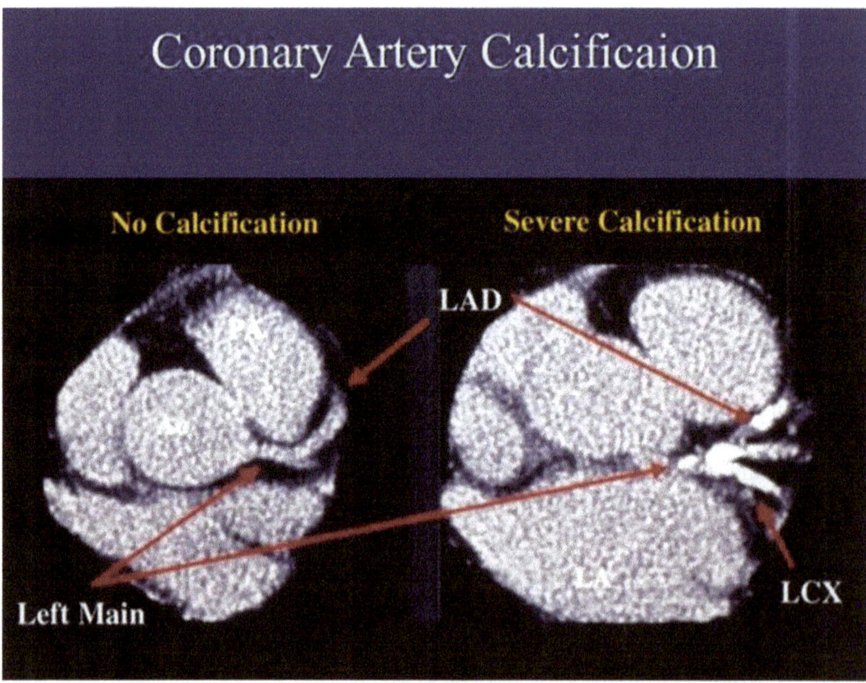

FIGURE 9.5 Coronary artery calcium in the main coronary arteries, including the left anterior descending (LAD), left main and left circumflex arteries (LCX).

The calcium in the coronary arteries calcification (CACs) is increased as you age and is related to all the risk factors such as hypertension, high cholesterol, diabetes mellitus, obesity, or smoking. The higher the score based on age and gender, the greater the risk for a heart attack. A normal score is zero. A baseline CAC score predicts heart attack and coronary heart disease risk beyond traditional risk factors. A CAC score of over 300 has a risk of a heart attack that is increased tenfold. (37–40)

9.2.6 Echocardiography (Heart Ultrasound) (ECHO)

The ECHO or echocardiography is an ultrasound of the heart (Figure 9.6). (41) This noninvasive test can determine the size (dilation) of the atria and ventricle chambers, thickening, stiffness, and enlargement of the heart chamber muscle (hypertrophy), pressures in the heart, and heart valve damage (insufficiency or regurgitation and stenosis). The ECHO also shows the heart function and pumping action (ejection fraction), stiffness of the ventricles (diastolic dysfunction), and congestive heart failure. Hypertension can dilate the various chambers of the heart, make them stiff, and cause enlargement, hypertrophy, and heart failure. (41) Also, if a valve is leaking or stenotic, the ECHO will show it (Figure 9.6). Finally, the ECHO may show an aneurysm of the thoracic aorta (big artery in the chest as it comes out of the heart).

9.2.7 Aortic Ultrasound for Aneurysms and Kidney Size

An ultrasound of the abdomen can show the size of the aorta and if an aneurysm is present. An aneurysm is a weakened artery wall that enlarges and when a certain size is reached, it may rupture. In addition, a renal ultrasound will show the size of

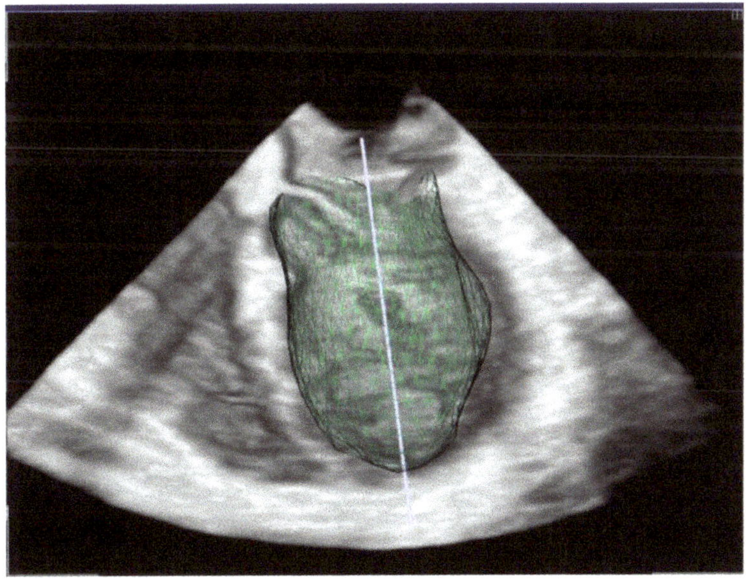

FIGURE 9.6 ECHO of the heart.

the kidneys. Small kidneys indicate damage from hypertension, with declining function and progression to end-stage renal disease.

9.2.8 Central Blood Pressure and Aortic Stiffness (Augmentation Index)

It is possible to measure the blood pressure centrally in the aorta just as it comes out of the heart. (42) This is a more accurate blood pressure reading than the one that we take in the arm. In addition, the **AtCor** machine measures the stiffness or elasticity of the aorta and the distal artery branches to predict the **augmentation index** (Figure 9.7). Hypertension causes the arteries to become stiff so that a wave of pressure in the artery wall bounces back to the aorta near the heart that further increases the systolic blood pressure and the risk for stroke, heart failure, and heart attack, and this is called the **augmentation index**. (42)

AtCor Medical SphygmoCor XCEL
PWA Clinical Report
Patient Data:
Patient Name:
Patient ID: 91458
Date Of Birth: 1/10/1951
Age, Gender: 68, Male
Height:
Brachial SYS/DIA: 175/108 mmHg
Measurement Data:
Date and Time: 3/28/2019 1:52 PM
Operator:
Visit:
Notes:
Quality Control:
Number Of Pulses: 4
Captured Peripheral Waveform
Aortic Pressure Waveform
Overlaid Peripheral Pulses
Aortic Clinical Parameters
Average Aortic Pressure Pulse
Aortic
SP: 157
DP: 109
PP: 48
MAP: 127
HR: 67 bpm
SphygmoCor Reference Age Not Calculated
Report Interpretation:
Physician:
Signature:

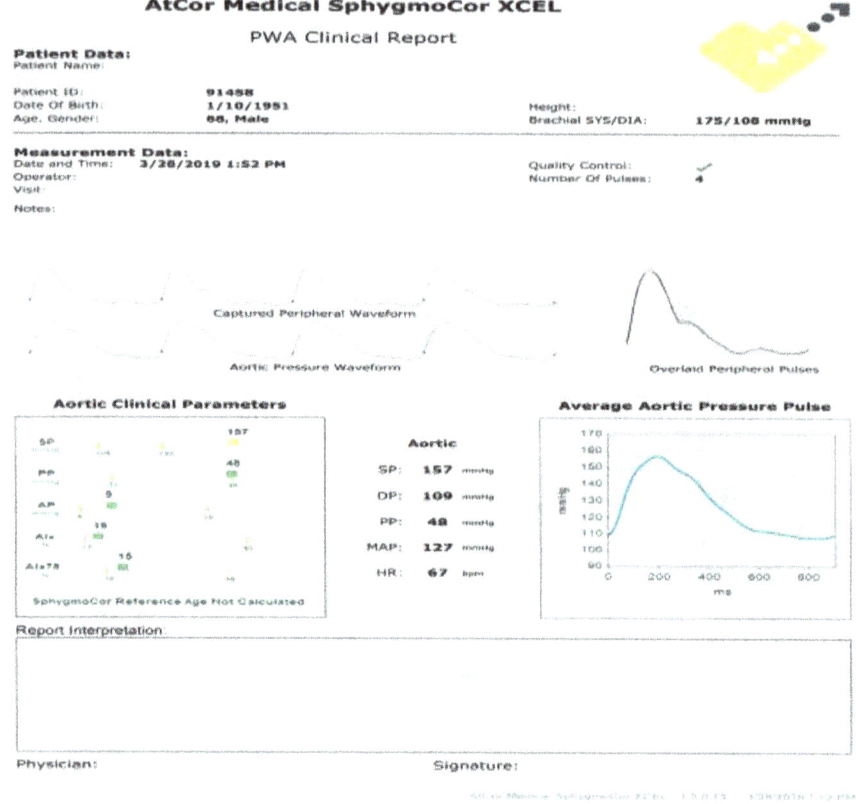

FIGURE 9.7 Central blood pressure and aortic stiffness. This AtCor test measures the central systolic and diastolic blood pressure, the pulse pressure, the heart rate, and the augmentation index. See the report.

9.2.9 Electrocardiogram and Cardiopulmonary Exercise Testing (CPET)

An electrocardiogram shows heart rate and rhythm, possible heart damage from a previous heart attack, types of electrical heart blocks, extra heart beats from the atria (premature atrial beats or PACs) and from the ventricle (premature ventricular beats or PVCs), other electrical problems, heart chamber enlargement, heart stress, and other problems due to hypertension. The **cardiopulmonary exercise testing** will determine risk for coronary heart disease with blockage in the arteries, spasm of the coronary arteries, extra heart beats with exercise, lung function, and blood pressure and heart rate response to exercise and recovery during exercise. These and other findings help one to predict cardiovascular events.

9.3 COMPLETE AND ADVANCED CARDIOVASCULAR LABORATORY TESTING

A complete cardiovascular blood panel with advanced testing should be done to evaluate cardiovascular and kidney damage from hypertension. These are listed in Table 9.1.

TABLE 9.1
Complete List of Advanced Cardiovascular Lab Tests

- Complete blood count (CBC) with differential.
- Urinalysis.
- Complete metabolic profile (CMP 12) that includes kidney function, creatinine and calculates effective glomerular filtration (eGFR) and electrolytes.
- Cystatin C and SDMA are measures of kidney function.
- Advanced lipid profile for particle size and particle number of all classes of lipids.
- Complete thyroid panel, including a free T4, T3, TSH, RT3, and thyroid antibodies.
- Magnesium.
- Iron, total iron-binding capacity (TIBC), and ferritin.
- Fibrinogen.
- hsCRP (C reactive protein).
- Homocysteine.
- Uric acid.
- Microalbuminuria.
- Gamma-glutamyl transpeptidase (GGTP) and hepatic profile.
- Myeloperoxidase (MPO).
- Cardiovascular genomics.
- Toxicology and heavy metal screen: spot or 24-hour urine or blood.
- Vitamin D_3.
- Fasting C peptide, hemoglobin AIC, insulin, proinsulin, 2-hour glucose tolerance test (GTT).
- Plasma renin activity (PRA) and aldosterone.
- Free testosterone, sex hormone-binding globulin (SHBG), estradiol, estriol, progesterone, dehydroepiandrosterone (DHEA and DHEAS).
- Omega 3 index.

9.4 SUMMARY AND KEY TAKEAWAY POINTS

1. Hypertension is a silent killer.
2. Most patients with hypertension have no clinical symptoms until the blood pressure is very high.
3. The first serious cardiovascular event may be a stroke, heart attack, rupture aneurysm, or kidney failure, or death.
4. There are many signs, blood tests, and noninvasive cardiovascular tests that your doctor can do to determine if your arteries, heart, brain, eyes, or kidneys are damaged.
5. Early detection and aggressive treatment will avoid cardiovascular complications.

REFERENCES

1. Whelton PK, et al. ACC/AHA/AAPA/ABC/ACPM/AGS/APhA/ASH/ASPC/NMA/PCNA Guideline for the prevention, detection, evaluation, and management of high blood pressure in adults: a report of the American College of Cardiology/American Heart Association Task Force on Clinical Practice Guidelines. Hypertension. Jun 2018;71(6):e13–e115.
2. Houston M. The role of nutrition and nutraceutical supplements in the treatment of hypertension. World J Cardiol. 2014;6(2):38–66.
3. Houston M. Nutrition and nutraceutical supplements for the treatment of hypertension: Part 1. J Clin Hypertens. 2013;15:752–757.
4. Houston M. Nutrition and nutraceutical supplements for the treatment of hypertension: Part II. J Clin Hypertens. 2013;15:845–851.
5. Houston M. Nutrition and nutraceutical supplements for the treatment of hypertension: Part III. J Clin Hypertens. 2013;15:931–937.
6. Borghi C, Cicero AF. Nutraceuticals with a clinically detectable blood pressure-lowering effect: a review of available randomized clinical trials and their meta-analyses. Br J Clin Pharmacol. 2017;83(1):163–171.
7. Sirtori CR, Arnoldi A, Cicero AF. Nutraceuticals for blood pressure control. Rev Ann Med. 2015;47(6):447–456.
8. Cicero AF, Colletti A. Nutraceuticals and blood pressure control: results from clinical trials and meta-analyses. High Blood Press Cardiovasc Prev. 2015;22(3):203–213.
9. Turner JM, Spatz ES. Nutritional supplements for the treatment of hypertension: a practical guide for clinicians. Curr Cardiol Rep. 2016;18(12):126. Review.
10. Caligiuri SP, Pierce GN. A review of the relative efficacy of dietary, nutritional supplements, lifestyle and drug therapies in the management of hypertension. Crit Rev Food Sci Nutr. 2017;57:3508–3527.
11. Houston MC, Fox B, Taylor N. What Your Doctor May Not Tell You About Hypertension. The Revolutionary Nutrition and Lifestyle Program to Help Fight High Blood Pressure. AOL Time Warner, Warner Books, New York, NY, 2003.
12. Houston M. Treatment of hypertension with nutrition and nutraceutical supplement: Part 1. Altern Complement Med. 2019;24:260–275.
13. Houston M. Treatment of hypertension with nutrition and nutraceutical supplement: Part 2. Altern Complement Med. 2019;25:23–36.
14. Sinatra S, Houston M, Editors. Nutrition and Integrative Strategies in Cardiovascular Medicine. CRC Press, 2015.
15. The seventh report of the Joint National Committee on prevention, detection, evaluation, and treatment of high blood pressure (JNC-7). JAMA. 2003;289:2560–2572.

16. Thomopoulos C, Parati G, Zanchetti A. Effects of blood pressure lowering on outcome incidence in hypertension: 7. Effects of more vs. less intensive blood pressure lowering and different achieved blood pressure levels – updated overview and meta-analyses of randomized trials. J Hypertens. 2016;34(4):613–622.
17. Ettehad D, Emdin CA, Kiran A, Anderson SG, Callender T, Emberson J, Chalmers J, Rodgers A, Rahimi K. Blood pressure lowering for prevention of cardiovascular disease and death: a systematic review and meta-analysis. Lancet. 2016;387(10022):957–967.
18. ESH/ESC Task Force for the Management of Arterial Hypertension. 2013 Practice guidelines for the management of arterial hypertension of the European Society of Hypertension (ESH) and the European Society of Cardiology (ESC): ESH/ESC Task Force for the Management of Arterial Hypertension. J Hypertens. 2013;31:1925–1938.
19. Flack JM, Calhoun D, Schiffrin EL. The new ACC/AHA hypertension guidelines for the prevention, detection, evaluation, and management of high blood pressure in adults. Am J Hypertens. 2018;31(2):133–135.
20. Matsuzawa Y, Sugiyama S, Sumida H, Sugamura K, Nozaki T, Ohba K, Matsubara J, Kurokawa H, Fujisue K, Konishi M, Akiyama E, Suzuki H, Nagayoshi Y, Yamamuro M, Sakamoto K, Iwashita S, Jinnouchi H, Taguri M, Morita S, Matsui K, Kimura K, Umemura S, Ogawa H. Peripheral endothelial function and cardiovascular events in high-risk patients. J Am Heart Assoc. Nov 25, 2013;2(6):e000426.
21. Prisant LM, Pasi M, Jupin D, Prisant ME. Assessment of repeatability and correlates of arterial compliance. Blood Press Monit. 2002;7(4):231–235.
22. Cohn JN, Hoke L, Whitwam W, Sommers PA, Taylor AL, Duprez D, Roessler R, Florea N. Screening for early detection of cardiovascular disease in asymptomatic individuals. Am Heart J. 2003;146(4):679–685.
23. Nelson MR, Stepanek J, Cevette M, Covalciuc M, Hurst RT, Tajik AJ. Noninvasive measurement of central vascular pressures with arterial tonometry: clinical revival of the pulse pressure waveform?. Mayo Clin Proc. 2010;85(5):460–472.
24. Hashimoto J, Ito S. Some mechanical aspects of arterial aging: physiological overview based on pulse wave analysis. Ther Adv Cardiovasc Dis. 2009;3(5):367–378.
25. Matsuzawa Y, Sugiyama S, Sugamura K, Nozaki T, Ohba K, Konishi M, Matsubara J, Sumida H, Kaikita K, Kojima S, Nagayoshi Y, Yamamuro M, Izumiya Y, Iwashita S, Matsui K, Jinnouchi H, Kimura K, Umemura S, Ogawa H. Digital assessment of endothelial function and ischemic heart disease in women. J Am Coll Cardiol. 2010;55(16):1688–1696.
26. Bonetti PO, Pumper GM, Higano ST, Holmes DR Jr, Kuvin JT, Lerman A. Noninvasive identification of patients with early coronary atherosclerosis by assessment of digital reactive hyperemia. J Am Coll Cardiol. 2004;44(11):2137–2141.
27. Hamburg NM, Keyes MJ, Larson MG, Vasan RS, Schnabel R, Pryde MM, Mitchell GF, Sheffy J, Vita JA, Benjamin EJ. Cross-sectional relations of digital vascular function to cardiovascular risk factors in the Framingham Heart Study. Circulation. 2008;117(19):2467–2474.
28. Schoenenberger AW, Urbanek N, Bergner M, Toggweiler S, Resink TJ, Erne P. Associations of reactive hyperemia index and intravascular ultrasound-assessed coronary plaque morphology in patients with coronary artery disease. Am J Cardiol. 2012;109(12):1711–1716.
29. Matsuzawa Y, Sugiyama S, Sumida H, Sugamura K, Nozaki T, Ohba K, Matsubara J, Kurokawa H, Fujisue K, Konishi M, Akiyama E, Suzuki H, Nagayoshi Y, Yamamuro M, Sakamoto K, Iwashita S, Jinnouchi H, Taguri M, Morita S, Matsui K, Kimura K, Umemura S, Ogawa H. Peripheral endothelial function and cardiovascular events in high-risk patients. J Am Heart Assoc. Nov 25, 2013;2(6):e000426.
30. Johnsen SH, Mathiesen EB. Carotid plaque compared with intima-media thickness as a predictor of coronary and cerebrovascular disease. Curr Cardiol Rep. 2009;11(1):21–27.

31. Bots ML, Taylor AJ, Kastelein JJ, Peters SA, den Ruijter HM, Tegeler CH, Baldassarre D, Stein JH, O'Leary DH, Revkin JH, Grobbee DE. Rate of change in carotid intima-media thickness and vascular events: meta-analyses cannot solve all the issues. A point of view. J Hypertens. 2012;30(9):1690–1696.
32. Lorenz MW, Markus HS, Bots ML, Rosvall M, Sitzer M. Prediction of clinical cardiovascular events with carotid intima-media thickness: a systematic review and meta-analysis. Circulation. 2007;115(4):459–467.
33. Rizzoni D, Porteri E, Duse S, De Ciuceis C, Rosei CA, La Boria E, Semeraro F, Costagliola C, Sebastiani A, Danzi P, Tiberio GA, Giulini SM, Docchio F, Sansoni G, Sarkar A, Rosei EA. Relationship between media-to-lumen ratio of subcutaneous small arteries and wall-to-lumen ratio of retinal arterioles evaluated noninvasively by scanning laser Doppler flowmetry. J Hypertens. 2012;30(6):1169–1175.
34. Ying GS, Maguire M, Pistilli M, Daniel E, Alexander J, Whittock-Martin R, Parker C, Mohler E, Lo JC, Townsend R, Gadegbeku CA, Lash JP, Fink JC, Rahman M, Feldman H, Kusek JW, Xie D, Coleman M, Keane MG; Chronic Renal Insufficiency Cohort (CRIC) Study Group. Association between retinopathy and cardiovascular disease in patients with chronic kidney disease (from the Chronic Renal Insufficiency Cohort [CRIC] Study). Am J Cardiol. 2012;110(2):246–253.
35. Virdis A, Savoia C, Grassi G, Lembo G, Vecchione C, Seravalle G, Taddei S, Volpe M, Rosei EA, Rizzoni D. Evaluation of microvascular structure in humans: a 'state-of-the-art' document of the Working Group on Macrovascular and Microvascular Alterations of the Italian Society of Arterial Hypertension. J Hypertens. 2014;32(11):2120–2129.
36. Al-Fiadh AH, Wong TY, Kawasaki R, Clark DJ, Patel SK, Freeman M, Wilson A, Burrell LM, Farouque O. Usefulness of retinal microvascular endothelial dysfunction as a predictor of coronary artery disease. Am J Cardiol. 2015;115(5):609–613.
37. Choi Y, Chang Y, Ryu S, Cho J, Kim MK, Ahn Y, Lee JE, Sung E, Kim B, Ahn J, Kim CW, Rampal S, Zhao D, Zhang Y, Pastor-Barriuso R, Lima JA, Chung EC, Shin H, Guallar E. Relation of dietary glycemic index and glycemic load to coronary artery calcium in asymptomatic Korean adults. Am J Cardiol. 2015;116(4):520–526.
38. Ahmadi N, Tsimikas S, Hajsadeghi F, Saeed A, Nabavi V, Bevinal MA, Kadakia J, Flores F, Ebrahimi R, Budoff MJ. Relation of oxidative biomarkers, vascular dysfunction, and progression of coronary artery calcium. Am J Cardiol. 2010;105(4):459–466.
39. Raggi P, Callister TQ, Shaw LJ. Progression of coronary artery calcium and risk of first myocardial infarction in patients receiving cholesterol-lowering therapy. Arterioscler Thromb Vasc Biol. 2004;24(7):1272–1277.
40. Criqui MH, Denenberg JO, Ix JH, McClelland RL, Wassel CL, Rifkin DE, Carr JJ, Budoff MJ, Allison MA. Calcium density of coronary artery plaque and risk of incident cardiovascular events. JAMA. 2014;311(3):271–278.
41. Cheitlin MD, AW. ACC/AHA/ASE 2003 guideline update for the clinical application of echocardiography—summary article. J Am Coll Cardiol. 2003;42:954–970.
42. Park CM, Korolkova O, Davies JE, et al. Arterial pressure: agreement between a brachial cuff-based device and radial tonometry. J Hypertens. Apr 2014;32(4):865–872.

10 Genes, Gene Expression, Environment, and Hypertension

What You Can Expect When Your Blood Pressure Is Reduced

The human genome (all of your genes and DNA) is 99.9% identical to your Paleolithic ancestors, but the changes in modern nutrition, macronutrient (types of fats, proteins, and carbohydrates), and micronutrient (vitamins, minerals) intake have impaired our ability to prevent and to maintain a normal blood pressure during our lifetime and optimally reduce cardiovascular disease related to hypertension (Table 10.1). (20) There are many genes that have been identified to cause hypertension. However, in many cases, a specific gene may not be found, and we are left with the family history as the risk. Vibrant America Lab has the best genetic testing for hypertension and cardiovascular disease. The gene test is called **CARDIA-X** (see sources). We will discuss this in more detail in the next chapter. Vascular biology (the way the arteries respond to our environment) assumes a pivotal role in the initiation and perpetuation of hypertension (1–31). Radical oxygen species, coupled with impaired oxidative defense, inflammation, vascular immune dysfunction, endothelial dysfunction, and loss of nitric oxide bioavailability contribute to hypertension through complex nutrient–gene interactions (Figure 10.1). (1–33) This is called **gene expression.** Gene expression means that the gene may respond in a good or bad way depending on the message it receives. That response could be an increase in blood pressure with high dietary sodium intake, for example, or a reduction in blood pressure with an increase in dietary potassium and magnesium. It could also result in a beneficial or a detrimental change in blood sugar, serum cholesterol, or a cardiovascular outcome. Food is like the input into your computer. Food communicates with and directs your genes to perform. This performance may good with good nutrition, but it may be bad with bad nutrition. (1–33)

The modern diet consists of a high dietary sodium intake with increased sodium-to-potassium (Na^+/K^+) ratio, a decrease in dietary potassium, and reduced consumption of magnesium. In addition, there is a lower dietary intake of fiber and complex carbohydrates (vegetables), decreased consumption of fruits and vegetables, lower quality and quantity of protein, omega-3 fatty acids (FA) (fish, nuts), and monounsaturated fats (MUFA) (nuts, olive products, and avocado). Also, there is an increased consumption of inflammatory omega-6 FA (hydrogenated fats, fried foods, and

TABLE 10.1
Contrasting the Intake of Nutrients Involved in Vascular Biology. Evolutionary Nutritional Impositions

Nutrient	Paleolithic Intake	Modern Intake
Potassium (g)	>256	6
Sodium (g)	<1.2	4
Sodium/potassium ratio (/day)	<0.13	>0.67
Fiber (g/day)	>100	9
Protein (%)	37	20
Carbohydrate (%)	41	40–50
Fat (%)	22	30–40
Polyunsaturated/saturated fat ratio	1.4	0.4

processed foods), saturated fat (SFA) and trans FA (TFA), and a high sugar (simple/refined carbohydrate) containing foods. All of these nutritional changes have contributed to hypertension. (1–31) In addition, obesity and our sedentary lifestyle with inadequate exercise, stress, excess alcohol, and smoking will increase the risk of hypertension.

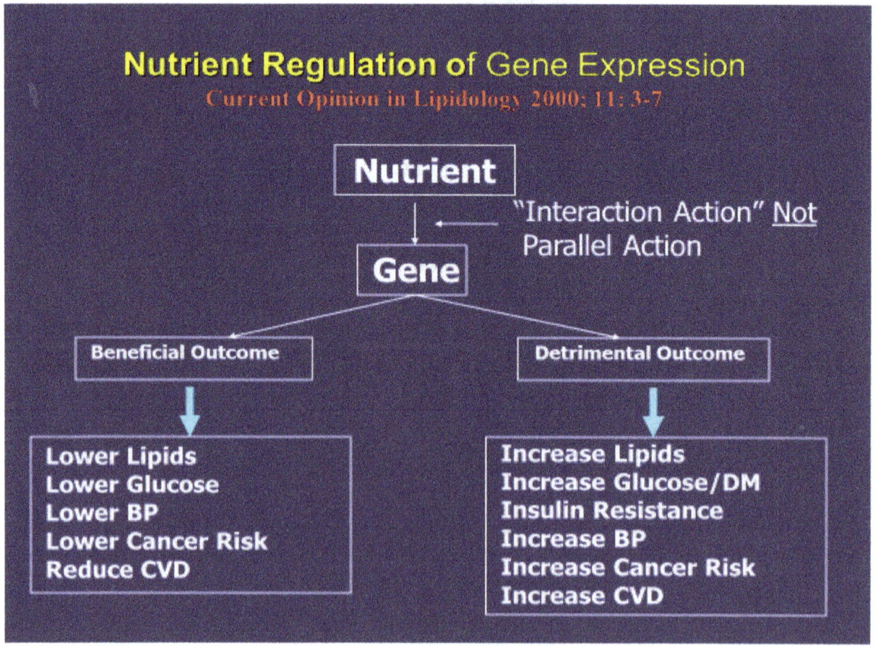

FIGURE 10.1 Nutrient–Gene Interactions and Gene Expression.

The implications of the genetic-nutrition/environmental connections mentioned earlier are enormous related to the prevention and treatment of hypertension and the associated cardiovascular disease. In the United States and other Western/industrialized countries, the blood pressure tends to increase with age. Notably, the systolic blood pressure increases more than the diastolic blood pressure as we age due to stiffening of our arteries. However, in nonindustrialized countries, the blood pressure does not increase much with aging. The Yanomamo Indians in South America consume a diet that is very low in sodium, high in potassium and magnesium and they exercise daily, maintain a healthy diet and optimal weight with age. At the age of 50–60 years, the average blood pressure in this population is 110/65 mm Hg and does not increase as they become older. (33)

Here are some important facts that you should know about your blood pressure: (1–4, 10, 11, 32)

- For every 1-mm Hg increase in your blood pressure over 120/80 mm Hg, the risk of cardiovascular events for stroke, coronary heart disease, heart attack, and kidney failure increases, whereas for every 1-mm Hg decrease in your blood pressure, the cardiovascular events decrease.
- If your blood pressure is only mildly elevated chronically to 140/90 mm Hg, you will reduce your life expectancy by 10–15 years.
- A normal blood pressure is 120/80 mm Hg, but the risk for a cardiovascular event may start at as low as 110/70 mm Hg.
- Both the systolic and the diastolic blood pressures are a continuum of risk for a cardiovascular event for each 1 mm Hg, starting at 120/80 mm Hg.
- For example, if the blood pressure increases by 20/10 mm Hg beyond 120/80 mm Hg, the risk for a cardiovascular event is doubled. However, for every 20/10-mm Hg reduction in blood pressure, your risk for a cardiovascular event is cut in half.
- If you lower your diastolic blood pressure by just 5 mm Hg, your risk for coronary heart disease or heart attack is decreased by 16%, the risk for a stroke is reduced by 38%, and the risk for congestive heart failure is down by 52%.
- If you lower your systolic blood pressure only 3 mm Hg, you decrease your risk for coronary heart disease or heart attack by 5%, the risk of a stroke is reduced by 8%, and the risk of congestive heart failure is lowered by 32%.

Later in this book, we will discuss all the various treatments to prevent and lower blood pressure. What is important to understand is that a large percentage of patients who have hypertension (60–70%) can lower their blood pressure to normal using these lifestyle changes of nutrition, supplements, exercise, weight management, stress reduction, stopping smoking, and limiting alcohol. In a clinical trial at the Hypertension Institute, 69% of hypertensive patients evaluated over 1 year were able to stop or reduce their blood pressure medications (34).

10.1 SUMMARY AND KEY TAKEAWAY POINTS

1. Our modern nutrition is not healthy. We consume too much of sodium, refined sugars, bad fats (trans fats and some SFA), and omega-6 FA but not enough potassium, magnesium, fruit, fiber, vegetables, high-quality protein, omega-3 FA, and MUFA. These nutritional habits contribute to hypertension and cardiovascular disease.
2. Your genes interact with your nutrition and your environment (gene expression) to determine your risk for hypertension and cardiovascular disease. You can test many of your blood pressure and cardiovascular genes with CARDIA X from Vibrant America Labs in the sources section.
3. Each 1-mm Hg increase in blood pressure increases the risk of cardiovascular events of stroke, coronary heart disease, heart attack, kidney failure, and early death. This risk starts above a blood pressure of 120/80 mm Hg.
4. Reduction in blood pressure reduces the risk of cardiovascular events of stroke, coronary heart disease, heart attack, and kidney failure proportional to the reduction in blood pressure.

REFERENCES

1. Houston M. The role of nutrition and nutraceutical supplements in the treatment of hypertension. World J Cardiol. 2014;6(2):38–66.
2. Houston M. Nutrition and nutraceutical supplements for the treatment of hypertension: Part 1. J Clin Hypertens. 2013;15:752–757.
3. Houston M. Nutrition and nutraceutical supplements for the treatment of hypertension: Part II. J Clin Hypertens. 2013;15:845–851.
4. Houston M. Nutrition and nutraceutical supplements for the treatment of hypertension: Part III. J Clin Hypertens. 2013;15:931–937.
5. Borghi C, Cicero AF. Nutraceuticals with a clinically detectable blood pressure-lowering effect: a review of available randomized clinical trials and their meta-analyses. Br J Clin Pharmacol. 2017;83(1):163–171.
6. Sirtori CR, Arnoldi A, Cicero AF. Nutraceuticals for blood pressure control. Review. Ann Med. 2015;47(6):447–456.
7. Cicero AF, Colletti A. Nutraceuticals and blood pressure control: results from clinical trials and meta-analyses. High Blood Press Cardiovasc Prev. 2015; 22(3):203–213.
8. Turner JM, Spatz ES. Nutritional supplements for the treatment of hypertension: a practical guide for clinicians. Curr Cardiol Rep. 2016;18(12):126. Review
9. Caligiuri SP, Pierce GN. A review of the relative efficacy of dietary, nutritional supplements, lifestyle and drug therapies in the management of hypertension. Crit Rev Food Sci Nutr. 2016 Aug 5:0. [Epub ahead of print].
10. Houston MC, Fox B, Taylor N. What Your Doctor May Not Tell You About Hypertension. The Revolutionary Nutrition and Lifestyle Program to Help Fight High Blood Pressure. AOL Time Warner, Warner Books, New York, NY, 2003.
11. Houston MC. Handbook of Hypertension. Wiley-Blackwell, Oxford, UK, 2009.
12. Houston MC. What Your Doctor May Not Tell You About Heart Disease. Grand Central Press, New York, NY, 2012.
13. Sinatra S, Houston M, Editors. Nutrition and Integrative Strategies in Cardiovascular Medicine. CRC Press, 2015.

14. The Seventh Report of the Joint National Committee on Prevention, Detection, Evaluation, and Treatment of High Blood Pressure (JNC-7). JAMA 2003;289: 2560–2572.
15. Thomopoulos C, Parati G, Zanchetti A. Effects of blood pressure lowering on outcome incidence in hypertension: 7. Effects of more vs. less intensive blood pressure lowering and different achieved blood pressure levels – updated overview and meta-analyses of randomized trials. J Hypertens. 2016; 34(4):613–622.
16. Ettehad D, Emdin CA, Kiran A, Anderson SG, Callender T, Emberson J, Chalmers J, Rodgers A, Rahimi K. Blood pressure lowering for prevention of cardiovascular disease and death: a systematic review and meta-analysis. Lancet. 2016;387(10022):957–967.
17. ESH/ESC Task Force for the Management of Arterial Hypertension. 2013 Practice guidelines for the management of arterial hypertension of the European Society of Hypertension (ESH) and the European Society of Cardiology (ESC): ESH/ESC Task Force for the Management of Arterial Hypertension. J Hypertens. 2013;31:1925–1938.
18. Flack JM, Calhoun D, Schiffrin EL. The new ACC/AHA hypertension guidelines for the prevention, detection, evaluation, and management of high blood pressure in adults. Am J Hypertens. 2018;31(2):133–135.
19. Appel LJ; American Society of Hypertension Writing Group. ASH position paper: dietary approaches to lower blood pressure. J Am Soc Hypertens. 2009; 3: 321–331.
20. Eaton SB, Eaton SB III, Konner MJ. Paleolithic nutrition revisited: a twelve-year retrospective on its nature and implications. Eur J Clin Nutr. 1997;51:207–216.
21. Layne J, Majkova Z, Smart EJ, Toborek M, Hennig B. Caveolae: a regulatory platform for nutritional modulation of inflammatory diseases. J Nutr Biochem. 2011;22:807–811.
22. Dandona P, Ghanim H, Chaudhuri A, Dhindsa S, Kim SS. Macronutrient intake induces oxidative and inflammatory stress: potential relevance to atherosclerosis and insulin resistance. Exp Mol Med. 2010;42(4):245–253.
23. Kizhakekuttu TJ, Widlansky ME. Natural antioxidants and hypertension: promise and challenges. Cardiovasc Ther. 2010;28(4):e20–e32.
24. Houston MC. New insights and approaches to reduce end organ damage in the treatment of hypertension: subsets of hypertension approach. Am Heart J. 1992;123:1337–1367.
25. Nayak DU, Karmen C, Frishman WH, Vakili BA. Antioxidant vitamins and enzymatic and synthetic oxygen-derived free radical scavengers in the prevention and treatment of cardiovascular disease. Heart Dis. 2001;3:28–45.
26. Ritchie RH, Drummond GR Sobey CG, De Silva TM, Kemp-Harper BK. The opposing roles of NO and oxidative stress in cardiovascular disease. Pharmacol Res. 2017;116:57–69
27. Russo C, Olivieri O, Girelli D, Faccini G, Zenari ML, Lombardi S, Corrocher R. Antioxidant status and lipid peroxidation in patients with essential hypertension. J Hypertens. 1998;16:1267–1271.
28. Tse WY, Maxwell SR, Thomason H, Blann A, Thorpe GH, Waite M, Holder R. Antioxidant status in controlled and uncontrolled hypertension and its relationship to endothelial damage. J Hum Hypertens. 1994;8:843–849.
29. Galley HF, Thornton J, Howdle PD, Walker BE, Webster NR. Combination oral antioxidant supplementation reduces blood pressure. Clin Sci. 1997;92:361–365.
30. Dhalla NS, Temsah RM, Netticadam T. The role of oxidative stress in cardiovascular diseases. J Hypertens. 2000;18:655–673.
31. Loperena R, Harrison DG. Oxidative stress and hypertensive diseases. Med Clin North Am. 2017;101(1):169–193.

32. Whelton PK, et al. ACC/AHA/AAPA/ABC/ACPM/AGS/APhA/ASH/ASPC/NMA/PCNA guideline for the prevention, detection, evaluation, and management of high blood pressure in adults: a report of the American College of Cardiology/American Heart Association Task Force on Clinical Practice Guidelines. Hypertension. 2018;71(6):e13-e115.
33. Oliver WJ, Cohen EL, Neel JV Blood pressure, sodium intake, and sodium related hormones in the Yanomamo Indians, a "no-salt" culture. Circulation. 1975;52(1):146–151.
34. Houston MC. The role of cellular micronutrient analysis and minerals in the prevention and treatment of hypertension and cardiovascular disease. Ther Adv Cardiovasc Dis. 2010;4:165–183.

11 Genetics, Hypertension, and Cardiovascular Disease

If one of your parents had high blood pressure, you have a 25% chance of developing high blood pressure yourself. If both parents had high blood pressure then the risk is about 50% that you will have high blood pressure. If your parents or a sibling developed high blood pressure before the age of 50 years then your risk is even higher to develop high blood pressure, but it will also occur at an earlier age. Numerous genes that cause hypertension can be specific for treatment with a drug, a supplement, an electrolyte, and with a diet or nutrition. There are numerous genes for hypertension that have now been discovered that help us to understand the previous unknown details and causes underlying the concept of "family history of hypertension." This genetic testing will allow your doctor to measure many of the genes that cause hypertension and provide a more direct, personalized, and precision treatment program without any of the guess work. This means that your blood pressure will be controlled sooner, better, with fewer drugs, less cost, and better cardiovascular outcomes. The **Cardia X genetic profile from Vibrant Labs America** in San Francisco measures 25 genes related to cardiovascular disease and hypertension. The "family history" is your primary risk factor to develop high blood pressure and now you can find out what the specific genes are in many cases. (1–85)

Genetics and nutrigenomics (the effect of nutrition and supplements on genes) provide us with an expanded perspective on the prevention and treatment of hypertension and cardiovascular disease. In cardiovascular management, nutrigenomics encompasses genetic testing and the identification of single nucleotide polymorphisms (SNPs), nutrient-genetic interactions, and how the genes express themselves. The genes may be "turned on" or "turned off" by nutrition, supplements, drugs, and other environmental factors. This is referred to as **gene expression**. (1–85)

Most genetic expression is driven by inflammation, and the majority of the genes, once turned on, promote an inflammatory response. Most of the active areas on genes associated with hypertension, heart attack, heart failure, and coronary heart disease are expressed through inflammation, oxidative stress, and immune-vascular dysfunction. A similar dynamic is evident in the vascular system. Regardless of the type of insult, blood vessels respond to insults via these same three mechanisms: inflammation, oxidative stress, and immune-vascular dysfunction. (1–85)

Consequently, the inflammatory pathways have become the primary focus in the management of genetic expression and of genetic risk for hypertension and cardiovascular disease. The prevention and the reduction of cardiovascular disease hypertension are not likely to improve without using genetic testing. Let us look at some of these influences on your genes such as nutrients, diet and nutrition, electrolytes, supplements, and drugs. (1–85)

Nutrients. Nutritional factors provide information that determines whether our genes are turned on or turned off, with a corresponding beneficial or detrimental outcome. One change in a single nutrient such as magnesium may cause 300 different changes in downstream mediators related to cardiovascular function and health. This is just one example of environmental influences and the importance of genetic expression. When there is interference with a metabolic pathway, a single area of abnormality can result in a myriad of defects and a spoke-like effect, resulting in a ripple of downstream changes in many metabolic pathways.

Epigenetics. There are several issues we want to define in patients. One is their genetic profile, the genes they were dealt. There are also epigenetic influences that are not genetic that alter the function of DNA that are termed methylation, histone modification, and non-coded messenger RNA function. These influences are not in the genetic code but can be passed on from mother to fetus and from generation to generation. For example, a mother that is malnourished during pregnancy is more likely to have a child that develops hypertension later in life. This risk for hypertension can then be passed on "epigenetically" to future generations. The final aspect is gene expression, as genes express themselves in response to nourishment or insults from different types of information coming in from the environment. Genetics have become important in determining not only dietary intake but also medication use in many patients, based on their genetic profile.

11.1 DIET

Mediterranean diet. We know the Mediterranean diet (MedDiet) turns on numerous beneficial genetic pathways that can reduce the risk for hypertension, cardiovascular disease, as well as the risk for type II diabetes. If you consume a Western diet, it will result in totally different outcomes in terms of gene expression, since most of the foods included in a Western dietary pattern have been shown to express 30–40 different inflammatory and immune pathways.

The MedDiet has an advantageous effect on many genes. In a clinical trial of this diet, other prevalent beneficial effects were related to atherosclerosis and hypertension. The MedDiet, in combination with CoEnyme Q 10 (CoQ10), has been shown to be the most beneficial intervention for healthy aging, preventing processes and diseases related to chronic oxidative stress, hypertension, and coronary heart disease. Changes in genetic expression toward a protective mode were often associated with improvement in systemic markers for inflammation, immune function, oxidative stress, hypertension, and coronary heart disease.

Pritikin and DASH diets. The Pritikin diet is one of the most effective ways to turn off the gene expression that increases the risk for hypertension and cardiovascular disease. The Pritikin diet can reduce risk of cardiovascular disease by as much as 30–35%. That benefit is directly correlated with the diet itself but is also enhanced when supplementing with nutrients such as CoQ10. The DASH-1 and DASH-2 diets have also been found beneficial in relation to changes in inflammatory genes, reducing the blood pressure, and improving the response to the types of medications prescribed for hypertension.

11.2 SPECIFIC NUTRIENTS

Electrolytes. The electrolytes, particularly sodium, potassium, and magnesium, can change genetic expression, salt sensitivity, intravascular volume, blood pressure, risk for coronary heart disease, heart attack, cardiac arrhythmias, and congestive heart failure. In terms of salt sensitivity, one of the most important is cytochrome P4A11 (expressed as **CYP4A11**), which relates to sodium and water diuresis and the role of the epithelial sodium channel (ENaC) function in the kidney tubules. Patients who have resistant hypertension due to CYP4A11 and are treated with the drug amiloride have dramatic reductions in blood pressure and often can discontinue or reduce the dose of other antihypertensive drugs.

Omega 3 fatty acids. Omega 3 fatty acids affect a large number of genes that reverse changes in our metabolic profile and in our genes that can improve mitochondrial health. As a result, adenosine tri-phosphate (ATP) production goes up, cells are healthier, and patients live longer. ATP is the energy produced by the mitochondria in our cells from metabolism of our food. The mitochondria are like small "nuclear power plants". We know that omega 3 fatty acids by themselves have dramatic effects on many receptors that can have enormous influences, reversing inflammation, oxidative stress, blood pressure, and risk for heart disease. In specific studies, omega 3 fats changed expression of 610 genes in men and 250 genes in women.

Monounsaturated fats. Olive oil and nuts contain monounsaturated fat that will have a positive impact on different SNPs and receptors, improving hypertension, coronary heart disease, and diabetes mellitus. Even without the MedDiet, olive oil and nuts given as a supplement can have dramatic and highly beneficial influences on genetic expression related to the three finite vascular responses for reducing blood pressure and cardiovascular disease.

11.3 GENES RELEVANT TO CARDIOVASCULAR RISK

Every patient should have their cardiovascular genetics testing by their physician (Tables 11.1 and 11.2). The recommended lab is Vibrant America Labs (see sources section). The genes are as follows:

Gene 9p21. One of the primary genes we are now measuring is the 9p21 gene that increases the risk of atherosclerosis, coronary heart disease, and heart attack. Patients who have a heterozygote SNP (1/2 of the gene) for 9p21 have a risk for

TABLE 11.1
Recommended Genetic Testing (Vibrant America Labs)

1. 9p21 (GG/CC) (inflammation, plaque rupture, thrombosis, aortic aneurysms atherosclerosis, coronary heart disease, heart attack, and diabetes mellitus)
2. 6p24.1 (coronary heart disease)
3. 4q25 (atrial fibrillation)
4. ACE I/D (DD allele) (hypertension, left ventricular hypertrophy, renal failure, coronary heart disease, heart attack, carotid disease, kidney failure, and microalbuminuria)
5. COMT: Val/Val or Met/Met allele (coronary heart disease, heart attack hypertension)
6. 1q25 (GLUL) (coronary heart disease in diabetes)
7. APO E (E4/E4) (coronary heart disease, lipids, dietary response to fats)
8. MTHFR (A1298C and C677T) for methylation (endothelial dysfunction, hypertension, thrombosis, coronary heart disease, heart attack, stroke, and hyper-homocysteinemia).
9. CYP 1A2 (IF/IF) and caffeine (hypertension, heart attack)
10. Corin (hypertension, volume and sodium, heart failure, and preeclampsia and eclampsia)
11. CYP 11 B2 (TT allele) (hypertension and aldosterone)
12. GSH-Px (glutathione peroxidase) (ALA-6 alleles, selenium) (CHD and MI)
13. NOS 3 (nitric oxide, HBP, and CHD)
14. ADR B2 (AA allele vs GG allele) (HBP and DASH diet and drugs)
15. APO A1 and A2 (lipids)
16. CYP4AII and CYP4F2 (HBP, sodium and volume overload, and ENac) (amiloride)
17. MMP-2, MMP-9, and TIMP-1 (cardiovascular remodeling, DD, LVH, CHF, and hypertension)
18. AGTR1, NR3C2, HSD11B1, and B2 (HBP, potassium) and AGTR1 (AA/AC) and ARB response
19. AT1R-AA (AT1R autoantibodies); hypertension (ARB vs ACEI)
20. Blood group type A, B, and AB (vWF and thrombosis)

heart attack that is increased by 50%. When a patient has a homozygote SNP (both halves of the gene), the risk goes up to approximately 100%. However, there are many other genes that should also be evaluated, not just for coronary heart disease but also for hypertension and dyslipidemia (abnormal cholesterol).

TABLE 11.2
Additional Hypertension Genes

ADD 1,2,3: Adducin
ADM: Adrenomedullin
ADORA2A: Adenosine
NEDD4L
PPARG
STK39
CALCA
GNA 12 and S1: G protein
GNB3: G Protein
GRK 4: G protein coupled receptor kinase type 4
M235T: Angiotensinogen gene

GLU 1q25 increases the risk of heart disease and heart attack in diabetes mellitus.

Apo E4 genotype. The Apo E4 genotype increases risk for coronary heart disease and heart attack. Management of risk factors for patients with the APO E4 allele, especially with the homozygote E4/E4 type, addresses issues such as:

- Increased cholesterol absorption and delayed clearance, resulting in higher serum LDL cholesterol (the bad form of cholesterol).
- Increased coronary heart disease risk with smoking and alcohol intake and overall increased incidence of heart attack, Alzheimer's disease, and dementia.
- Inability to repair the vascular endothelium to produce nitric oxide, which may increase blood pressure.
- Less response to statins to lower cholesterol.
- Best reduction of LDL occurs through dietary restriction of carbohydrates, with low fat diets, and omega 3 fatty acids.

COMT polymorphisms. One of the newest genes that we're looking at is COMT (catechol-*O*-methyltransferase), which provides instructions for the breakdown of norepinephrine and epinephrine (adrenalin from the adrenal glands). If this genetic SNP is present, the patient will have higher levels of norepinephrine and epinephrine in the blood and urine and an increased risk of hypertension, coronary heart disease, and heart attack. There is a variation in response depending on which of the specific COMT SNPs the patient carries; for example, aspirin or vitamin E may be beneficial for patients with one type of COMT SNP but detrimental if one of the other SNPs is present.

Glutathione-related SNPs. The risk of myocardial infarction can be increased by 71% if a SNP affecting glutathione metabolism (**GSH-Px, glutathione peroxidase**) is present. This selenium-dependent enzyme expresses different capacities to neutralize oxidative molecules related to increases in oxidative stress and cardiovascular disease. For these patients, glutathione peroxidase and selenium levels would be key measurements to track for the risk of heart attack:

- Low GSH-Px is a major coronary heart disease risk factor.
- Higher levels of glutathione peroxidase support more rapid recycling of glutathione, resulting in higher availability of glutathione that is one of the most important antioxidants inside the cell.
- Increased glutathione peroxidase (GSH-Px) decreases blood pressure and heart attack.

11.4 GENES RELEVANT TO HYPERTENSION

There is a whole host of genetic influences on blood pressure, probably over 30 different genes that we have recognized to date, all of which are helpful in determining both risk for hypertension and risk for cardiovascular target organ damage (Tables 11.1 and 11.2).

These genes are also helpful to determine the response to diet and nutrition, various nutrients, supplements, electrolytes, caffeine, and medications.

P-450-1A2: We know, for example, that someone who consumes caffeine in the form of caffeinated coffee and tea, and has the SNP, cytochrome **P-450-1A2** and is a slow metabolizer of caffeine, will increase their risk of tachycardia, hypertension, aortic stiffness, and myocardial infarction. Of course, one could have the right type of SNP for caffeine detoxification and that will reduce their risk. The risk of having this gene is about 50% of the population. The 50% of the population with this gene are slow metabolizers of caffeine, and their risk for hypertension and heart attack actually go up directly based on the amount of caffeine consumption and their age. Before you drink caffeine (coffee, tea), you need to check the gene for cytochrome P-450 function.

CYP 11 B2: The **CYP 11 B2** is related to resistant hypertension, salt and water retention, increased blood volume, high aldosterone levels, and low blood potassium that can be treated with the drugs spironolactone or eplerenone. These patients may be on four or more drugs for hypertension, and it is still not controlled. This may be a cause of hypertension in 20% of the population that is resistant to other drugs. Once the correct blood pressure medication (spironolactone or eplerenone) and dose is started, in about 6–8 weeks, the blood pressure will decrease often to normal and the previous medications can be stopped. We will review these blood pressure–lowering drugs later in this book.

CYP4A11: Also, in terms of salt sensitivity and resistant hypertension, one of the most important is cytochrome P4A11 (expressed as **CYP4A11**), which relates to sodium and water diuresis and the role of the ENaC function in the kidney. These patients have an avid reabsorption of sodium in the kidney tubules from the ENaC, which increases the blood volume and blood pressure. Most of these patients have resistant hypertension and are taking three or four drugs, and their blood pressure remains elevated. Patients who have resistant hypertension due to CYP4A11 and treated with the drug amiloride have dramatic reductions in blood pressure and often can discontinue or reduce the dose of other antihypertensive drugs within 2 months. We will review these blood pressure–lowering drugs later in this book.

ACE I/D: The **ACE I/D** (DD allele) is associated with hypertension, left ventricular hypertrophy (enlargement of the heart), coronary heart disease, heart attack, carotid disease, kidney failure, and microalbuminuria (loss of the protein, albumin, in the urine due to damage of the kidney) These patients respond well to the blood pressure–lowering class called **ACEI, or angiotensin-converting enzyme inhibitors**. We will review these blood pressure–lowering drugs later in this book.

COMT (Val/Val or Met/Met allele) is causative of hypertension due to high levels of norepinephrine and epinephrine (adrenalin). These hormones cause the arteries to constrict, become inflamed with an increase in blood pressure

MTHFR gene is related to methylation and folic acid and other B vitamins and if defective will cause hypertension

GSH-Px (glutathione peroxidase) if abnormal, increases oxidative stress in the artery and causes hypertension.

NOS 3 is an important enzyme in the production of nitric oxide that improves vascular health and lowers blood pressure. If the NOS 3 is defective then blood pressure increases as does cardiovascular disease. Treatment with high a nitrate/nitrite diet with dark green leafy vegetables, like kale and spinach and with beets or some beet root extracts like NEO 40 will improve nitric oxide levels. We will discuss these treatments in the nutrition section of this book later.

ADR B2 gene is related to how effective the DASH diet will be in lowering blood pressure. If you have a defect in this gene then the DASH 2 diet results in a reflex increase in the enzyme, renin, with increases the formation of the potent vasoconstrictor angiotensin II that increases blood pressure. If this happens, giving an ACEI or ARB (angiotensin receptor blocker) will lower the blood pressure effectively with the DASH diet. We will review these blood pressure–lowering drugs later in this book.

AGTR1 (AT1R-AA) is related to autoantibodies and hypertension. An autoantibody is an abnormal antibody (part of your immune system that attacks your own organs, i.e., attacks "the self"). This autoantibody attaches to and stimulates a receptor called AT1R (angiotensin receptor I) that causes hypertension. ARBs are the most effective treatment to lower blood pressure in patients with this defective gene. We will review these blood pressure–lowering drugs later in this book.

As you can see, there are numerous genes for hypertension that have now been discovered that help us to understand the previous unknown details and causes with the idea of "family history of hypertension". This will allow your doctor to measure many of the genes that cause hypertension and provide a more direct, personalized, and precision treatment program without the guess work. This means that your blood pressure will be controlled sooner, better, with fewer drugs, less cost, and better cardiovascular outcomes.

Cardiovascular SNPs. Obviously, there are large numbers of cardiovascular SNPs that we could check. At this point, I recommend testing for those that have the best validation, the highest correlation with risk prediction, and those that are easily attainable and have implications for a specific treatment. The genetic tests listed in Table 11.1 define risk for coronary heart disease, arrhythmias, heart failure, and hypertension; these are the genetic factors I recommend that you evaluate. From these tests, you will be able to determine the nutritional programs, medications, and other interventions that are the best.

Response to specific blood pressure–lowering drug classes

Beta Blockers: rs1801253, GNA S1, ADR B1 GRK4

Diuretics: ADD 1, GNB3, NOS 3, ACE, ADRBK1, CYP4A11 (amiloride) CYP11B2 (spironolactone and eplerenone), or GRK2

ACEI: ACE I/D, ADR B1, and M235T

ARB: ACE I/D, ADR B, AGTR1, and M235T
Clonidine: GNB3
CCB (calcium channel blockers): ACE I/D
Salt sensitivity: GRK4, M235T

11.5 SUMMARY AND KEY TAKEAWAY POINTS

1. If one of your parents had high blood pressure, you have a 25% chance of developing high blood pressure yourself. If both parents had high blood pressure then the risk is 50% that you will have high blood pressure. If your parents or a sibling developed high blood pressure before the age of 50 years then your risk is even higher to develop high blood pressure, but also at an earlier age.
2. Numerous genes that cause hypertension are specific for treatment with a drug, a supplement, an electrolyte, or with a diet and nutrition. There are numerous genes for hypertension that have now been discovered that help us to understand the previous unknown details and causes underlying the concept of "family history of hypertension." This will allow your doctor to measure many of the genes that cause hypertension and provide a more direct, personalized and precision treatment program without any guess work. This means that your blood pressure will be controlled sooner, better, with fewer drugs and less cost.
3. Evaluate specific genetic SNP's, for cardiovascular disease and hypertension, The **Cardia X genetic profile from Vibrant Labs** in San Francisco measures 25 genes related to cardiovascular disease and hypertension.
4. Traditional MedDiet with five tablespoons EVOO/day (50 g) and nuts and CoQ10 lowers blood pressure, cardiovascular disease, and diabetes mellitus.
5. Modified low-glycemic DASH 2 for hypertension is recommended. These patients especially respond related to the B2-AR AA/GG alleles.
6. Omega 3 fatty acids should be given to all patients, dose dependent (1–5 g/day to lower blood pressure and reduce cardiovascular disease.
7. Recommended intake of electrolytes is 2 g sodium, 5–10 g of potassium, and 1000 mg of magnesium per day.
8. Avoid caffeine in CYP 1A2 SNP (IF/IF and IF/IA alleles).
9. Selective use of ASA, vitamin E depending on COMT phenotype.
10. 20.5 methylfolate and B vitamins depending on MTHFR genotype for methylation.
11. Selenium should be given with GSH-Px gene if defective
12. Specific antihypertensive drug selection based on genotypes such as ACE I/D, CYPII B2, CYP 4A11, ADRB2, AGTR1, and AGTAA.

REFERENCES

1. Sinatra ST, Houston MC, Editors. Nutritional and Integrative Strategies in Cardiovascular Medicine. CRC Press, Boca Raton, FL, 2015.
2. Price PT, Nelson CM, Clarke SD. Omega-3 polyunsaturated fatty acid regulation of gene expression. Curr Opin Lipidol. 2000;11(1):3–7.

3. McNiven EM, German JB, Slupsky CM. Analytical metabolomics: nutritional opportunities for personalized health. J Nutr Biochem. 2011;22(11):995–1002.
4. O'Donnell CJ, Nabel EG. Genomics of cardiovascular disease. N Engl J Med. 2011;365(22):2098–2109.
5. Nuno NB, Heuberger R. Nutrigenetic associations with cardiovascular disease. Rev Cardiovasc Med. 2014;15(3):217–225.
6. Holdt LM, Teupser D. From genotype to phenotype in human atherosclerosis–recent findings. Curr Opin Lipidol. 2013;24(5):410–418.
7. Roberts R, Stewart AF. Genetics of coronary artery disease in the 21st century. Clin Cardiol. 2012;35(9):536–540.
8. Houston MC. What Your Doctor May Not Tell You About Heart Disease. Grand Central Press, New York, NY, 2012.
9. Houston M. The role of noninvasive cardiovascular testing, applied clinical nutrition and nutritional supplements in the prevention and treatment of coronary heart disease. Ther Adv Cardiovasc Dis. 2018;12(3):85–108.
10. Houston MC. New concepts in cardiovascular disease. J Restor Med. 2013;2:30–44.
11. Webster AL, Yan MS, Marsden PA. Epigenetics and cardiovascular disease. Can J Cardiol. 2013;29(1):46–57.
12. Castañer O, Corella D, Covas MI, Sorlí JV, Subirana I, Flores-Mateo G, Nonell L, Bulló M, de la Torre R, Portolés O, Fitó M; PREDIMED study investigators. In vivo transcriptomic profile after a Mediterranean diet in high-cardiovascular risk patients: a randomized controlled trial. Am J Clin Nutr. 2013;98(3):845–853.
13. Konstantinidou V, Covas MI, Sola R, Fitó M. Up-to date knowledge on the in vivo transcriptomic effect of the Mediterranean diet in humans. Mol Nutr Food Res. 2013;57(5):772–783.
14. Corella D, Ordovás JM. How does the Mediterranean diet promote cardiovascular health? Current progress toward molecular mechanisms: gene-diet interactions at the genomic, transcriptomic, and epigenomic levels provide novel insights into new mechanisms. Bioessays. 2014;36(5):526–537.
15. Estruch R, Ros E, Salas-Salvadó J, Covas MI, Corella D, Arós F, Gómez-Gracia E, Ruiz-Gutiérrez V, Fiol M, Lapetra J, Lamuela-Raventos RM, Serra-Majem L, Pintó X, Basora J, Muñoz MA, Sorlí JV, Martínez JA, Martínez-González MA; PREDIMED Study Investigators. Primary prevention of cardiovascular disease with a Mediterranean diet. N Engl J Med. 2013;368(14):1279–1290.
16. González-Guardia L, Yubero-Serrano EM, Delgado-Lista J, Perez-Martinez P, Garcia-Rios A, Marin C, Camargo A, Delgado-Casado N Roche HM, Perez-Jimenez F, Brennan L, López-Miranda J. Effects of the Mediterranean diet supplemented with coenzyme q10 on metabolomic profiles in elderly men and women. J Gerontol A Biol Sci Med Sci. 2015;70(1):78–84.
17. Appel LJ, Moore TJ, Obarzanek E, Vollmer WM, Svetkey LP, Sacks FM, Bray GA, Vogt TM, Cutler JA, Windhauser MM, Lin PH, Karanja N. A clinical trial of the effects of dietary patterns on blood pressure. DASH Collaborative Research Group. N Engl J Med. 1997;336(16):1117–1124.
18. Sacks FM, Svetkey LP, Vollmer WM, Appel LJ, Bray GA, Harsha D, Obarzanek E, Conlin PR, Miller ER 3rd, Simons-Morton DG, Karanja N, Lin PH; DASH-Sodium Collaborative Research Group. Effects on blood pressure of reduced dietary sodium and the Dietary Approaches to Stop Hypertension (DASH) diet. DASH-Sodium Collaborative Research Group. N Engl J Med. 2001;344(1):3–10.
19. Ornish D, Scherwitz LW, Billings JH, Brown SE, Gould KL, Merritt TA, Sparler S, Armstrong WT, Ports TA, Kirkeeide RL, Hogeboom C, Brand RJ. Intensive lifestyle changes for reversal of coronary heart disease. JAMA. 1998 Dec 16;280(23):2001–2007.

20. Laffer CL, Elijovich F, Eckert GJ, Tu W Pratt JH, Brown NJ. Genetic variation in CYP4A11 and blood pressure response to mineralocorticoid receptor antagonism or ENaC inhibition: an exploratory pilot study in African Americans. J Am Soc Hypertens. 2014;8(7):475–480.
21. Vanden Heuvel JP. Nutrigenomics and nutrigenetics of ω3 polyunsaturated fatty acids. Prog Mol Biol Transl Sci.2012;108:75–112.
22. Varela LM, Ortega-Gomez A, Lopez S, Abia R, Muriana FJ, Bermudez B. The effects of dietary fatty acids on the postprandial triglyceride-rich lipoprotein/apoB48 receptor axis in human monocyte/macrophage cells. J Nutr Biochem. 2013;24(12):2031–2039.
23. Silva S, Bronze MR, Figueira ME, Siwy J, Mischak H, Combet E, Mullen W. Impact of a 6-wk olive oil supplementation in healthy adults on urinary proteomic biomarkers of coronary artery disease, chronic kidney disease, and diabetes (types 1 and 2): a randomized, parallel, controlled, double-blind study. Am J Clin Nutr. 2015;101(1):44–54.
24. Costanza AC, Moscavitch SD Faria Neto HC Mesquita ET. Probiotic therapy with *Saccharomyces boulardii* for heart failure patients: a randomized, double-blind, placebo-controlled pilot trial. Int J Cardiol. 2015;179:348–350.
25. Khalesi S, Sun J, Buys N Jayasinghe R. Effect of probiotics on blood pressure: a systematic review and meta-analysis of. randomized, controlled trials. Hypertension. 2014 Oct;64(4):897–903.
26. Tuohy KM, Fava F, Viola R. The way to a man's heart is through his gut microbiota'–dietary pro- and prebiotics for the management of cardiovascular risk. Proc Nutr Soc. 2014 May;73(2):172–185.
27. Khanna S, Tosh PK. A clinician's primer on the role of the microbiome in human health and disease. Mayo Clin Proc. 2014 Jan;89(1):107–114.
28. O'Donnell CJ, Nabel EG. Genomics of cardiovascular disease. N Engl J Med. 2011; 365(22):2098–2109.
29. Paloaki GE, Melillo S, Bradley LA. Association between 9p21 genomic markers and heart disease: a meta-analysis. JAMA. 2010;303:648–656.
30. Qi L, Qi Q, Prudente S, Mendonca C, Andreozzi F, di Pietro N Sturma M, Novelli V. Association between a genetic variant related to glutamic acid metabolism and coronary heart disease in individuals with type 2 diabetes. JAMA. 2013 Aug 28;310(8):821–828.
31. Schaefer EJ. Lipoproteins, nutrition, and heart disease. Am J Clin Nutr. 2002;75(2):191–212.
32. Skulas-Ray AC, Kris-Etherton PM, Harris WS, Vanden Heuvel JP, Wagner PR, West SG. Dose-response effects of omega-3 fatty acids on triglycerides, inflammation, and endothelial function in healthy persons with moderate hypertriglyceridemia. Am J Clin Nutr. 2011;93(2):243–252.
33. Hall KT, Nelson CP, Davis RB, Buring JE, Kirsch I Mittleman MA, Loscalzo J, Samani NJ, Ridker PM, Kaptchuk TJ, Chasman DI. Polymorphisms in catechol-O-methyltransferase modify treatment effects of aspirin on risk of cardiovascular disease. Arterioscler Thromb Vasc Biol. 2014;34(9):2160–2167.
34. Winter JP, Gong Y, Grant PJ, Wild CP. Glutathione peroxidase 1 genotype is associated with an increased risk of coronary artery disease. Coron Artery Dis. 2003;14(2):149–153.
35. Blankenberg S, Rupprecht HJ, Bickel C, Torzewski M, Hafner G, Tiret L, Smieja M, Cambien F, Meyer J, Lackner KJ; AtheroGene Investigators. Glutathione peroxidase 1 activity and cardiovascular events in patients with coronary artery disease. N Engl J Med. 2003;349(17):1605–1613.
36. Korkor MT, Meng FB, Xing SY, Zhang MC, Guo JR, Zhu XX, Yang P. Microarray analysis of differential gene expression profile in peripheral blood cells of patients with human essential hypertension. Int J Med Sci. 2011;8(2):168–179.
37. Harrap SB. Blood pressure genetics: time to focus. J Am Soc Hypertens. 2009;3(4):231–237.

38. Zhou L, Xi B, Wei Y, Shen W, Li Y. Meta-analysis of the association between the insertion/deletion polymorphism in ACE gene and coronary heart disease among the Chinese population. J Renin Angiotensin Aldosterone Syst. 2012;13(2):296–304.
39. Fernández-Llama P Poch E, Oriola J, Botey A, Coll E, Darnell A, Rivera F, Revert L. Angiotensin converting enzyme gene I/D polymorphism in essential hypertension and nephroangiosclerosis. Kidney Int. 1998;53(6):1743–1747.
40. Gardemann A, Fink M, Stricker J, Nguyen QD, Humme J, Katz N, Tillmanns H, Hehrlein FW, Rau M, Haberbosch W. ACE I/D gene polymorphism: presence of the ACE D allele increases the risk of coronary artery disease in younger individuals. Atherosclerosis. 1998;139(1):153–159.
42. Castellano M, Muiesan ML, Rizzoni D, Beschi M, Pasini G, Cinelli A, Salvetti M, Porteri E, Bettoni G, Kreutz R. Angiotensin-converting enzyme I/D polymorphism and arterial wall thickness in a general population. The Vobarno Study. Circulation. 1995;91(11):2721–2724.
43. Mesas AE, Leon-Muñoz LM, Rodriguez-Artalejo F, Lopez-Garcia E. The effect of coffee on blood pressure and cardiovascular disease in hypertensive individuals: a systematic review and meta-analysis. Am J Clin Nutr. 2011;94(4):1113–1126.
44. Palatini P, Ceolotto G, Ragazzo F, Dorigatti F, Saladini F, Papparella I, Mos L, Zanata G, Santonastaso M. CYP1A2 genotype modifies the association between coffee intake and the risk of hypertension. J Hypertens. 2009;27(8):1594–1601.
45. Armaly Z, Assady S, Abassi Z. Corin: a new player in the regulation of salt-water balance and blood pressure. Curr Opin Nephrol Hypertens. 2013;22(6):713–720.
46. Zhou Y, Wu Q. Corin in natriuretic peptide processing and hypertension. Curr Hypertens Rep. 2014;16(2):415.
47. Peng H, Zhang Q, Cai X, Liu Y, Ding J, Tian H, Chao X, Shen H, Jiang L, Jin J, Zhang Y. Association between high serum soluble corin and hypertension: a cross-sectional study in a general population of China. Am J Hypertens. 2015;28(9):1141–1149.
48. Fontana V, de Faria AP, Barbaro NR, Sabbatini AR, Modolo R, Lacchini R, Moreno H. Modulation of aldosterone levels by -344 C/T CYP11B2 polymorphism and spironolactone use in resistant hypertension. J Am Soc Hypertens. 2014;8(3):146–151.
49. Levinsson A, Olin AC, Björck L, Rosengren A, Nyberg F. Nitric oxide synthase (NOS) single nucleotide polymorphisms are associated with coronary heart disease and hypertension in the INTERGENE study. Nitric Oxide. 2014;39:1–7.
50. Sun B, Williams JS, Svetkey LP, Kolatkar NS, Conlin PR. Beta2-adrenergic receptor genotype affects the renin-angiotensin-aldosterone system response to the Dietary Approaches to Stop Hypertension (DASH) dietary pattern. Am J Clin Nutr. 2010;92(2):444–449.
51. Chen Q, Turban S, Miller ER, Appel LJ. The effects of dietary patterns on plasma renin activity: results from the Dietary Approaches to Stop Hypertension trial. J Hum Hypertens. 2012;26(11):664–669.
52. Laffer CL, Elijovich F, Eckert GJ, Tu W, Pratt JH, Brown NJ. Genetic variation in CYP4A11 and blood pressure response to mineralocorticoid receptor antagonism or ENaC inhibition: an exploratory pilot study in African Americans. J Am Soc Hypertens. 2014;8(7):475–480.
53. Ward NC, Tsai IJ, Barden A, van Bockxmeer FM, Puddey IB, Hodgson JM, Croft KD. A single nucleotide polymorphism in the CYP4F2 but not CYP4A11 gene is associated with increased 20-HETE excretion and blood pressure. Hypertension. 2008;51(5):1393–1398.
54. Sun Y, Liao Y, Yuan Y, Feng L, Ma S, Wei F, Wang M, Zhu F. Influence of autoantibodies against AT1 receptor and AGTR1 polymorphisms on candesartan-based antihypertensive regimen: results from the study of optimal treatment in hypertensive patients with anti-AT1-receptor autoantibodies trial. J Am Soc Hypertens. 2014;8(1):21–27.

55. Yang X, Sethi A, Yanek LR, Knapper C, Nordestgaard BG, Tybjærg-Hansen A, Becker DM, Mathias RA, Remaley AT, Becker LC. SCARB1 gene variants are associated with the phenotype of combined high high-density lipoprotein cholesterol and high lipoprotein (a). Circ Cardiovasc Genet. 2016;9(5):408–418.
56. Mendoza S, Trenchevska O King SM, Nelson RW, Nedelkov D, Krauss RM, Yassine HN. Changes in low-density lipoprotein size phenotypes associate with changes in apolipoprotein C-III glycoforms after dietary interventions. J Clin Lipidol. 2017;11(1):224–233.
57. Wyler von Ballmoos MC, Haring B, Sacks FM. The risk of cardiovascular events with increased apolipoprotein CIII: A systematic review and meta-analysis. J Clin Lipidol. 2015;9(4):498–510.
58. Zheng C. Updates on apolipoprotein CIII: fulfilling promise as a therapeutic target for hypertriglyceridemia and cardiovascular disease. Curr Opin Lipidol. 2014;25(1):35–39.
59. Thomas GS, Voros S, McPherson JA, Lansky AJ, Winn ME, Bateman TM, Elashoff MR, Lieu HD, Johnson AM, Daniels SE, Ladapo JA, Phelps CE, Douglas PS, Rosenberg S. A blood-based gene expression test for obstructive coronary artery disease tested in symptomatic nondiabetic patients referred for myocardial perfusion imaging the COMPASS study. Circ Cardiovasc Genet. 2013;6(2):154–162.
60. McPherson JA, Davis K, Yau M, Beineke P, Rosenberg S, Monane M, Fredi JL. The clinical utility of gene expression testing on the diagnostic evaluation of patients presenting to the cardiologist with symptoms of suspected obstructive coronary artery disease: results from the IMPACT (Investigation of a Molecular Personalized Coronary Gene Expression Test on Cardiology Practice Pattern) trial. Pathw Cardiol. 2013;12(2):37–42.
61. Wingrove JA, Daniels SE, Sehnert AJ, Tingley W, Elashoff MR, Rosenberg S, Buellesfeld L, Grube E, Newby LK, Ginsburg GS, Kraus WE. Correlation of peripheral-blood gene expression with the extent of coronary artery stenosis. Circ Cardiovasc Genet. 2008;1(1):31–38.
62. Rosenberg S, Elashoff MR, Lieu HD, Brown BO, Kraus WE, Schwartz RS, Voros S, Ellis SG, J Waksman R, McPherson JA, Lansky AJ, Topol EJ; PREDICT Investigators. Whole blood gene expression testing for coronary artery disease in nondiabetic patients: major adverse cardiovascular events and interventions in the PREDICT trial. Cardiovasc Transl Res. 2012;5(3):366–374.
63. Ganna A, Salihovic S, Sundström J Broeckling CD, Hedman AK, Magnusson PK, Pedersen NL, Larsson A, Siegbahn A, Zilmer M, Prenni J, Arnlöv J, Lind L, Fall T, Ingelsson E. Large-scale metabolomic profiling identifies novel biomarkers for incident coronary heart disease. PLoS Genet. 2014;10(12): e1004801.
64. Granger CB, Newgard CB, Califf RM, Newby LK.Shah SH, Sun JL, Stevens RD, Bain JR, Muehlbauer MJ, Pieper KS, Haynes C, Hauser ER, Kraus WE. Baseline metabolomic profiles predict cardiovascular events in patients at risk for coronary artery disease. Am Heart J. 2012;163(5):844–850.
65. Rizza S, Copetti M, Rossi C, Cianfarani MA Zucchelli M, Luzi A, Pecchioli C, Porzio O, Di Cola G, Urbani A, Pellegrini F, Federici M. Metabolomics signature improves the prediction of cardiovascular events in elderly subjects. Atherosclerosis. 2014;232(2):260–264.

12 Guidelines for the Treatment of Hypertension and the Hypertension Institute Program and Approach

The official guidelines for the Treatment of Hypertension – published in 2017 by the ACC (American College of Cardiology)/AHA (American Heart Association) and other organizations – are listed in Table 12.1. Although we agree with most of these recommendations, we have some major differences in our recommendations regarding **diet, nutrition and specific drug** therapies such as **thiazide diuretics and older types of beta-blockers.** Where we also differ dramatically from these guidelines are our recommendations on the use of **nutritional supplements** that have strong scientific rationale with an extensive body of peer reviewed medical publications. In the chapters on nutrition, nutritional supplements, and drug therapy, we will point out these differences. The chapter on nutritional supplements and nutrition form the "heart" of this book, as these treatments are the most overlooked and effective treatments for hypertension that are not being applied by most doctors for lowering the blood pressure (BP) in their patients. Finally, more recent conferences by the AHA and the American Society of Hypertension have revised and updated some of the 2017 recommendations about drug therapy that are more consistent with the recommendations in this book.

The consequence of not using the **Hypertension Institute Program** is that many patients take too many drugs to lower their BP, have too many side effects, and do not feel well. These side effects may include fatigue, memory loss, dizziness, headache, constipation, diarrhea, nausea, depression, anxiety, dry mouth, sedation, low heart rate, and inability to exercise. In addition, other problems may occur, including erectile dysfunction, loss of libido, gout, muscle cramps and aches, cold hands, dehydration, cough, edema in the legs, flushing, fast heart rate, palpitations, shortness of breath or wheezing, and weakness, loss of taste or appetite. Also, the drugs may induce metabolic changes that are not healthy for the cardiovascular system, such as high blood sugar, insulin resistance, metabolic syndrome, high cholesterol, high homocysteine, high uric acid, kidney dysfunction, electrolyte abnormalities, nutrient deficiencies, drug-nutrient interactions, and drug-drug interactions.

TABLE 12.1
2017 Guideline for High Blood Pressure in Adults in the United States

The following are key points to remember from the 2017 Guideline for the Prevention, Detection, Evaluation, and Management of High Blood Pressure in Adults:

Part 1: General Approach, Screening, and Follow-up

1. The 2017 guideline is an update of the "Seventh Report of the Joint National Committee on Prevention, Detection, Evaluation and Treatment of High Blood Pressure" (JNC 7), published in 2003. The 2017 guideline is a comprehensive guideline incorporating new information from studies regarding blood pressure (BP)-related risk of cardiovascular disease (CVD), ambulatory BP monitoring (ABPM), home BP monitoring (HBPM), BP thresholds to initiate antihypertensive drug treatment, BP goals of treatment, strategies to improve hypertension treatment and control, and various other important issues.
2. It is critical that health-care providers must follow the standards for accurate BP measurement. BP should be categorized as normal, elevated, or stages 1 or 2 hypertension to prevent and treat high BP. Normal BP is defined as <120/<80 mm Hg; elevated BP 120–129/<80 mm Hg; hypertension stage 1 is 130–139 or 80–89 mm Hg, and hypertension stage 2 is ≥140 or ≥90 mm Hg. Prior to labeling a person with hypertension, it is important to use an average based on ≥2 readings obtained on ≥2 occasions to estimate the individual's level of BP. Out-of-office and self-monitoring of BP measurements are recommended to confirm the diagnosis of hypertension and for titration of BP-lowering medication, in conjunction with clinical interventions and telehealth counseling. Corresponding BPs based on site/methods are office/clinic 140/90, HBPM 135/85, daytime ABPM 135/85, nighttime ABPM 120/70, and 24-hour ABPM 130/80 mm Hg. In adults with an untreated systolic BP (SBP) > 130 but < 160 mm Hg or diastolic BP (DBP) > 80 but < 100 mm Hg, it is reasonable to screen for the presence of white coat hypertension using either daytime ABPM or HBPM prior to diagnosis of hypertension. In adults with elevated office BP (120–129/<80) but not meeting the criteria for hypertension, screening for masked hypertension with daytime ABPM or HBPM is reasonable.
3. For an adult 45 years of age without hypertension, the 40-year risk for developing hypertension is 93% for African-Americans, 92% for Hispanics, 86% for whites, and 84% for Chinese adults. In 2010, hypertension was the leading cause of death and disability-adjusted life-years worldwide, and a greater contributor to events in women and African-Americans compared with whites. Often overlooked, the risk for CVD increases in a log-linear fashion; from SBP levels <115 to >180 mm Hg, and from DBP levels <75 to >105 mm Hg. A 20 mm Hg higher SBP and 10 mm Hg higher DBP are each associated with a doubling in the risk of death from stroke, heart disease, or other vascular diseases. In persons ≥30 years of age, higher SBP and DBP are associated with increased risk for CVD, angina, myocardial infarction (MI), heart failure (HF), stroke, peripheral arterial disease, and abdominal aortic aneurysm. SBP has consistently been associated with increased CVD risk after adjustment for, or within strata of, SBP; this is not true for DBP.
4. It is important to screen for and manage other CVD risk factors in adults with hypertension: smoking, diabetes, dyslipidemia, excessive weight, low fitness, unhealthy diet, psychosocial stress, and sleep apnea. Basic testing for primary hypertension includes fasting blood glucose, complete blood cell count, lipids, basic metabolic panel, thyroid-stimulating hormone, urinalysis, electrocardiogram with optional echocardiogram, uric acid, and urinary albumin-to-creatinine ratio.

TABLE 12.1 (*Continued*)

2017 Guideline for High Blood Pressure in Adults in the United States

5. Screening for secondary causes of hypertension is necessary for new-onset or uncontrolled hypertension in adults, including drug-resistant (≥3 drugs), abrupt onset, age <30 years, excessive target organ damage (cerebral vascular disease, retinopathy, left ventricular hypertrophy, HF with preserved ejection fraction [HFpEF] and HF with reduced EF [HFrEF], coronary artery disease [CAD], chronic kidney disease [CKD], peripheral artery disease, albuminuria) or for the onset of diastolic hypertension in older adults or in the presence of unprovoked or excessive hypokalemia. Screening includes testing for CKD, renovascular disease, primary aldosteronism, obstructive sleep apnea, drug-induced hypertension (nonsteroidal anti-inflammatory drugs, steroids/androgens, decongestants, caffeine, monoamine oxidase inhibitors), and alcohol-induced hypertension. If more specific clinical characteristics are present, screening for uncommon causes of secondary hypertension is indicated (pheochromocytoma, Cushing's syndrome, congenital adrenal hyperplasia, hypothyroidism, hyperthyroidism, and aortic coarctation). Physicians are advised to refer patients screening positive for these conditions to a clinician with specific expertise in the condition.
6. Nonpharmacologic interventions to reduce BP include weight loss for overweight or obese patients with a heart-healthy diet, sodium restriction, and potassium supplementation within the diet, and increased physical activity with a structured exercise program. Men should be limited to no more than two and women no more than one standard alcohol drink(s) per day. The usual impact of each lifestyle change is a 4–5 mm Hg decrease in SBP and 2–4 mm Hg decrease in DBP; but a diet low in sodium, saturated fat, and total fat and an increase in fruits, vegetables, and grains may decrease SBP by approximately 11 mm Hg.
7. The benefit of pharmacologic treatment for BP reduction is related to atherosclerotic CVD (ASCVD) risk. For a given magnitude reduction of BP, fewer individuals with high ASCVD risk would need to be treated to prevent a CVD event (i.e., lower number needed to treat), such as in older persons, those with coronary disease, diabetes, hyperlipidemia, smokers, and CKD. Use of BP-lowering medications is recommended for secondary prevention of recurrent CVD events in patients with clinical CVD and an average SBP ≥ 130 mm Hg or a DBP ≥ 80 mm Hg, or for primary prevention in adults with no history of CVD but with an estimated 10-year ASCVD risk of ≥10% and SBP ≥ 130 mm Hg or DBP ≥ 80 mm Hg. Use of BP-lowering medication is also recommended for primary prevention of CVD in adults with no history of CVD and with an estimated 10-year ASCVD risk <10% and an SBP ≥ 140 mm Hg or a DBP ≥ 90 mm Hg. The prevalence of hypertension is lower in women compared with men until about the fifth decade but is higher later in life. While no randomized controlled trials have been powered to assess outcome specifically in women (e.g., SPRINT), other than special recommendations for the management of hypertension during pregnancy, there is no evidence that the BP threshold for initiating drug treatment, the treatment target, the choice of initial antihypertensive medication, or the combination of medications for lowering BP differs for women compared with men. For adults with confirmed hypertension and known CVD or 10-year ASCVD event risk of 10% or higher, a BP target of <130/80 mm Hg is recommended. For adults with confirmed hypertension, but without additional markers of increased CVD risk, a BP target of <130/80 mm Hg is recommended as reasonable.

(*Continued*)

TABLE 12.1 (*Continued*)

2017 Guideline for High Blood Pressure in Adults in the United States

8. Follow-up: In low-risk adults with elevated BP or stage 1 hypertension with low ASCVD risk, BP should be repeated after 3–6 months of nonpharmacologic therapy. Adults with stage 1 hypertension and high ASCVD risk (≥10% 10-year ASCVD risk) should be managed with both nonpharmacologic and antihypertensive drug therapy with repeat BP in 1 month. Adults with stage 2 hypertension should be evaluated by a primary care provider within 1 month of initial diagnosis and be treated with a combination of nonpharmacologic therapy and two antihypertensive drugs of different classes with repeat BP evaluation in 1 month. For adults with a very high average BP (e.g., ≥160 mm Hg or DBP ≥100 mm Hg), prompt evaluation and drug treatment followed by careful monitoring and upward dose adjustment is recommended.

   Part 2: Principles of Drug Therapy and Special Populations

9. Principles of drug therapy: Chlorthalidone (12.5–25 mg) is the preferred diuretic because of long half-life and proven reduction of CVD risk. Angiotensin-converting enzyme (ACE) inhibitors, angiotensin-receptor blockers (ARBs), and direct renin inhibitors should not be used in combination. ACE inhibitors and ARBs increase the risk of hyperkalemia in CKD and with supplemental K^+ or K^+ sparing drugs. ACE inhibitors and ARBs should be discontinued during pregnancy. Calcium channel blocker (CCB) dihydropyridines cause edema. Non-dihydropyridine CCBs are associated with bradycardia and heart block and should be avoided in HFrEF. Loop diuretics are preferred in HF and when glomerular filtration rate (GFR) is <30 ml/min. Amiloride and triamterene can be used with thiazides in adults with low serum K^+ but should be avoided with GFR < 45 ml/min.

   Spironolactone or eplerenone is preferred for the treatment of primary aldosteronism and in resistant hypertension. Beta-blockers are not first-line therapy except in CAD and HFrEF. Abrupt cessation of beta-blockers should be avoided. Bisoprolol and metoprolol succinate are preferred in hypertension with HFrEF and bisoprolol when needed for hypertension in the setting of bronchospastic airway disease. Beta-blockers with both alpha- and beta-receptor activity such as carvedilol are preferred in HFrEF.

   Alpha-1 blockers are associated with orthostatic hypotension; this drug class maybe considered in men with symptoms of benign prostatic hyperplasia. Central acting $alpha_2$-agonists should be avoided and are reserved as last-line due to side effects and the need to avoid sudden discontinuation. Direct-acting vasodilators are associated with sodium and water retention and must be used with a diuretic and beta-blocker.

10. Initial first-line therapy for stage 1 hypertension includes thiazide diuretics, CCBs, and ACE inhibitors or ARBs. Two first-line drugs of different classes are recommended with stage 2 hypertension and an average BP of 20/10 mm Hg above the BP target. Improved adherence can be achieved with once-daily drug dosing, rather than multiple dosing, and with combination therapy rather than administration of the free individual components.

    For adults with confirmed hypertension and known stable CVD or ≥10% 10-year ASCVD risk, a BP target of <130/80 mm Hg is recommended. The strategy is to first follow standard treatment guidelines for CAD, HFrEF, previous MI, and stable angina, with the addition of other drugs as needed to further control BP. In HFpEF with symptoms of volume overload, diuretics should be used to control hypertension, following which ACE inhibitors or ARBs and beta-blockers should be titrated to SBP < 130 mm Hg. Treatment of hypertension with an ARB can be useful for the prevention of recurrence of atrial fibrillation.

11. CKD: BP goal should be <130/80 mm Hg. In those with stage 3 or higher CKD or stage 1 or 2 CKD with albuminuria (>300 mg/day), treatment with an ACE inhibitor is reasonable to slow the progression of kidney disease. An ARB is reasonable if an ACE inhibitor is not tolerated.

TABLE 12.1 (*Continued*)
2017 Guideline for High Blood Pressure in Adults in the United States

12. Adults with stroke and cerebral vascular disease are complex. To accommodate the variety of important issues pertaining to BP management in the stroke patient, treatment recommendations require recognition of stroke acuity, stroke type, and therapeutic objectives, which along with ideal antihypertensive therapeutic class have not been fully studied in clinical trials. In adults with acute intracranial hemorrhage and SBP > 220 mm Hg, it maybe reasonable to use continuous intravenous drug infusion with close BP monitoring to lower SBP. Immediate lowering of SBP to <140 mm Hg from 150 to 220 mm Hg is not of benefit to reduce death and may cause harm. In acute ischemic stroke, BP should be lowered slowly to <185/110 mm Hg prior to thrombolytic therapy and maintained to <180/105 mm Hg for at least the first 24 hours after initiating drug therapy. Starting or restarting antihypertensive therapy during the hospitalization when patients with ischemic stroke are stable with BP > 140/90 mm Hg is reasonable. In those who do not undergo reperfusion therapy with thrombolytic or endovascular treatment, if the BP is ≥220/120 mm Hg, the benefit of lowering BP is not clear, but it is reasonable to consider lowering BP by 15% during the first 24 hours post onset of stroke. However, initiating or restarting treatment when BP is <220/120 mm Hg within the first 48–72 hours post-acute ischemic stroke is not effective.
    Secondary prevention following a stroke or transient ischemic attack (TIA) should begin by restarting treatment after the first few days of the index event to reduce recurrence. Treatment with ACE inhibitor or ARB with thiazide diuretic is useful. Those not previously treated for hypertension and who have a BP ≥ 140/90 mm Hg should begin antihypertensive therapy a few days after the index event. The selection of drugs should be based on comorbidities. A goal of <130/80 mm Hg maybe reasonable for those with a stroke or TIA. For those with an ischemic stroke and no previous treatment for hypertension, there is no evidence of treatment benefit if the BP is <140/90 mm Hg.
13. Diabetes mellitus (DM) and hypertension: Antihypertensive drug treatment should be initiated at a BP ≥ 130/80 mm Hg with a treatment goal of <130/80 mm Hg. In adults with DM and hypertension, all first-line classes of antihypertensive agents (i.e., diuretics, ACE inhibitors, ARBs, and CCBs) are useful and effective. ACE inhibitors or ARBs maybe considered in the presence of albuminuria.
14. Metabolic syndrome: Lifestyle modification with an emphasis on improving insulin sensitivity by means of dietary modification, weight reduction, and exercise is the foundation of treatment of the metabolic syndrome. The optimal antihypertensive drug therapy for patients with hypertension in the setting of the metabolic syndrome has not been clearly defined. Chlorthalidone was at least as effective for reducing CV events as the other antihypertensive agents in the ALLHAT study. Traditional beta-blockers should be avoided unless used for ischemic heart disease.
15. Valvular heart disease: Asymptomatic aortic stenosis with hypertension should be treated with pharmacotherapy, starting at a low dose, and gradually titrated upward as needed. In patients with chronic aortic insufficiency, treatment of systolic hypertension is reasonable with agents that do not slow the heart rate (e.g., avoid beta-blockers).
16. Aortic disease: Beta-blockers are recommended as the preferred antihypertensive drug class in patients with hypertension and thoracic aortic disease.
17. Race/ethnicity: In African-American adults with hypertension but without HF or CKD, including those with DM, initial antihypertensive treatment should include a thiazide-type diuretic or CCB. Two or more antihypertensive medications are recommended to achieve a BP target of <130/80 mm Hg in most adults, especially in African-American adults, with hypertension.

(*Continued*)

TABLE 12.1 (*Continued*)
2017 Guideline for High Blood Pressure in Adults in the United States

18. Age-related issues: Treatment of hypertension is recommended for noninstitutionalized ambulatory community-dwelling adults (≥65 years of age), with an average SBP ≥ 130 mm Hg with SBP treatment goal of <130 mm Hg. For older adults (≥65 years of age) with hypertension and a high burden of comorbidity and/or limited life expectancy, clinical judgment, patient preference, and a team-based approach to assess risk/benefit is reasonable for decisions regarding intensity of BP lowering and choice of antihypertensive drugs. BP lowering is reasonable to prevent cognitive decline and dementia.
19. Preoperative surgical procedures: Beta-blockers should be continued in persons with hypertension undergoing major surgery, as should other antihypertensive drug therapy until surgery. Discontinuation of ACE inhibitors and ARBs preoperative maybe considered. For patients with planned elective major surgery and SBP ≥ 180 mm Hg or DBP ≥ 110 mm Hg, deferring surgery maybe considered. Abrupt preoperative discontinuation of beta-blockers or clonidine maybe harmful. Intraoperative hypertension should be managed with intravenous medication until oral medications are resumed.
20. For discussion regarding hypertensive crises with and without comorbidities, refer to Section 11.2: Hypertensive Crises – Emergencies and Urgencies in the Guideline.
21. Every adult with hypertension should have a clear, detailed, and current evidence-based plan of care that ensures the achievement of treatment and self-management goals; effective management of comorbid conditions; timely follow-up with the healthcare team; and adheres to CVD evidence-based guidelines. Effective behavioral and motivational strategies are recommended to promote lifestyle modification. A structured team-based approach, including a physician, nurse, and pharmacist collaborative model, is recommended, along with integrating home-based monitoring and telehealth interventions. Outcome maybe improved with quality improvement strategies at the health system, provider, and patient level. Financial incentives paid to providers can be useful.

Whelton PK, Carey RM, Aronow WS, et al. 2017 ACC/AHA/AAPA/ABC/ACPM/AGS/APhA/ASH/ASPC/NMA/PCNA Guideline for the prevention, detection, evaluation, and management of high blood pressure in adults: a report of the American College of Cardiology/American Heart Association Task Force on Clinical Practice Guidelines. J Am Coll Cardiol. 2018;71: e127–e248.

12.1 HYPERTENSION INSTITUTE PROGRAM AND APPROACH TO HYPERTENSION DIAGNOSIS AND TREATMENT

12.1.1 Understand the Problem

Hypertension is a process and maybe more of a marker for a damaged and unhealthy artery (endothelium, glycocalyx, and artery). Hypertension is a disease of the artery and the increase in BP is really a "marker" for the abnormal artery. Abnormalities of arterial and heart function and structure may precede the development of hypertension by decades. Certainly, once hypertension occurs, it will inflict more damage on the arteries such that hypertension becomes a "bidirectional process." (1–20) This new concept is shown in Figure 12.1. The best approach is to select optimal nutrition, nutraceutical supplements, lifestyle changes, and drugs to improve arterial function and structure and lower BP.

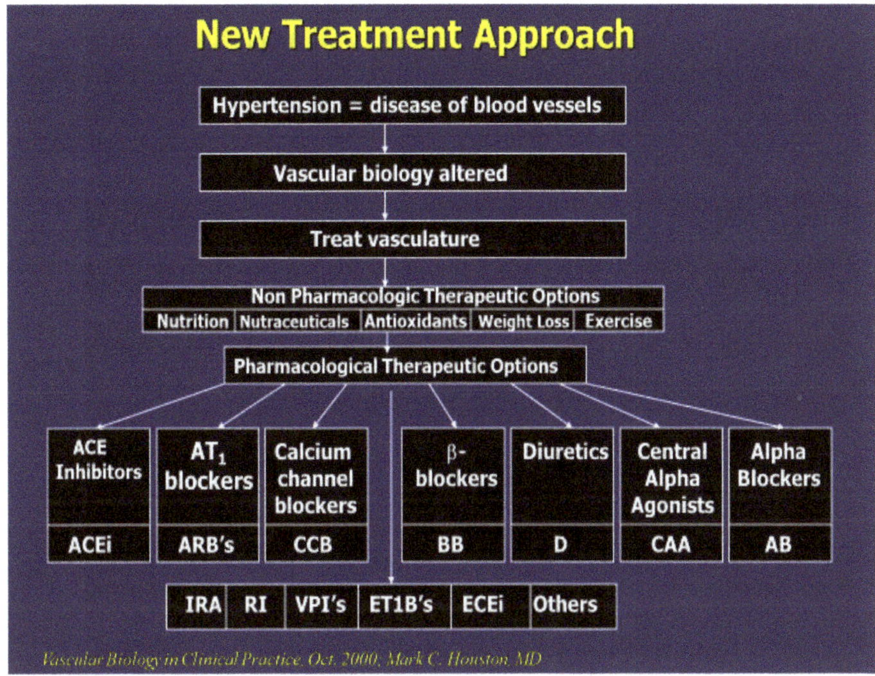

FIGURE 12.1 New approach to the treatment of hypertension based on vascular biology and that hypertension is a disease of the artery.

The arterial damage and dysfunction occur early leading to an abnormal vasculature. Nondrug treatment combined with the best BP-lowering medications that address both the function and structure of the artery and reduce the BP is the best approach.

12.1.2 Institute the Hypertension Institute Programs for Diagnosis and Treatment (1–20) Ask Your Doctor to Determine All of the Items Listed in the Following for You.

1. Determine the BP level and other important measurements using a 24-hour ambulatory BP monitoring device (24-hour ABPM) in conjunction with regular office BPs measured correctly using the AHA criteria and instruct the patient in the proper use of home BP readings with the best validated BP monitors.
2. Measure in the blood your micronutrient and macronutrient status and optimally replace all of those deficiencies with proper nutrition and supplements, antioxidants, and minerals. We recommend the **Spectracell Labs Micronutrient Test, (MNT), Houston, Tx.** for nutrient testing **(see sources).**

3. Measure blood tests that determine the type of hypertension that is present. The two forms are called **high-renin hypertension and low-renin hypertension.** The blood tests include a plasma renin activity or PRA, (a hormone that controls BP and aldosterone (a hormone that controls BP and blood volume. This will be discussed in detail later in this book.
4. Measure the genetics that determines your BP and risk for coronary heart disease, heart attack, BP, diabetes mellitus, cholesterol, and other blood fats. We recommend **Vibrant Labs in San Francisco for the Cardia X cardiovascular genomic profile (see sources).**
5. Assess the presence and severity of the artery function, structure, and damage, artery elasticity and stiffness, endothelial function, glycocalyx function, nitric oxide levels, heart function and stiffness, heart size (enlargement), risk for coronary heart disease, coronary artery calcification, rest and exercise BP, heart rate and its variability, the function of your nervous system, and how it relates to BP and your overall cardiovascular risk with various noninvasive cardiovascular testing (**see** Chapter 9).
6. Exclude all of the secondary causes of hypertension (**see** Chapter 3, Table 12.1).
7. Assess all of the new and emerging blood and urine tests, which are called cardiovascular risk factors, in addition to the usual measured risk factors, such as blood fats and cholesterol, blood sugar (diabetes mellitus), homocysteine, inflammation markers, and many more (**see** Chapter 9, Table 12.1).
8. Properly measure obesity, total and regional body fat with a special machine called **body impedance analysis. Maintain your ideal body weight, BMI, and body fat.**
9. Determine the need for early and aggressive control of BP based on the information listed earlier.
10. Start the Hypertension Institute BP nutrition program (**see Nutrition** Chapters 14 and 15).
11. Use specific BP-lowering nutritional supplements (**see** Chapter 16).
12. Exercise regularly with both resistance and aerobic exercises using guidelines that are recommended in this book (ABCT) and by your physician (**see** Chapter 17).
13. De-stress your life with meditation, relaxation, and breathing exercises and more (**see** Chapter 17).
14. Stop all tobacco products (**see** Chapter 17).
15. Reduce or stop alcohol (**see** Chapter 17).
16. Stop caffeine if your genetics show that you cannot break down caffeine rapidly (slow metabolizer) (**see** Chapter 17).
17. Stop or reduce all medications, if possible, that may increase your BP (**see** Chapter 3, Table 12.1).
18. Use the best medications to lower BP, improve arterial function and structure, and decrease cardiovascular events (Chapter 18).

12.1.3 The Criteria to Start Early and Aggressive Treatment of Hypertension" (1–20)

1. Level of BP. The higher the level the greater the risk for cardiovascular disease and the more urgent and aggressive the treatment should be.
2. Presence of other coronary heart risk factors, such as diabetes mellitus, high cholesterol, smoking, obesity, and others.
3. Calculation of coronary heart risk with one of the new risk scoring system that indicates high risk for heart attack or other cardiovascular complications.
4. Presence of cardiovascular target organ damage, such as retinal damage, heart enlargement, known coronary heart disease, previous stroke or heart attack, kidney damage, protein in the urine, arteriosclerosis, atherosclerosis, carotid artery blockage or increase in carotid IMT, endothelial dysfunction, arterial stiffness, and heart stiffness.
5. Presence of other preclinical tests for vascular damage such as EndoPAT, CAPWA, central BP, augmentation index, ECHO, CPET, CAC as previously discussed in Chapter 9.
6. Presence of clinical symptoms related to BP, such as headache, chest pain at rest or with exercise, and dyspnea.

12.1.4 Proof that the Hypertension Institute Program Works. Published Clinical Trial (20)

A clinical trial was performed at the Hypertension Institute in Nashville and published in 2010. The design and details of that study are described as follows:

1. A total of 671 hypertensive patients with BPs of 140/90–210/115 mm Hg at baseline BP measurement were studied.
2. MNT (micronutrient testing) and plasma renin activity and aldosterone blood levels were done in all patients.
3. Treatment was with antihypertensive drugs, repletion of nutritional deficiencies, therapeutic doses of appropriate nutritional supplements, DASH 2 diet, combined aerobic and resistance exercise, and ideal body weight and composition.
4. A composite nutritional program included proprietary nutraceutical supplement combinations for vascular protection, BP.
5. Hypertensive patients had significantly more micronutrient deficiencies compared to normal patients ($n = 2667$) ($p < 0.0017$).
6. These deficiencies included biotin, serine, asparagine, calcium, and vitamin D ($p < 0.0017$) and for vitamin B1, choline, insulin, magnesium, coenzyme Q-10, lipoic acid, and total antioxidant level with Spectrox ($p < 0.05$).
7. Repeat testing at 6 months showed a significantly improved antioxidant profile by 8.47% ($p = 0.03$) and over 97% complete repletion rate of micronutrients with the supplement and nutrition program.
8. A total of 62% of the hypertensive patients over a period of 6 months (average) range 4–12 months were able to taper and discontinue antihypertensive drugs with a controlled BP range of 120/80–126/84 mm Hg.

In other words, *62% of those patients* who followed the Hypertension Institute Program were able to gradually discontinue their BP medications on 1 year and maintain a normal BP of about 120/80 mm Hg! Even more patients, who had less severe BP levels of less than 160 mm Hg systolic and less than 95 mm Hg diastolic at their baseline evaluations, were able to stop BP medications in 1 year (**almost 75%**)!

12.2 SUMMARY AND KEY POINTS

1. Hypertension is a process of vascular dysfunction that occurs early in life based on genetics and other environmental factors.
2. Hypertension is a marker of vascular dysfunction.
3. Once the BP is elevated, there is bidirectional vascular damage.
4. Aggressive diagnostic testing should be done to identify vascular and heart damage, risk factors, nutrient status, type of hypertension, genetics, and BP levels.
5. Early and aggressive treatments to improve vascular function, structure, and BP are key to reduce cardiovascular disease.
6. Many classes of BP-lowering medications have adverse effects others are better tolerated.
7. Nutrition and nutritional supplements with lifestyle changes and optimal drug therapy provide a personalized, precise, and integrative approach to control BP, reduce cardiovascular damage, decrease drug side effects, and cost.

REFERENCES

1. Whelton PK, et al. ACC/AHA/AAPA/ABC/ACPM/AGS/APhA/ASH/ASPC/NMA/PCNA Guideline for the prevention, detection, evaluation, and management of high blood pressure in adults: a report of the American College of Cardiology/American Heart Association Task Force on Clinical Practice Guidelines. Hypertension. 2018 Jun;71(6):e13–e115.
2. Houston M. The role of nutrition and nutraceutical supplements in the treatment of hypertension. World J Cardiol. 2014;6(2):38–66.
3. Houston M. Nutrition and nutraceutical supplements for the treatment of hypertension: Part 1. J Clin Hypertens. 2013;15:752–757.
4. Houston M. Nutrition and nutraceutical supplements for the treatment of hypertension: Part II. J Clin Hypertens. 2013;15:845–851.
5. Houston M. Nutrition and nutraceutical supplements for the treatment of hypertension: Part III J Clin Hypertens. 2013;15:931–937.
6. Borghi C, Cicero AF. Nutraceuticals with a clinically detectable blood pressure-lowering effect: a review of available randomized clinical trials and their meta-analyses. Br J Clin Pharmacol. 2017;83(1):163–171.
7. Sirtori CR, Arnoldi A, Cicero AF. Nutraceuticals for blood pressure control. Rev Ann Med. 2015;47(6):447–456.
8. Cicero AF, Colletti A. Nutraceuticals and blood pressure control: results from clinical trials and meta-analyses. High Blood Press Cardiovasc Prev. 2015;22(3):203–213.
9. Turner JM, Spatz ES. Nutritional supplements for the treatment of hypertension: a practical guide for clinicians. Curr Cardiol Rep. 2016;18(12):126.

10. Caligiuri SP, Pierce GN. A review of the relative efficacy of dietary, nutritional supplements, lifestyle and drug therapies in the management of hypertension. Crit Rev Food Sci Nutr. 2017;57:3508–3527.
11. Houston MC, Fox B, Taylor N. What Your Doctor May Not Tell You About Hypertension. The Revolutionary Nutrition and Lifestyle Program to Help Fight High Blood Pressure. AOL Time Warner, Warner Books, New York, NY, 2003.
12. Houston M. Treatment of hypertension with nutrition and nutraceutical supplement: Part 1. Altern Compliment Med. 2019;24:260–275.
13. Houston M. Treatment of hypertension with nutrition and nutraceutical supplement: Part 2. Altern Compliment Med. 2019;25:23–36.
14. Sinatra S, Houston M, Editors. Nutrition and Integrative Strategies in Cardiovascular Medicine. CRC Press, 2015.
15. The seventh report of the Joint National Committee on prevention, detection, evaluation, and treatment of high blood pressure (JNC-7). JAMA. 2003;289:2560–2572.
16. Thomopoulos C, Parati G, Zanchetti A. Effects of blood pressure lowering on outcome incidence in hypertension: 7. Effects of more vs. less intensive blood pressure lowering and different achieved blood pressure levels – updated overview and meta-analyses of randomized trials. J Hypertens. 2016;34(4):613–622.
17. Ettehad D, Emdin CA, Kiran A, Anderson SG, Callender T, Emberson J, Chalmers J, Rodgers A, Rahimi K. Blood pressure lowering for prevention of cardiovascular disease and death: a systematic review and meta-analysis. Lancet. 2016;387(10022):957–967.
18. ESH/ESC Task Force for the Management of Arterial Hypertension. 2013 Practice guidelines for the management of arterial hypertension of the European Society of Hypertension (ESH) and the European Society of Cardiology (ESC): ESH/ESC Task Force for the Management of Arterial Hypertension. J Hypertens. 2013;31:1925–1938.
19. Flack JM, Calhoun D, Schiffrin EL. The New ACC/AHA hypertension guidelines for the prevention, detection, evaluation, and management of high blood pressure in adults. Am J Hypertens. 2018;31(2):133–135.
20. Houston MC. The role of cellular micronutrient analysis and minerals in the prevention and treatment of hypertension and cardiovascular disease. Ther Adv Cardiovasc Dis. 2010;4:165–183.

13 Beyond The Dash I and Dash II Diets

Making the case for the HIP (Hypertension Institute Plan) – A paradigm for the modern age

Given the multitude of dietary approaches to mitigate hypertension and cardiovascular disease, why the need for another option? Simple. Diets in practice are different than diets in theory. Every day, my clinical experience corroborates a simple idea that should be obvious, but is not – patients have far better outcomes when a dietary strategy is tailored to their individual needs. After all, there is no such thing as an average patient and thus, it is bad practice to take an isolated view of diet based solely on the need to control high blood pressure, or any health condition for that matter.

There are many components that influence the formulation of the most advantageous diets. These include age, gender, health history, health goals, health conditions, current body composition, hormone status, level of activity, palate preferences, and, likely the most important factor, a patient's response to a diagnosis and whether that serves as the catalyst for changing current dietary and lifestyle choices.

My clinical approach has always been very goal oriented. Having spent most of my adult life in urban environments, I have observed that those who live in cities where they battle daily traffic, compete for parking spots, and wait in lines for almost everything, do not have patience for a program, or anything else, that does not yield results. In the words of the immortal Zig Ziglar, "If you aim at nothing, you will hit it every time." To that end, I have never understood the point of handing a patient a sheet of paper with an outline for a diet without a blueprint for how to actually put it into practice and make it stick. Compliance counts. Starting a new program is easy, but making it a permanent part of your lifestyle takes a comprehensive strategy.

Prior to moving to Nashville, I was the Director of Nutrition for the former clinical chiefs of rheumatology at Cedars-Sinai in Los Angeles. During my time there, I had designed a comprehensive program for our patients that was at its core a gut healing, anti-inflammatory, glucose regulating diet, coupled with cognitive behavioral therapy, more succinctly known as CBT. The addition of this critical feature into the program supported the need to bridge the gap between a patient knowing what to do, and actually being able to do it. Based on formal education, but more importantly the experience in clinical work, it became clear to me that wellness was best achieved through a multifaceted approach that drew heavily from the principles of integrative medicine, or what some refer to today as functional medicine.

The principles of my practice have always been seen through the prism of functional medicine, which is essentially a systems-oriented approach (as opposed to a reductionist view). This approach takes into account the whole person: the influence of genetics, environment, daily habits, integrity of sleep, stress reduction rituals, and health history, as well as the science behind specific conditions. Once aligned with a program to develop the concrete skills needed to achieve long-lasting results, we hit the sweet spot – no pun intended.

And thus, the question on the table was, could this successful protocol designed for autoimmune patients be updated and modified for the individual needs of hypertension patients? And could we diminish not only the risks associated with hypertension and cardiovascular disease but also address many of the common attendant issues such as obesity, type II diabetes, high inflammatory status, and gut issues? The short answer was heck yeah. And thus, the *H*ypertension *I*nstitute *P*rotocol, or *HIP*, was conceived and put into practice. Since its implementation approximately 2 years ago, the results have been unprecedented for our patient population, as well as for us as practitioners.

The following are but three of countless success stories that highlight the transformative impact HIP has had on patient lives and well-being. In these narratives, it should be clear that these interventions took a bespoke approach that considered the holistic patient and not a particular health issue.

Case Study #1 – PAUL

Paul was a 61-year-old, successful record company executive with a rigorous travel schedule. At 5′10″ and weighing in at 302 lbs., his primary health concerns were his weight, hypertension, dyslipidemia, psoriatic arthritis, and the long list of medications that he was on to keep his chronic health conditions under control and the potential side effects of those meds. He had tried numerous dietary strategies over the years and most recently adopted a vegan diet for almost a year with no long-lasting success. At the time of our consult, he was eating roughly half of his meals at home and the other half at restaurants. He drank 3 to 4 cups of coffee daily and reported abundant cravings for carb-rich foods. His goals were simple — drop some weight, normalize blood pressure, taper down on medications, feel lighter and most importantly, realize his commitment to establishing a ‘new normal’ way of life. As committed as Paul was to adopting new rituals that would improve the quality of his life, I was committed to Paul for the long haul. He started the HIP and within a two-week period, Paul had dropped 12 lbs. and had seen his daily, morning blood pressure readings drop from an average of 150/85 to 130/78; and, he began to report an almost total elimination of food cravings, along with a greater sense of well-being and optimism that he would achieve his goals, specifically getting down to the 220 lb. range, a weight he hadn’t seen on his scale since his mid 20s. After a year, he has maintained over 100 lbs. weight loss and is on the lowest dosage of only one medication.

Case Study #2 – DORIS

Doris came to see me as a two-time survivor of breast and colon cancer. In her early 60s, she's 5′7″ at a weight of 205 lbs. Her primary health concerns were keeping her inflammatory markers down and thereby improving her chances of being cancer free, addressing hypertension, achieving an optimum body weight, and, at all cost, avoiding type II diabetes. What's interesting about Doris is that she was far from consuming the SAD, or the Standard American Diet. She was convinced she had as clean a diet as she could muster, given her understanding of food groups, and told me during our consult that she would be shocked if a dietary change would elicit any real improvement in her weight or biomarkers. Six months into the HIP, Doris is down 45 lbs., her HbA1c has dropped from 6.8 to 5.1, and she is enjoying preparing glucose regulating meals for her friends and family.

Case Study #3 – KERRY

Kerry, at 50, was defeated and depleted when we first met. At 225 lbs., she was on two hypertension medications, was deeply concerned about her weight and her lack of mobility and had taken a sizeable hit to her self-esteem and health. Overall, she was experiencing a diminished quality of life and sense of hopelessness. She fondly recalled better times in her life when she felt good about herself, her health prospects, and also expressed concern over what kind of role model she was for her daughters once she 'let herself go.' After 5 months almost to the day on the HIP, she's down 70 lbs., off of all hypertension medications, has a renewed interest in exercise, and has a newfound sense of vitality and optimism.

These success stories speak to the strengths of the HIP approach, but more importantly, they provide insight into why treating the holistic patient *and* engaging that patient in the therapeutic process are so essential. Especially when it comes to food, a primary driver for all of us, this two-pronged approach creates a more likely scenario for success. While Paul, Doris, and Kerry had unique needs, they also shared certain characteristics that improved their odds of successfully navigating the HIP. First and foremost, they were motivated by health goals, not weight. That is not to say that dropping weight was not a source of motivation and gratification, but it was not the primary driver. Second, they were all coachable. In other words, they were invested and genuinely interested in unraveling the mystery of their individual biochemistry, but they were all open to and willing to implement new ideas and strategies in order to facilitate a different outcome. Third, they embraced the temporary discomfort of changing habits in order to achieve greater health and go all-in on the HIP.

13.1 THE ROLE OF FOOD IN HEALTH AND WELLNESS

So, what is food and why does it matter so much? According to dictionary.com, food is "any nourishing substance that is eaten, drunk, or otherwise taken into the body to sustain life, provide energy, promote growth, etc.." That same source defines "nourishing" as, "(of food) containing substances necessary for growth, health, and good condition". Needless to say, I am a little suspicious about the inclusion of "etc.," but let us let that slide for the time being.

In the simplest terms, food is **information**. In other words, what are you telling your body when you opt for kale versus an average trip through the drive-thru? According to the National Institutes of Health (NIH), four of the six leading causes of death in the United States are linked to unhealthy diet. What you choose to eat has tremendous influence over your health status.

Perhaps, part of the problem facing so many Americans relates to the shift toward prioritizing exercise that has happened since the 1980s. The preeminence of exercise in the American psyche has worked to almost make food an afterthought. While we give lip service to diet, most of us think that exercise is the primary driver in achieving health and wellness goals. To flip that around, diet correlates in our minds with restriction and/or weight loss and is not conceived of as *adding value to our lives.* In a recent Gallup poll looking at American perceptions of weight loss, 31% of Americans said that exercising was their main tool in losing weight, while 23% cited "eating less." Only a handful of respondents referenced improving the *quality* of what they eat, such as removing sugars from their diet. The American paradigm today is to restrict and amp up the exercise while leaving toxins and sugars to do their dirty work.

This is not to say that exercise is not essential and relevant to health and wellness. Although exercise is a vital part of well-being for a variety of reasons, diet still accounts for roughly 80% of your health, while movement contributes somewhere near the remaining 20%. This may explain why you may have noticed that when you amped up your exercise regimen in the past, but did not reshape your diet, your scale did not move much. There are dire consequences for disregarding the importance of how you feed yourself. (3) According to the Centers for Disease Control and Prevention (CDC), for 2018, these are the leading causes of death in the United States: heart disease, cancer, accidents, chronic lower respiratory diseases, stroke, Alzheimer's disease, diabetes, influenza, and pneumonia.

13.1.1 SAD Eating – An American Way of Life

It is said that as a nation we are overfed and undernourished. This is played out every day in the Standard American Diet, sadly referred to as, well, SAD. The SAD is a modern dietary construct built for an age that has put a premium on convenience, low cost, and mindless acquisition. These low-nutrient density, highly processed, often prepackaged foods tend to be high in animal fats, high in sugar, high in hydrogenated vegetable oils, and high sodium and can be found almost anywhere at almost any time. It is not only the *quality* of our food selections. According to Pew Research, Americans eat a greater *quantity* than we did historically. In 2010, the average American consumed 23% more calories than we did in 1970, which in terms of calorie intake, means most adults are taking in more than they need to maintain their current weight.

Nearly half of those additional calories come from only two food groups: flours and grains, and fats and oils. And while meats, dairy products, and sweeteners account for smaller shares of our daily caloric intake than they did four decades ago, we have also reduced the degree to which we consume fruits and vegetables.

Why are we eating like this? The Industrial Revolution, which kicked in about 200 years ago, dramatically altered the way, as a society, we eat. For the first time in human history, with the advent of factory farming, processing, mass distribution, and marketing to the consumer, food became a product. Now, instead of nourishing us, food the commodity had to constantly strive is to be made faster, cheaper, and "better." The holy grail of processing is to lower the cost of food. No one would dispute the nobility in the endeavor to get calories into the masses. For most of human history, food scarcity was a primary concern as was the specter of malnutrition. No one could have predicted the consequences of moving our society into a world of abundance.

Popular thinking today (as promoted by the CDC's body mass index standards) is that America's weight began ticking up in the 1980s (ironically, during the uptick in the exercise craze.). Research conducted in the European Union suggests a much longer and slower trend, a march toward obesity that paced itself from the Industrial Revolution to the 1980s:

> *"The lifestyle changes of the 20th century affected the four groups under study somewhat differently. Identifying the deep causes of the long-run trends is outside of the scope of this study, but the "creeping" nature of the epidemic, as well as its persistence, does suggest that its roots are embedded deep in the social fabric and are nourished by a network of disparate slowly changing sources as the 20th-century US population responded to a vast array of irresistible and impersonal socio-economic and technological forces.*

The most obviously persistent among these were:

- *the major labour-saving technological changes of the 20th century,*
- *the industrial processing of food and with it the spread of fast-food eateries (To illustrate the spread of fast food culture, consider that White Castle, the first drive-in restaurant, was founded in 1921. McDonald started operation in the late 1940s, Kentucky Fried Chicken in 1952, Burger King in 1954, Pizza Hut in 1958, Taco Bell in 1962, and Subway in 1962.),*
- *the associated culture of consumption,*
- *the rise of an automobile-based way of life,*
- *the introduction of radio and television broadcasting,*
- *the increasing participation of women in the work force, and*
- *the IT revolution.*

> *These elements – taken together – virtually defined American society in the 20th century*
>
> *Chou et al. 2008, Cutler et al. 2003, Hamermesh 2010, Lakdawalla and Philipson 2009, Offer 2006, Philipson and Posner 2003, Popkin, 2004."*[1]

In modern times, the big food industry, whether it is trickled down to your local grocery store or manufacturers, offers abundant incentives such as coupons and sales for these foods that have already been aggressively marketed to consumers. According to a report from BIA Advisory Services, the fast-food industry was on track to spend $4 billion on advertising in 2019. When is the last time you spotted a sultry ad for watercress? According to the CDC, only one in ten Americans meets the requirement for fruit and vegetables daily.

The consequences of the SAD have been devastating on Americans and the American health-care system. Over 40% of adults are overweight or obese along with one-third of children. **This diet is a disease manual.**

The SAD maintains a focus on processed, artificially sweetened, and fast foods and is high in sodium, cheese, and low-quality animal proteins with a minimal intake of whole foods such as vegetables, fruits, clean-sourced animal proteins, and healthy fats. Fifty percent of the diet focused on flour and grain products, in essence, foods that are high in sugar and that convert to sugar in the body. Consumption of corn is also higher than it has been ever before in human history.

At some point in the late 1980s, too, foods promoted as "healthy" began to appear on grocery store shelves. These deceptive products focused on fat intake and America's fear of its increasing waistline. While they may have been low on fat or even entirely fat-free, these foods were chock-full of one thing – sugar. Thus, not only were the general foods in the American diet heavy on cheap carbs but also the foods purporting to be "good for you."

All this being said, why have we been doing it? Why has America been indulging in a diet that is so destructive?

THERE ARE TWO PRIMARY BENEFITS OF THE STANDARD AMERICAN DIET:

1. It is easy to comply with because there is no thought needed to eat high processed food and it can be found anywhere at any time. From fast food to local grocery stores to convenience markets, airports, sporting events. It is always available.
2. It is CHEAP. Processed foods with ingredients you cannot pronounce are cheap to produce, and grocers offer loads of incentives through coupons and sales on these items, but not too often for the fresh food.

According to the Journal of the American Heart Association, it is estimated that 30–50% of all US adults have hypertension. Data suggests hypertension is the costliest of all cardiovascular diseases, and it is estimated that the current state of healthcare expenditures related to hypertension cost is about $131 billion dollars annually. This merits a concerted effort on behalf of practitioners and patients to focus on treatment and prevention.

Diabetes costs Americans $327 billion annually according to the American Diabetes Association. More than 30 million are with type II diabetes. CAN WE AFFORD THIS HEALTH CONDITIONS??? These are staggering costs and the solutions require deep deliberation on what we have been doing, and what can be done.

13.2 THE HIP – A TRANSFORMATIONAL ALTERNATIVE TO SAD

Why did other diets fail and the Hypertension Institute Plan (HIP) sail? HIP is a program that was borne out of the need to radically improve patient outcomes in a world that wants to throw a Band-Aid on health conditions. A pill for every ill, rather than start from the ground up and ask patients a hard question: What have you done to contribute to your metabolic conditions, and are you willing to make the changes needed to improve your life? It is said that we do not have "health care" in America, we have "disease management." This rings true to me. A significant part of that comes through how medicine performed as "disease management" eliminates the patient from the equation. HIP, as an alternative, gives the patient agency and makes them a stakeholder in the process.

HIP adheres to three central principles:

- Education
- Empowerment
- Patient responsibility

To this end, each patient participating in the HIP process asks themselves, "Do I understand what I've been diagnosed with, and do I know the consequences of that diagnosis?" I ask every patient, "What does it mean to be hypertensive? What does it mean that you're insulin resistant, pre-diabetic, or have type II diabetes?" Less than 10% know what either of those diagnoses actually means. In studies run on both diabetes patients and patients with heart conditions, patients who had more dialogue with their doctors and had a better understanding of their conditions fared better in treatment. Even without the science, each of us can understand the experience of doing better when we have more clarity and more agency.

This is at the heart, too, of the CBT process, in which the patient is engaged in identifying triggers and invited to participate in the development of their own interventions. As a form of nutritional intervention that incorporates the protocols of CBT, HIP is predicated on patient participation and asks them to create their own change.

So, HOW do patients create permanent change? HIP is a multidimensional approach. At its heart, it is a dietary strategy, natch. Like other interventions in the traditional nutritional counseling framework, HIP addresses **what to eat** and **how to eat**. Beyond that, however, it is an approach to **lifestyle modification**.

For one, we use technology to track patients and make them accountable. Holding them accountable is done constructively, and they are engaged in the process of correcting missteps and holding themselves accountable. All along the way, patients can and are encouraged to ask questions. They get answers quickly and then course correct for their needs.

It is through this combination of patient engagement and dietary modifications that HIP achieves its goal – it *works*.

Almost anyone can give you a sheet of paper with a plan for a diet, medications, supplements, and some lifestyle modifications that would benefit a patient; but, more often than not, there is a chasm between knowing what to do and actually being able to facilitate it. That is where the real work lies. Time and time again, through HIP, it is been proven that when we can bridge that gap, success is found.

13.2.1 Creating an Environment of Collaboration Through HIP

The HIP is not a sheet of paper with a set of instructions but rather a living, breathing, collaborative approach to educating patients and shifting the responsibility of care. It cannot be said enough – HIP requires patient involvement.

I used the term "accountable" earlier. Accountability is, really, an oversimplification of what we do in HIP. HIP is about creating an environment in which patients can learn about their condition, collaborate on a strategy to address their individual needs, go through trial and error, connect with us in (ART) almost real time, and afford us (and themselves!) the opportunity to course correct.

Societal norms in health care have historically limited patient participation, across medical disciplines. A medical culture that dictates a passive role on the part of the patient has left the patient incapable of and unwilling to assert themselves or participate. Patient participation does not only give them agency, it can actually affect the quality of medical care. Research done at NIH showed that an increase in patient participation could potentially limit the occurrence of medical errors. When patients are given the power to speak up and participate, they can spot human error and machine error, for example. In the context of HIP, they can speak to their quality of care, what is working and not working, and develop coping mechanisms and execute adjustments, as they would in a CBT setting.

I am HIP, we teach you the practical strategies you need when you want to master your rituals and create permanent change and remarkable results…if we cannot find a path to compliance, no diet will help you. The patient is invited to create their own change.

If you are not able to change a habit that will lead to the results you are after, it is not YOU, it is your rituals. What we do is to help you engage in the repetition necessary to hard-wire results. Changing habits is never easy for anyone. As practiced in CBT, changing habits requires three steps:

1. Acknowledgment: The patient needs to acknowledge that they want to change. Their attention then shifts toward the behavior that needs to change. Similar to the practice of mindfulness in Buddhism, this attention shift focuses the mind with clarity and specificity on the change that needs to happen.
2. Focus: With the patient's attention now on the habit that needs to change, the patient maintains focus, honing in on the reasons change is necessary and weighing both the assets and deficits of continuing this type of behavior. In this way, the patient gets a motivator in the form of a "why" that can drive them toward more positive behaviors.
3. Intentional Repetition: Repetition is key to creating real change in our minds, and the only way to rewire neural pathways. The patient is encouraged to replace the old habit with the new in an ongoing and mindful way. Eventually, the new habit should become second nature and supplant the negative habit.

Through these three steps, the HIP patient learns to align themselves with healthier habits and engage in a more productive relationship with food. While other dietary plans address only the what, HIP gives the patient a why and how.

13.2.2 Treating the Whole Patient in HIP

Another concern I have with multiple dietary interventions out there is that they do not treat the whole patient. Instead, they address a single aspect of a disease and do not consider the multiple factors that inform a patient's individual relationship with nutrition. To understand this more clearly, let us consider how a patient with hypertension is typically handled.

If you have high blood pressure, chances are you have been advised to lose weight – if you are overweight or obese, the higher your blood pressure is likely to be. Furthermore, the presence of hypertension predicts a likelihood of a future diagnosis of type II diabetes, and the incidence of hypertension significantly increases the likelihood of type II diabetes. In other words, high blood pressure and type II diabetes are bidirectional. According to statistics from the CDC and National Health and Nutritional Examination Survey (NHANES), type II diabetes mellitus (T2DM) has risen sharply in the last few decades and it is estimated that T2DM affects more than 30 million people in the United States, and over 70% of individuals aged 18 years or more with diabetes have hypertension.[2]

With that in mind, would not it make sense that, if you are going to address hypertension with diet and lifestyle modifications, it would be prudent to also address glycemic control at a minimum? And yet, that is not done in the majority of nutritional interventions for patients like these. There is not a modicum of sense in addressing the issue of hypertension without looking at attendant conditions for individual patients. Thus, we need a comprehensive strategy that includes diet and lifestyle interventions to improve weight and other metabolic conditions and risk factors. That is good medicine.

That is HIP.

Standing in opposition to HIP is what has been the gold standard until now in addressing hypertension – DASH, or the Dietary Approach to Stop Hypertension.

13.2.3 The Disappointment of DASH

Since it originated in the 1990s, yes, as in 30 years ago give or take, the **D**ietary **A**pproach to **S**top **H**ypertension, more commonly known as, **DASH**, has been touted as the holy grail of guidelines for eating, designed to treat and/or prevent high blood pressure and reduce the risk of heart disease without the benefit of medication.

The DASH diet does NOT list specific foods to include in your diet. Instead, it is a dietary framework focused on servings of specific food groups that are listed in the following based on a 2000 calorie/day plan:

- Whole grains: 6–8 servings/day
- Vegetables: 4–5 servings/day
- Fruits: 4–5 servings/day

- Low-fat dairy products: 2–3 servings/day
- Lean chicken, meat, and fish: 6 or fewer servings per day
- Nuts, seeds, and legumes: 4–5 servings/week
- Fats and oils: 2–3 servings/day
- Candy and added sugars: 5 or fewer servings per week

In addition, there are guidelines pertaining to sodium intake as well as suggestions for limits on caffeine and alcohol. To comply with the original iteration of the DASH means you can consume up to 2300 mg of sodium per day, or one teaspoon. If you opt for the DASH II, there is a greater reduction in sodium intake to 1500 mg daily, or roughly 3/4 teaspoon. Both versions of the DASH have a lower sodium requirement when compared to the SAD, which can be higher than 3400 mg daily. That may sound cheering, but, to give these ranges some context, the American Heart Association recommends **1500 mg a day** as the upper limit for sodium daily.

So, what are the known benefits of the DASHs?

Like most things in life, context is the key and thus the real question here is how do the DASHs compare to what your current diet looks like and is it an improvement? For most Americans, the answer is – yes and/or no.

Yes, it is an improvement if you are like most people and have adopted the SAD. Anything, frankly, is an improvement from the SAD. Adopting the DASH in lieu of more health-conscious dietary choices, however, is **not** beneficial. DASH has some sizeable shortcomings when compared to a more bioindividualized dietary strategy such as HIP that takes into account the whole person rather than just the diagnosis.

DASH is considered a success for one reason and one reason alone – it reduces sodium intake. Think about that. What is the gold standard for dietary intervention in treating conditions as complex as hypertension? Instead, how could a patient benefit from a more whole foods-based, glucose regulating, gut healing, and low inflammatory diet?

Consider this, too: Evidence suggests that disrupted carbohydrate metabolism is more common in hypertensives, thereby indicating that the pathogenic relationship between type II diabetes and hypertension is actually **bidirectional**. Given the prevalence of T2DM and HPT, can you responsibly make dietary recommendations for one without taking the other into consideration? I do not think so. Consider, too, these downsides of the DASH plan.

Difficult to keep up

I cited a figure above that is jarring – the average American consumes around 3400 mg of sodium each day. Putting aside the terrifying implications that have for health, let us consider what that has done to the American palette. Simply put, people can no longer taste or enjoy food unless it is soaked in salt.

For this reason alone, DASH can be hard for patients to maintain in the long term. With palettes skewed toward high sodium intake, the DASH plan is unsatisfying and, as a result, harder to keep up and manifest as a true lifestyle change.

There have been some alternatives suggested. One variation on the DASH plan introduces more fat into the diet, theorizing that the uptick in fat will assuage the patient craving for sodium. This alternative managed to lower blood pressure without raising LDL significantly but there is no indication that it had a sizeable impact on patient compliance.

All in, the research has indicated that adhering to DASH is difficult for patients, and that more than nutritional counseling is needed for patients to keep the plan up in the long term.

To that end, DASH has no integrated, organized support for patients. There are registered dietitians who might provide coaching in tandem with the DASH plan, but there is no protocol in place within DASH to foment true behavioral change in patients, as is the case with HIP.

Another concern is the lack of individualization in the DASH plan. While calorie counting is not part of the plan, patients are required to adhere to certain calorie goals within each food group. This does not take into account any of the bioindividual characteristics of a patient. The NIH simply provides downloadable guidelines that are meant to serve as a "one-size-fits-all" for all DASH patients.

Finally, and astonishingly, DASH is not considered appropriate for patients **with many disorders that are typically comorbid with hypertension, such as diabetes mellitus type II.** A study that looked at the DASH plan in the context of specialized patient populations found that DASH was inadvisable for patients with chronic liver disease and kidney disease, and that modifications to DASH were necessary for patients with chronic heart failure, diabetes, lactose intolerance, and celiac disease.

Again, given the bidirectional pathogenic relationship between hypertension and diabetes, for example, how can DASH be the best answer or even a viable fit?

Given that, let us look in detail at the HIP approach and its benefits.

13.3 LET US GO: THE POWERFUL UTILITY OF LIVER DETOXIFICATION COUPLED WITH AN ELIMINATION DIET

So, where do we begin? According to the principles of Traditional Chinese Medicine, the liver has been deemed the "master organ" and is believed to be the root cause of the majority of imbalances in the body. Due to the influence of the SAD and a more sedentary modern lifestyle, our livers are often overburdened and therefore cannot function in the way they were designed. The liver has a big job. In addition to determining what nutrients we need to absorb and the dangerous or unnecessary substances that have to be filtered out, the liver stores vitamins and minerals, produces bile, supports detoxification, and is also the site of immune cell activation and hormone production. (1) According to the Mayo Clinic, nonalcoholic fatty liver disease, or NAFLD, is one of the most prevalent diseases in the United States, affecting an estimated 80–100 million people. This silent killer is defined as inflammation of the liver caused by a saturation of fat in the liver tissue of those who consume very little or no alcohol.

In my estimation, an elimination diet is still the gold standard for identifying food sensitivities. Many lean on lab tests but I find them to be costly and unreliable. There are notable differences between food allergies, intolerances, and sensitivities although the terms are often erroneously used interchangeably.

In brief, the differences are as follows:

1. A food allergy is an immune response to a substance, usually a protein found in a food or food group. This triggers a histamine reaction that often results in hives, rashes, or, sometimes, a more severe reaction like anaphylaxis. The reaction to a food allergy is often within a short window of time following exposure.
2. A food intolerance is a digestive response when you lack an enzyme to break down a certain food or additives. An example would be lactose intolerance, which is characterized by a lack or insufficient supply of lactose, the enzyme needed to break down the sugar, lactase, found in milk.
3. A food sensitivity is common, yet poorly defined. It can be a reaction to a food or food group that may be associated with an elevation in a particular IgG subclass that is sensitive to a specific food. Unlike a food allergy, the reaction can be immediate but is often delayed after the ingestion of the trigger food.

The HIP begins by redirecting your diet. This involves a two-stage process. Phase One entails the elimination of a variety of potentially inflammatory foods and food groups, as well as a list of substances that are known to be toxic to your body. This includes the following:

- Gluten
- Dairy
- Eggs
- Corn
- Peanuts
- Soy
- All grains (rice, quinoa, millet, wheat, barley, rye, etc.)
- All legumes (peas, beans, lentils)
- Nuts and seeds
- Nightshade vegetables (tomatoes, white potatoes, all peppers from sweet to spicy, eggplant.)
- Alcohol
- Caffeine
- Processed food
- Fast food
- Sugar
- Recreational drugs
- Tobacco

Research suggests that these foods contribute to intestinal permeability, or what is more commonly referred to as "leaky gut." This elimination phase in HIP will signal the beginning of both body and gut healing and allow the immune system an opportunity to relax and find greater calm.

The consequences of food sensitivities are often linked to chronic inflammation, so for anyone who has a hypertension diagnosis, it is of vital importance to know which foods are incompatible with your biochemistry so you can select foods/food groups that will optimize your health and well-being.

Phase Two is where you will reintroduce the foods you eliminated in Phase One. You have gone through all of the trouble of eliminating foods/food groups from your diet but it is this phase of the program that offers the real KEY to your success. This will require a bit of patience.

During Phase Two, you will embark on a worthwhile process of discovery to determine which foods/food groups prompt any reactive response, and which ones do not. Further, this process may bring to light that you are able to tolerate non-autoimmune foods such as dairy, eggs, seeds, and nuts that can significantly enhance your enjoyment of food at home and when you dine out.

An elimination diet followed by food reintroductions is still the best way to determine the broadest possible diet that will suit your individual needs. While there are lab tests for food sensitivities, I have found them to be largely unreliable with both a high incidence of false negatives and false positives. The gold standard is still the elimination diet.

As we get the aforementioned elimination phase underway, we also begin the liver detox program. I have found over the years that coordinating a detox plus an elimination diet concurrently makes both easier to comply with and will increase the speed in which patients reap results such as a boost to weight loss, greater mental clarity, improved energy and sleep, and a reduction in inflammatory response and blood pressure.

After a diagnosis of cardiovascular disease, such as hypertension (HPT), coronary artery disease, and congestive heart failure, if you want to improve the quality of your life, it is important to commit to changes in your diet and lifestyle. Now that you have read through the information on how to prepare during the pre-cleanse week and your refrigerator, pantry, and psyche are all set to embark on a new direction – this begs the question – what does a typical day on the detox + elimination phase of this program look like? Take a peek in the following.

13.4 OPTION ONE: THE TRADITIONAL APPROACH TO A GIVEN DAY

The following are protocols that you might adhere to on a typical day on the HIP. This combination of steps allows your body to reset to a healthier baseline while revving up your metabolism. On a typical day on the HIP, you will:

- Consume 8–16-oz of water upon waking. This will help to rev up your metabolism as well as quell any residual dehydration from the night before. This will also help with your morning bowel movement.
- Within an hour or so, you will compose your first shake. You can opt to use the manual shaker you received along with your 14-day detox kit; however, I think the texture is greatly improved when you toss all of the ingredients into a blender.

With regards to making your shakes, you can **mix and match shake ingredients. This is NOT a recipe but rather a list of options:**

- 8–16 oz of filtered water, cold herbal tea, coconut water, coconut milk.
- 1/2 cup frozen berries. COSTCO has a great frozen antioxidant blend that includes strawberries, blackberries, blueberries, cherries, and pomegranate. Organic.
- 1/2 frozen banana.
- Coconut milk, unsweetened coconut milk yogurt, or unsweetened shredded coconut.
- 1 cup frozen spinach, kale, or any raw vegetables. Unexpected, but adds great texture.
- 1/2 small avocado. Adds richness and leads to a sense of fullness.
- Frozen or refrigerated unsweetened coconut milk yogurt.
- Dash of cinnamon and cloves.
- Crushed ice.
- About 3/4 hours later, you will blend another shake. Please note, you can opt to have the shake at dinner and have a proper meal for lunch if that better suits your dietary preference or lifestyle. If you have a lunch plan at a restaurant, then a shake for dinner makes more sense.
- What is for dinner (or lunch)? Lots of flavorful and satisfying choices to be found here.

Rather than setting your sights on all the foods/food groups you are eliminating, focus on what you CAN have. If you were to visualize an ideal plate, it would be 70–75% non-starchy veg, 10–15% clean-sourced animal proteins, 10–15% healthy fats, and 1/2 cup of starch. Simple. Clean. Delicious.

Remember, use the allowed spices and herbs to amp up the flavor. Your meals need not be dull, and there is no reason to think you have to suffer when it comes to taste with HIP!

13.5 WHAT IS ON YOUR PLATE?

Now that we have looked at a typical day and gone through what you **will not** have on your plate, let us look at all the healthy foods you **can** include on your plate with HIP. The following highlight what you can consume in each category of food:

- **PROTEINS:** Your plate may include 4–6 oz of clean-sourced proteins such as grass-fed beef bison or lamb, pasture-raised poultry, organic pork, wild-caught fish, and shellfish.
- **VEGETABLES:** Any non-starchy vegetables included within the framework of the program such as leafy greens, broccoli, cauliflower, asparagus, Brussels sprouts, onions, cabbage, spaghetti squash, zucchini, and turnips
- **HEALTHY FATS:** Avocado, avocado oil, olives, olive oil, and coconut.

- **STARCH:** 1/2 cup of root vegetables such as sweet potato, yams, mashed celeriac, roasted beets, rutabaga, Jerusalem artichokes, or winter squashes such as acorn, banana, Hubbard, butternut, kabocha, and delicata

As you can see, there is still a wealth of tasty options available to you. As you progress in your relationship with HIP, you will find your body resetting to a new normal and able to access all the satisfaction and value out of these whole foods.

13.6 LIFE IN THE FAST LANE – FINDING A FASTING PATH THAT WORKS FOR YOU

Ben Franklin said a number of clever things, but one of my favorites is this: "The best of all medicines are resting and fasting."

WHAT you eat matters, but of equal importance is HOW you eat – in other words, how much space do you put in between meals. In simple terms, intermittent fasting (IF) is making the conscious choice to restrict eating to a specified window of time with no regard for calorie counting or altering the macronutrient ratios (proteins, fats, carbs) of your diet. According to a survey by the International Food Information Council Foundation in 2019, IF was the most popular approach to diet in 2018 that translates to one out of ten people following some version of fasting; but, make no mistake, fasting is the antithesis of a fad diet. The idea of refraining from eating has been around for millennia both in the realms of the secular or part of religious customs. So why has the idea of fasting withstood the test of time? Throughout the overwhelming majority of human history, as a species, we have been shaped by food scarcity, the specter of famine which could last a few days or an entire season and being at the mercy of an unreliable food supply. One could make the argument that humans are wired for protracted periods of fasting. From an evolutionary perspective, animals, who could retain strength and vitality during times of scarcity, would have the best odds of survival as opposed to those who became fatigued and dysfunctional due to a skipped meal or two. Requiring mini meals or snacks every 2 hours, as many of us have been wrongly indoctrinated into believing would benefit us, has been shown to be a recipe for obesity and a host of metabolic issues that plague us. According to the American Journal of Clinical Nutrition, during the past 30 years, the space between meals has gotten shorter and shorter for adults and children and thus we are more food, more often, throughout the day which has resulted in the establishment of a "new normal" approach to food which includes essentially means three meals and snacking in between. It is likely not a coincidence that we have seen a dramatic rise in Americans who are overweight and obese.

13.7 THE BENEFITS OF FASTING

What are the benefits or fasting? There are numerous advantages for those who engage in fasting, from reduced insulin resistance and inflammation to enhanced brain function.

1. Fasting and blood sugar
   Multiple studies have shown that fasting may improve the way in which the body controls blood sugar. This benefits a wide array of patients, but most especially those at risk of developing diabetes. IF, as well as alternate day fasting, has the potential to decrease sugar levels in the blood while reducing insulin resistance.
2. Fasting and inflammation
   Inflammation is, of course, a natural and sometimes useful process in the immune system. Chronic inflammation, however, can seriously impact health and wellness. Studies have found that IF has the potential to decrease various inflammation markers in the body.
3. Fasting, cholesterol, and blood pressure
   In multiple studies, fasting has been associated with lower instances of coronary heart disease and has been shown to potentially lower triglycerides and cholesterol, as well as blood pressure.
4. Fasting and brain function
   Research into the links between fasting and brain function in humans is ongoing, but there has been significant research into the same with animals. What this research has shown is that fasting correlates with improved brain function, an increase in the synthesis of nerve cells and potentially protects against neurodegenerative conditions.
5. Fasting and your metabolism
   Fasting has also been shown to boost the metabolism and aid in weight loss. One study found that fasting in the short term may rev up the metabolism by raising norepinephrine in the body, a neurotransmitter that can affect weight loss. Fasting has also been shown to help preserve muscle tissue while reducing body fat.
6. Fasting and longevity
   Animal studies into fasting have shown a delayed rate of aging in animals that fasted every other day. While the human research is still thin, these animal studies have promising implications for human fasting as it relates to life span.

   As you can see, the benefits of fasting are myriad and can impact many aspects of your health and wellness. With this in mind, then, how can you approach fasting in a sustainable way that delivers the biggest impact on your health?

13.8 FINDING THE RIGHT BALANCE WITH FASTING

With the right frame of mind, IF can make your life easier while allowing you to more rapidly lose weight, improve body composition, and maintain an optimum body weight. For many, making a habit of IF is far less challenging than it sounds and may be worth a try. Throughout history, fasting has been a commonplace practice but it is been the present-day research that suggests the following benefits:

- Promotes insulin sensitivity. Optimizing glucose regulation is vital for your health as insulin resistance (IR), which is the path to type II diabetes, contributes to nearly all chronic diseases.

- Lowers triglycerides.
- Normalizes ghrelin, also known as your hunger hormone and thus reduces appetite.
- Suppresses inflammation.
- Increases energy production.
- Increases growth hormone which has a vital role in overall health and the aging process.
- Exercising in a fasting state boosts fat burning.
- Autophagy, a metabolic pathway which purges waste material from cell, is triggered with fasting.
- Research suggests that IF extends life span because it mimics caloric restriction.
- IF makes it easier to eat fewer calories and is a very effective strategy to lose belly fat.
- Your taste buds may change so that you no longer crave sugary foods.
- You may find you have a diminished appetite the day after a fast day. There is no need to eat if you do not have the desire. It is prudent to wait until you are hungry before eating on a non-fast day.
- You should endeavor to eat "normally" on non-fast days. One of the many benefits of IF is that it encourages breaking free of anxiety about food while controlling your weight.

13.9 THE MOST POPULAR APPROACH TO FASTING IS THE 16/8 METHOD

This involves daily fasts of 16 hours and restricting your eating to an 8-hour window of time.

It is best to focus on when you CAN eat rather than when you cannot. Most commonly, the fast is broken roughly 6 hours after waking. Consistency counts with your daily eating window as hormones can be disrupted and make compliance more difficult. Further, it is important to note that because our bodies are designed to rest and repair at the end of the day, it is prudent to close your eating window relatively early, say at 6:00 or 7:00 pm. Late-night eating can interfere with hormone rhythm thus adversely affecting sleep, which influences overall health and wellness.

Men and women differ in how they should begin the practice of IF as fasting can cause hormonal imbalances in women if done too quickly or too often. When a women's body senses the signals of starvation, it can increase production of the hunger hormones, leptin and ghrelin, thereby derailing some of the potential benefits that you seek to experience. To maximize your outcome with IF, women can:

- Fast on 2–3 nonconsecutive days per week, such as Monday, Wednesday, and Saturday.
- Begin fasting for only 12 hours, and then gradually expand your "eating window" to a maximum of 16 hours. Easing into the hours that you fast will help to avoid unnecessary, excessive hunger, commonly referred to as "starving animal syndrome."

- Get adequate fluids from filtered water, broths, and herbal teas. Limit coffee to one cup daily.
- After a couple of weeks when you have established a routine, feel free to add 1 more day of fasting to your week and expand your food window.
- On fasting days, add 5–8 g of branched-chain amino acids (BCAA supplement). By providing fuel for muscles, this can help to diminish hunger and increase energy.

Other fasting strategies that you may want to try – I look at fasting options like rungs on a ladder that we can climb based on desire

- 12-hour fast that means if you finish eating at 7:00 pm, no food until 7:00 am.
- 16/8 which means 16 hours of fasting followed by an 8-hour feeding window.
- 18/6 which means 18 hours of fasting followed by a 6-hour feeding window.
- 20/4 which means 20 hours of fasting followed by a 4-hour feeding window. This is essentially a meal and a snack.
- 22/2 which means 22 hours of fasting followed by a 2-hour feeding window. This is essentially one meal a day.
- 24-hour water fast. I recommend doing this no more than 1 day/week.
- One day green juice fast. (8) 16 oz, green juices without ANY fruit, over the course of 1 day/week.
- The 5:2 diet is a type of fasting where followers eat about 25% of their recommended calorie needs (about 500–600 calories) on two scheduled fasting days and then eat normally the other 5 days that week.
- ProLon Fasting Mimicking Diet. prolonmd.com.
- Multiday liquid fasts.

13.10 KEY TAKEAWAY POINTS

1. Long-term societal change has created unhealthy food paradigms for the American public vis-a-vis the SAD.
2. While considered the gold standard for three decades, the DASH plan does not address the patient as a whole and focuses solely on the reduction of sodium in the diet.
3. The HIP serves as a viable alternative to DASH and other traditional methods, focusing on holistic health and addressing multiple, comorbid conditions.
4. HIP combines nutritional protocols with therapeutic intervention grounded in the principles of CBT to encourage patient adoption of newer, more productive eating habits and lifestyle changes.
5. IF can offer long-term benefits to HIP patients, impacting both body and mind.

NOTES

1. https://voxeu.org/article/100-years-us-obesity
2. https://www.ahajournals.org/doi/full/10.1161/hypertensionaha.117.10546

REFERENCES

1. https://www.ahajournals.org/doi/10.1161/JAHA.118.008731
2. https://www.ncbi.nlm.nih.gov/books/NBK279027/#:~:text=It%20is%20estimated%20that%20diabetes,more%20with%20diabetes%2C%20have%20hypertension.
3. No significant improvement in insulin sensitivity
4. https://www.ncbi.nlm.nih.gov/pubmed/21058045
5. https://care.diabetesjournals.org/content/40/9/1273
6. https://www.cdc.gov/nchs/fastats/deaths.htm
7. https://www.pewresearch.org/fact-tank/2016/12/13/whats-on-your-table-how-americas-diet-has-changed-over-the-decades/

14 Putting Nutrition to Work to Lower Your Blood Pressure
The Practical Steps and Solutions

Now that we have looked at an overview of the Hypertension Institute Plan (HIP) and how it compares to other dietary approaches, let us look at how the HIP works in real terms in the daily lives of our patients. By addressing everything from ritual to recipes, the HIP provides patients with a truly comprehensive way to reframe and rethink their relationship to food, health, and wellness.

14.1 THE IMPORTANCE OF RITUALS

"Rituals are the formulas by which harmony is restored."
Terry Tempest Williams

What is counterintuitive about motivation is that it is often sparked AFTER starting a new behavior, not BEFORE. So many of us seek inspiration in order to get off the starting blocks but, when success is actually found, it is the other way around...getting started is the activated form of inspiration that naturally leads to momentum.

By understanding the rituals that are included in a patient's typical day/week/month, I can often gain some insight into what contributed to their current health condition/s and where the avenues for change can be identified. Right at the top, I want to make a distinction between routine and ritual, which are often conflated. These two are actually quite distinct, and what we will be discussing here is "ritual," a process that becomes deeply embedded in our psyches, and not routine, which is quotidian.

Routine has value. We need routines. After all, brushing our teeth is important to our health and a valued part of self-care. While performed iteratively as routine is, rituals are something very different. They are actions that **express our values** – things that we do **with intent**. According to one of my favorite authors and fellow student of the ancients Stoics, Ryan Holiday, while routines are different for everyone, the practice of ritual is nearly universal. They include journaling, setting a wake time, quiet moments of reflection or mediation, exercise, reading, and long walks.

Here are but two rituals that I would swiftly add to that list that are at once simple and yet effective. The first is, I insist that patients pick a "throne" in their house, in other words, a favorite chair in the kitchen, dining room, or wherever they eat most of their meals. There is NO food consumed unless they are seated on their throne. That eliminates the numerous opportunities for a bite here and there, samples of this or that, and handfuls of eating while preparing food, clearing the table, washing dishes, or cruising the refrigerator or pantry. The second is that when sitting down to a meal, we pay full attention to our food. That means getting rid of the modern distractions of watching TV, looking or looking at a computer screen, and slowing down, chewing our food thoroughly, and embracing a practice of gratitude for what we have.

Summary: Rituals are at the heart of reframing thinking around food in the HIP.

14.2 WHAT STANDS IN THE WAY OF CHANGE – IDENTIFYING THE ENEMY

"Know thy enemy and know yourself; in a hundred battles, you will never be defeated."
Sun Tsu

Anecdotally, we have all known the dirty secret about diets all along – they do not work. People end up losing weight at first, but then regaining more than they lost within a few short years. The science is there to back this up. A meta-analysis of 29 long-term weight-loss studies done in 2019 found that **half of dieters regained weight lost after 2 years and 80% of dieters regained their lost weight after 5 years**. Dieting consistently (and ironically!) predicts weight gain.

What is getting in the way? What is the adversary causing all this havoc on our best laid plans to lose weight? Well, what makes dieting such a failure for so many is that there are multiple enemies, and each of them has a pretty sneaky agenda.

For one, as we have established, we live in an **obesogenic environment**. An expansive array of cultural developments, urban planning, and the inexhaustible availability of **highly processed foods and sweetened drinks** in the United States is pushing us toward weight gain and the attendant health consequences. This is not only from the staggering consumption of sugars and the foods that convert to sugar, processed foods, and a sedentary lifestyle but also includes junk food marketing, and the fact that cheaper food is associated with a higher intake of calories. So, **culture counts**.

Beyond that, however, and as we discussed in the previous chapter, patients cannot champion real change in their lives unless they do some serious work inside themselves. A patient's own expectations can be a huge challenge in this process, as well. For our part, I work to manage expectations for patients. I start them off with a realistic baseline – where are you in your health and wellness journey? Together with the patient, we assess where the patient is and where they want to be.

Finally, ask any military strategist and they will tell you the need to understand your adversary and determine what you are really up against. In the case of appetite control and weight loss, unbeknownst to many, the opposition is...evolution.

Is the patient's own biology working against them? Beyond our metabolisms. As a species, **our brains are hardwired to compel us to eat almost everything we see**. For our ancient ancestors, the calorie-seeking brain was a huge asset and improved the odds that our species would survive and thrive because we lived in a world of scarcity. But for modern-day people who live in a world of abundance, coupled with the bombardment of marketing and effortless access to high-reward foods, that same calorie-seeking brain is now a big, big, big liability. Scientists refer to this as an **evolutionary mismatch** – traits that were at one time considered an advantage become a disadvantage once they materialize in a different environment.

From this truthful starting point, we then develop a game plan. We know where you are and where you want to go – how can we build a bridge to get you there?

A bridge may not be the most apt analogy, however, because the journey from A to B with the HIP is never linear. Given the level of self-assessment and self-awareness required, it often involves fits and starts, and a few steps forward, followed by a step back. By preparing the patients to understand that this is a process, patients can sidestep frustration and stay focused on goals. **A significant part of how we do this comes through cognitive behavioral therapy (CBT).**

Summary: Cultural norms and our own biological and evolutionary traits work against us in dieting. Understanding this and managing expectations around these issues is central to the HIP.

14.3 COGNITIVE BEHAVIOR STRATEGIES WHEN WE WANT LONG-TERM CHANGE

One of the main reasons CBT has gained so much momentum over the last several decades is that it **allows patients to make long-term change**. How does it do this?

When developing CBT in the 1960s, Dr. Aaron Beck noticed something interesting during sessions – patients were engaging in an ongoing interior monologue. The rub was this: they were not necessarily telling him about it. They were leaving out significant parts of this internal narrative, leaving him to address only a handful of the issues at hand.

More importantly, this realization led Beck to the understanding that thoughts and feelings were deeply connected. He conceived of the idea of "automatic thoughts" to define the feelings-rich thoughts that pop up in our minds on a regular basis. Beck saw that his patients were not always aware that these thoughts were affecting them. So, he developed a method whereby patients could learn to spot these thoughts and report on them to their practitioner. By externalizing this internal narrative and making it part of a proactive action plan, patients could better understand and overcome their difficulties. The result of this, CBT, brings together two things:

the importance of personal meaning and patterns of thought
with
our behaviors and our relationship to our behaviors

Hopefully, it is clear to you from this how this relates to the HIP journey but let us spell it out in detail.

Why do most people who lose weight gain it back? Because losing weight can be easy at first but sticking to new eating habits after the first few weeks or months, and **continuing to lose weight, can be VERY difficult**. That is, unless you have learned how to identify and anticipate the challenges that you are CERTAIN to encounter and develop strategies to address them as they arise. The uncertainties and stressors of modern life, food pimps, vacations, celebrations, work parties, and holidays, to name a few, pose unique challenges. What happens when your motivation wanes and you simply want to coat your nerves with food and revert back to old habits? Without a method to address these real-life situations, keeping weight off can be a constant and frustrating battle and studies show that most of us will fail in the long run. I take a dim view of the word diet as it implies there is a beginning and an end, that essentially, you are embarking on a journey that is temporary. I am going on a diet? Where are you actually going and when do you get there?

An **effective way to bridge the gap** between knowing what to do and actually being able to put it into practice is **achieved through CBT**. According to the American Psychological Association, CBT is based on several core principles, including:

- Psychological problems are based, in part, on faulty or unhelpful ways of thinking.
- Psychological problems are based, in part, on learned patterns of unhelpful behavior.
- People suffering from psychological problems can learn better ways of coping with them, thereby relieving their symptoms and becoming more effective in their lives.

CBT treatment usually involves efforts to change thinking patterns. These strategies might include the following:

- Learning to recognize one's distortions in thinking that are creating obstacles, and then to reevaluate them in light of reality.
- Gaining a better understanding of the behavior and motivation of others.
- Using problem-solving skills to cope with difficult situations.
- Learning to develop a greater sense of confidence is one's own abilities.

CBT treatment also usually involves efforts to change behavioral patterns. These strategies might include facing one's fears instead of avoiding them and learning to calm one's mind and relax one's body.

In the context of the HIP, patients need to be able to answer the question of "why" they want to make these changes, and I like the idea of concrete strategies when we want permanent change to dietary choices and lifestyle. Once on the HIP, we have patients identify their deeper motivations for wanting to achieve change. Be specific. What do patients find comfort in that has nothing to do with food?

A simple and yet highly effective tool I use is this: I ask each patient to keep an index card with them at all times. On the front of the card, they jot down their reasons for wanting to achieve their health and weight-loss goals. This, in effect, impels patients to define WHY they are here. In other words, what are their personal reasons for wanting to achieve a greater sense of well-being? Is it to be fully present for their children? To avoid the pitfalls of the modern health-care system and stay off of, or taper down on, medications. Is it wanting to look better in clothing? On the back of that very index card, I have patients make a list of six things they find genuine comfort in other than food.

Here is what is remarkable about that question…over half of the people I ask to answer that query, have no idea what they find comfort in outside of eating and drinking! This is a dispiriting state of affairs and one reason that I find it very useful for patients to have a physical reminder of WHY they are engaged in this process. Sometimes, when a craving strikes, taking a peek at those concrete reasons is all it takes to find that spark of motivation to make better choices and derail the impulse to find comfort in a handful of gummy bears.

We live in a world that is driven by social media and 24-hour a day connectivity and thus through the wizardry of easy transmission, we are overexposed to flawed ideas, half-truths, and distorted thinking. This is a major liability of the attention economy we are all steeped in. This aspect of modern times has fostered a fertile environment for the big food industry, and media influencers who often have financial incentives to promote products, to take their gargantuan research and development budgets to sway and manipulate research to publish results that reflect better on their brands and lobby the government or a variety of other influential institutions to defend their peddling of goods that are not in the interest of human health. With all that said, this makes an even more compelling case for the need to educate ourselves and see the far-reaching advantages of taking personal responsibility for the information we allow to guide our dietary and lifestyle choices.

14.4 IT DOES NOT MATTER WHAT YOU DO ON THANKSGIVING

When most of us undertake a new dietary approach, we focus largely on what we are going to eat in a given day. This week will it be vegan, paleo, low carb, high carb, low fat, keto, Mediterranean …these broad guidelines are a good start and well-intentioned; however, what do you do when you have a plan in place for what to eat and the day does not go off according to your plan? Like most, you declare the rest of the day is nullified in favor of "starting tomorrow"… or on Friday… or after your best friend's birthday party.

It is always been interesting to me that "starting a diet" never seems to include a strategy for how to manage the days when you have stepped out of the blueprint. Would anyone take up golf and not learn how to troubleshoot the inevitable frustration of an inconsistent swing? No. You would take a few lessons at the very least to assess your grip, stance, and alignment in order to be able to get back on track and achieve the results you are after. So, when we apply this principle to a new dietary approach, it seems that it would be essential to be able to assess your ability to manage your needs and your thinking around food on an ongoing basis if you want to achieve your goals.

There is also very little discussion around the importance of what I call, **recovery days**. I often find it is the development of these strategies that are the lynchpin in avoiding the inescapable creep up in body weight that confounds and frustrates so many. Recovery days matter in a nutritional program, just as they would in an athletic training program. **Recovery is defined as, "a return to a normal state of health, mind, or strength."**

When most of us begin a new approach to food, we do not formulate recovery strategies ahead of time in anticipation of the long-term endurance needed to achieve permanent change. I think of these skills as tools in a toolbox. **We rely too heavily on what the foods are rather than behavior modification.** We need different tools for different occasions. I do not care what patients do on Thanksgiving or birthdays, but I do care quite a bit about what they do the day after. To that end, I offer guidance and encourage experimentation and trial and error with different iterations of fasting, how to green juice without fruit on a given day, or drop the carb load to realign habits. One of my road rules is just say no to 2 days in a row of high-reward foods.

Summary: Techniques used in CBT help the HIP patient modify behavior to engage in more healthful and mindful eating. Additionally, techniques such as recovery days and fasting can help with long-term goals.

14.5 RECREATE YOUR FOOD ENVIRONMENT

Shortly after I arrived in Nashville, I drove to a local, big chain market to stock up on groceries. As this was a chain, I was not familiar with because they did not have this particular store in LA, I asked a sales associate where I might find fermented foods. She quickly responded, "Oh, that's found in the health food section which is two small aisles in the back of the store." Hmm, I thought…if "two small aisles in the back of the store" are deemed health food, what do you call the rest of the food found here?

Our culture engages in disordered thinking about food. To underscore the point, **all food is health food** when done correctly. What are these foods of which they speak that are not healthy and nourishing?

This disordered thinking around food has affected our relationship with food. Hunger is an important drive in humans, no doubt. But we turn to food, when we do not need it because our disordered thinking around it has confused us.

When we are hungry, we do not want to wait! It helps to have nutritious and satisfying options within reach when hunger strikes. Did you know that the way we store our groceries can influence what we eat? We are three times as likely to eat the first thing we see in the fridge or the pantry so keep nutrient-dense foods such as ready-to-eat foods that are compliant with the HIP in your line of sight!

Fewer people are eating at home with more and more meals being eaten at restaurants, fast-food, prepared foods. While restaurants are fun and necessary and can provide an important psychological break, they do prevent some of us from maintaining a conscious and conscientious relationship with food. When things are handed to you on a silver platter, so to speak, you lose agency and you may forget to think about what you are eating. When eating in restaurants or shopping in the grocery store, you need to do one thing:

> **Remind yourself that everything you eat is either health promoting or disease promoting, so choose consciously.**

Pick a day of the week (or two) to shop for local, seasonal produce such as peppers, mushrooms, onions, sweet potatoes, squash, fennel, berries, and melons. When you get home, wash, cut, and prep all of your items for roasting or to be refrigerated raw. On several cookie sheets, add a splash of olive oil, salt, and pepper, and perhaps some fresh herbs, such as basil or rosemary, and spices, such as cumin, turmeric, or chili powder. Roast on 350 until tender. Let cool, then store in glass containers. Keep in the fridge on hand for weekly lunches, snacks, and dinners. Try the same approach with chicken. Prep, cook, slice, and store for a quick and easy addition to a stir-fry or salad. Spending 2 hours or so prepping healthy foods makes short work of putting meals together for the whole week! Now that is fast food…and remember, when it comes to food prep, the biggest consumer of time is clean up! One solution is to prepare food in large batches.

Washed and bagged greens of all types are now widely available, including spinach, arugula, kale, mustard greens, and watercress, just to name a few. Lots of already prepped fruit and other vegetables are usually found in the same section of your market, so when time is tight, go for convenience. Spending extra money to make nutritious meals at home will almost always be more cost-effective than dining out…and you know exactly what is in your food.

Fall in love with your slow cooker or Instant Pot!! Both are convenient ways to make nutritious meals while saving time by being able to add all of your ingredients, put the lid on, and go about your day. Further, a slow cooker or Instant Pot tenderizes less expensive cuts of meats such as beef brisket and chicken thighs. And, it is a simple way to brew your weekly bone broth.

14.6 ADDITIONAL TIPS

- Remove all hydrogenated fats, anything labeled artificial, including flavors or colors, and high-fructose corn syrup. Toss any processed foods. Remember, real food does not have a label!
- Explore the alternatives to nonstick pans, which are lined with chemical coatings that are extremely toxic. Try stainless steel, enameled cast iron, and an innovative nonstick surface called Thermalon, which is developed from minerals rather than Teflon.
- Plastic containers are made from a variety of materials, many of which leach chemicals into your food. For food storage, opt for safe alternatives such as glass.
- Big retail chains now carry a variety of green cleaners that do not leave harmful chemicals behind on your dishes, floors, and counters.

Summary: Grocery stores and restaurants affect how we purchase and consume food. The HIP participant reframes their food purchasing, storage, and casual consumption with a focus on whole foods.

14.7 PUTTING IT ALL TOGETHER: HOW TO GET HIP

***"Take a simple idea and take it seriously."* Charlie Munger**

When a patient walks into the nutrition side of the clinic, our relationship begins with an extensive 1-hour assessment and consultation during which we review health history, health concerns, health goals, current diet and rituals, sleep challenges, gauge levels of daily stress, assess interest in preparing meals, and have an open discussion about a prospective patient's willingness to adopt a new approach to how they live their lives.

If they seem to be a suitable candidate, or more accurately, **collaborator for the HIP**, we outline what is involved in launching the program. Once we agree to work together, I disseminate information with our patients in three ways:

First, **a workbook that serves as our blueprint**. This is an easy to follow road map for the 6-week program. Included in that workbook are explicit guidelines for the initial detox and elimination phase and the subsequent reintroduction phase, shopping lists, surveys, outlines for a typical eating day complete with meal plans, recipes, logs to track progress, and educational handouts to offer written support for questions that inevitably arise. As the program unfolds and more information is added, this workbook will evolve into a personalized troubleshooting manual that our patients will have always have within reach to refer to as needed. Many patients report that they continue to refer to the pages in their workbook for many months, even years later, to refresh their memories, or to reinvigorate their enthusiasm, for the changes they have made.

Second, I set up a **call schedule** where we connect with our patients once per week to outline what is expected of them for the following 7 days as I am a big believer in setting short-term achievable goals. These calls are really the lynchpin in our process as this 30–60-minute weekly call affords the patient and me the opportunity to assess what is working and what is not and make any course corrections whether those are behavioral adaptations, medication changes, or fielding and addressing questions on the merits or liabilities of particular foods and food groups. This is often where we discuss disappointment, modify changes in thinking that can lead to poor compliance, and commit to the rituals that pave the way to success. According to a study funded by the National Institutes for Health in 2018 on long-term management of obesity, cognitive restructuring is a key element in achieving the, more often than not, fleeting outcomes patients so desperately seek to avoid:

> "Cycles of negative and maladaptive thoughts (e.g., "What's the point…I failed again and I'll never lose weight!") and coping patterns (e.g., binge eating in response to gaining a few pounds) are counterproductive and demotivating. Helping patients to recognize and restructure the core beliefs and thought processes that underlie these patterns helps minimize behavioral fatigue and prevent or productively manage slips and lapses."

An example of this would be the inevitable development of stalled progress, or what is commonly referred to as a plateau. This can be a frustrating and confounding part of weight loss if patients do not understand the basic physiologic principles behind this phenomenon.

If a satisfactory explanation and effective support are not available at this critical juncture, many patients will simply give up and use this as justification to revert back to old habits with all too familiar consequences. What a missed opportunity to keep a patient invested in their process by way of a simple explanation as to what is actually happening metabolically, why it is a natural part of the weight-loss process, and why it is no cause for concern. I also discuss the benefits they can expect if they stick with the program. It is this kind of interchange on the weekly calls that allows me to strengthen a patient's cognitive resilience and manage the discrepancies between expectations and realistic outcomes. Cognitive pliability, in other words, the ability to remain invested in the process when one's results are not what they had hoped for, is a core competency for long-term behavioral change.

Third, I utilize **technology**. Apps and online platforms increase connectivity, motivation, and accountability. At the Hypertension Institute, we use customized platforms that allow patients to log in their weights, blood pressure data, glucose readings, photos of their meals, and instant message any questions or concerns that may arise, including the need for possible medication adjustments. Simultaneously, we grant our patients access to an **online, interactive classroom with daily CBT modules** that cover a wide variety of challenges that one may have to confront on the road to establishing new habits. These topics include how to organize your food environment, how to differentiate the impulses to quell hunger from giving in to cravings, how to define a sense of fullness, how to manage discouragement, to name a few. Logging in daily and completing a 5-minute CBT module serves as a touchstone and keeps patients invested in our work together.

A detox program coupled with an elimination diet accomplishes several things concurrently:

- Realigns eating patterns in short order resulting in weight loss, more vitality, patient confidence.
- Reduces inflammation and, often, attendant pain.
- There is not an induction phase and then jarring shift into a maintenance phase as much as it is a launch followed by the budding of a more permanent approach to lifestyle and the resulting "new normal."

Once a patient has completed this initial, 14-day phase, we often move on to the reintroduction phase in which we systematically reintroduce foods and food groups in the service of ferreting out possible food sensitivities. As I stated early, our objective is to find the broadest possible, nutrient dense, diet that will work with a patient's palate, budget, and lifestyle while still allowing them to achieve their health objectives.

With all that being said, I am still frequently asked, "Do you like Paleo? Keto? Vegan?" The answer is…it depends who is asking. As a general principle, I prefer to formulate food parameters based on a wide range of possibilities of what to include, and what to avoid rather than a "brand" of diet. For example, it is prudent to avoid processed food, hydrogenated oils, foods in boxes, bags, or cans (there are some health-conscious exceptions), fruit juice, artificial sweeteners. As for what to include, I am inspired by the work of Michael Pollen who very succinctly proclaimed in his book, *In Defense of Food: An Eater's Manifesto*, that the simplest answer to the question of "What to Eat?" is "Eat Food. Not Too Much. Mostly Plants." In the spirit of common sense and simplicity, he further went on say....

1. Avoid food products that are:
   a. Unfamiliar,
   b. unpronounceable,
   c. more than five ingredients, and
   d. include high-fructose corn syrup.
2. Do not eat anything your great-grandmother would not recognize as food.
3. Avoid food products that make health claims.
4. Do not eat anything incapable of rotting.
5. Shop the peripheries of the supermarket and stay out of the middle.
6. Get out of the supermarket whenever possible.
7. Eat mostly plants, especially leaves.
8. You are what you eat eats, too.
9. Eat well-grown food from healthy soils.
10. Eat wild foods when you can.
11. Regard nontraditional foods with skepticism.
12. Do not look for the magic bullet in the traditional diet.
13. Eat meals.
14. Pay more, eat less.
15. Do all your eating at a table.
16. Do not get your fuel from the same place your car does.
17. Try not to eat alone, and eat slowly.
18. Cook and, if you can, plant a garden.

I admire Pollen. He makes sense on many levels. He asserts in the same book that "nutritionism" has become an ideology that has unnecessarily overcomplicated and actually done harm to American eating habits. I concur wholeheartedly for reasons of logic as well as what we know about the challenges associated with research in the field of nutrition. Not only does enormous variability in individual responses to diet and food exist, but as researchers, we are largely at the mercy of the data that is self-reported on human studies, which relies heavily on food frequency questionnaires or self-administered food journals or dietary recalls. The potential errors in that method of data collection should be self-evident. Underreporting of food intake remains a primary obstacle in the validity and accuracy of these studies that are then hijacked by the big food industry and the media to spread claims that have flimsy research behind them.

According to a study in the *European Journal of Clinical Nutrition,* a *whopping 46% of those in nutrition studies "either deliberately and knowingly or reluctantly" altered their prescribed diets and added false entries into their food logs.* Forty-six percent of the sample admitted altering their diet, either deliberately and knowingly or reluctantly due to difficult circumstances. Underreporting of dietary intakes remains one of the principal hurdles in the disclosure of valid habitual estimates of food eaten.[1]

My interpretation of Pollen's thesis is, at its core, something I advocate for our patients...most of the time, keep your diet simple. Uncomplicated. I would add to that, save the more exotic, high pleasure meals for what you do some of the time, not most of the time.

I know that at this point a template for a diet might be expected. But that is exactly the point, and why Pollen's approach resonates with the HIP philosophy. Despite the desire to discover one, there is no such thing as a "diet in a box." While there are key principles involved, each approach is customized to the individual. For example, tomatoes may work for some, and not for others. There are no 6–8 servings of this or that. While this may disappoint the reader – it is exactly this lack of specificity that illustrates why the HIP works. We assess daily results with our patients and provide individualized recommendations. This, in turn, empowers the patient to stay on course. Any and all intervention MUST be tailored to the individual's unique makeup. We are all defined by a unique panoply of genes, history, preferences, tolerances, and desired outcomes. The good news is that we can improve so much of what ails us, but it must be done on an individual basis.

The **principles of HIP** can provide insight and guidance. Let us take a look.

14.8 HIP IN PRACTICE – THE KEY POINTS

1. Liver detox, gut healing + elimination diet.
2. Reintroduction phase to uncover food sensitivities/intolerances.
3. Shift from sabotaging habits to productive habits.
4. Cognitive behavioral therapy.
5. Establish a culture of support through collaboration which leads to higher thinking and self-awareness.
6. Educate patients and engender greater self-confidence.
7. Greater understanding of how food selection influences overall health.
8. Improve sleep hygiene.
9. Encourage mind/body practice to reduce anxiety.
10. As needed, utilize targeted supplements.
11. Strive not for happiness, but what the ancient Greeks called, eudaimonia…a sense of fulfillment.
12. Keep a journal. Jot down level of energy, symptoms, and mood throughout the day to help identify any patterns with food intake. Remember, this requires you to be in tune with your body.
13. Most of the time, keep food simple, but robust.
14. If you eliminate or significantly reduce processed foods, you will naturally consume less sodium and when you dine out, be specific about how you want your food prepared. Most of the time, it is easy to ask that your dish be prepared without salt.

Summary: The HIP patient undergoes an initial assessment to determine suitability with the program. A combination of ongoing consultation, CBT modules, and support during key periods such as "plateau-ing" keeps the HIP patient motivated and on track. While individualized, there are central principles that define the HIP, including detox, a focus on holistic wellness, and the elimination of toxic foods and allergens.

Let us GO!

Week One

Structure: detox + elimination diet.

Plan: two shakes plus one meal.

Meal composition: Create Your Plate (see next).

Agenda for our call: how to get your household and your psyche set up the detox + elimination phase I.

Week Two

Structure: detox + elimination diet.

Plan: two shakes plus one meal.

Meal composition: Create Your Plate.

Agenda for our call: how to stay motivated for Week Two. Troubleshoot issues and acknowledge successes.

Week Three

Structure: begin reintroduction phase, if appropriate.

Plan: start to add foods that were eliminated during first phase for meal. One or two shake options.

Meal composition: Create Your Plate.

Agenda for our call: how to reintroduce foods and begin Phase II. Troubleshoot issues and acknowledge successes.

Week Four

Structure: continue to expand dietary options.

Plan: continue food reintroductions. Zero, one, or two shake options.

Meal composition: Create Your Plate.

Agenda for our call: intermittent fasting strategies. How to navigate dining out, holidays, and how to add "luxury" foods. Troubleshoot issues and acknowledge successes.

Week Five

Structure: continue to expand dietary options.

Plan: continue food reintroductions. Discuss shake options or meals only.

Meal composition: Create Your Plate.

Agenda for our call: how to understand and manage plateaus. Troubleshoot issues and acknowledge successes.

CREATE YOUR PLATE

70–75% non-starchy vegetables. The rest is negotiable.

10–15% clean-sourced animal proteins.

10–15% health-promoting fats.

1/2–1 cup starchy/root vegetables.

Non-Starchy Vegetables

Broccoli

Brussels sprouts

Bean sprouts

Cauliflower

Bok choy

Cabbage (green, red, Chinese, Napa)
Swiss chard
Kohlrabi
Mushrooms
Swiss chard
Arugula
Watercress
Microgreens
Salad greens (chicory, endive, escarole, lettuce, romaine, spinach, arugula, radicchio, watercress)
Sprouts
Squash (summer, crookneck, spaghetti, zucchini)
Greens (collard, kale, mustard, turnip)
Kale
Asparagus
Celery
Radishes
Hearts of palm
Jerusalem artichokes, sunchokes
Onions
Leeks
Scallions
Shallots

Clean-Sourced Proteins

Alaskan halibut
Alaskan salmon (fresh, canned)
Canned tuna
Freshwater bass
Hawaiian fish
Sardines
Whitefish
Chicken
Turkey
Duck
Beef
Bison
Lamb
Pork
Wild game (elk, venison, boar)

Health-Promoting Fats

Algae oil
Avocado
Avocado oil
Olives
Olive oil
Coconut, shredded, flakes, unsweetened

Coconut oil
Ghee
Grass-fed, cultured butter
Macadamia oil
MCT oil
Perilla oil
Walnut oil
Red palm oil
Sesame oil
Cod liver oil
Almonds
Chia seed
Macadamia nuts
Walnuts
Pistachios
Pecans
Hazelnuts
Flaxseeds
Hemp seeds
Pine nuts
Brazil nuts

Starchy/Root Vegetables to Consider

Cassava
Carrots
Sweet potatoes or yams
Winter squash (acorn, butternut, hubbard, kabocha, delicata)
Parsnips
Celery root
Green plantains
Green bananas
Siete brand tortillas
Jicama
Turnips
Tiger nuts
Green mango
Green papaya

Something Sweet

Allulose
Erythritol (Swerve)
Monk fruit, Luo Han Guo
Stevia
Xylitol

Fun Foods

Coconut aminos
Nomato sauce
Shirataki noodles

Palmini noodles
Smart coffee with L-theanine

Foods to Say "Yes" to

Wild-caught fish
Alaskan halibut
Alaskan salmon (fresh, canned)
Canned tuna
Freshwater bass
Hawaiian fish
Sardines
Whitefish
Pastured poultry
Chicken
Turkey
Duck
Grass-fed, grass-finished meat
Beef
Bison
Lamb
Pork
Wild game (elk, venison, boar)
Non-starchy, cruciferous vegetables
Broccoli
Brussels sprouts
Bean sprouts
Cauliflower
Bok choy
Cabbage (green, red, Chinese, Napa)
Swiss chard
Kohlrabi
Mushrooms
Swiss chard
Arugula
Watercress
Microgreens
Salad greens (chicory, endive, escarole, lettuce, romaine, spinach, arugula, radicchio, watercress)
Sprouts
Squash (summer, crookneck, spaghetti, zucchini)
Greens (collard, kale, mustard, turnip)
Kale
Asparagus
Celery
Radishes

Hearts of palm
Jerusalem artichokes, sunchokes
Onions
Leeks
Scallions
Shallots
Fats
Algae oil
Avocado
Avocado oil
Olives
Olive oil
Coconut, shredded, flakes, unsweetened
Coconut oil
Ghee
Grass-fed, cultured butter
Macadamia oil
MCT oil
Perilla oil
Walnut oil
Red palm oil
Sesame oil
Cod liver oil
Sweeteners
Allulose
Erythritol (Swerve)
Monk fruit, Luo Han Guo
Stevia
Xylitol
Vinegar
Any, without sugar
Flours
Coconut
Almond
Sweet potato
Cassava
Tiger nut
Arrowroot
Herbs
Basil
Mint
Parsley
Cilantro
Rosemary
Thyme
Sage

Chives
Dill
Oregano
Starch
Cassava
Carrots
Sweet potatoes or yams
Winter squash (acorn, butternut, hubbard, kabocha, delicata)
Parsnips
Celery root
Green plantains
Green bananas
Siete brand tortillas
Jicama
Turnips
Tiger nuts
Green mango
Green papaya
Fermented foods
Raw sauerkraut
Raw fermented vegetables
Kombucha
Coconut milk yogurt
Almond milk yogurt
Sheep and goat milk yogurt
Fun foods
Shirataki noodles
Kelp noodles
Palmini noodles
Nuts and seeds
Almonds, sprouted or raw
Macadamia nuts
Walnuts
Pistachios
Pecans
Hazelnuts
Flaxseeds
Hemp seeds
Pine nuts
Brazil nuts

Foods to Avoid or Moderate

Refined, starchy foods
Rice
Pasta

White potatoes
Potato chips
Bread
Pastry
Cookies
Crackers
Pretzels
Cereal
Products made from grain and pseudo-grain
Sweeteners
Agave
Splenda (sucralose)
Sweet One (acesulfame K)
Sugar
NutraSweet (aspartame)
Splenda (sucralose)
Sweet'n Low (saccharin)
Diet drinks
Crystal Light
Maltodextrin
Legumes
Alfalfa
Beans (pinto, black, white, navy)
Lentils
Peas
Chickpeas
Carob
Soybeans
Peanuts
Oils
Soy
Grapeseed
Corn
Peanut
Cottonseed
Safflower
Sunflower
Vegetable
Canola
Partially hydrogenated
Margarine
Plant-based "meats"
Nightshades
White potatoes
Tomatoes
Eggplant

Bell peppers
Cayenne pepper
Paprika

14.9 A WORD ABOUT SODIUM

As we have established, overconsumption of sodium can increase blood pressure and make the kidneys work harder. Because hypertension is a leading contributor to stroke, heart attack, and kidney diseases, to name a few, it seems sensible to identify the most likely sources of sodium in the diet. This requires an exploration of not only what we are eating, but where we are sourcing our meals.

According to the National Restaurant Association, there are 1 million restaurants in the United States which contribute to a whopping $900 billion dollar a year business sector. Almost 25% of Americans **eat three or more fast-food meals per week** and spend $200 billion annually on fast food. A total of 52% of consumers say **purchasing takeout or delivered food is essential to the way they live.** Studies show that "food away from home" (FAFH) at either fast-food or full-service restaurants resulted in diners consuming about 200 additional daily calories, along with a higher intake of sodium, sugar, and saturated fat.

Far be it from me to cast doubt on the need for convenience or the quest for nourishment without the labor involved in planning, shopping, prepping, cooking, and cleaning up. We live in an on-the-go world and so many of us have deep time constraints and thus struggle just to meet the demands of work, childcare, and financial obligations. When it comes to feeding ourselves and our families, convenience counts; but, it is also important to consider the potential hit to your health of having someone else in charge of the calories you put into your body, especially if you are like the majority of Americans who spend roughly 42% of their food budget on FAFH, which studies find, overall, to be less nutritious than food prepared at home. Studies show that, on the whole, **food purchased outside of the home has more saturated fat and sodium**, and far less fiber and fewer nutrients. In a recent study, Harvard researchers concluded that the cumulative effects of excess sodium accounted for roughly 2.3 million deaths each year, globally – that is, one in ten US deaths due to heart attacks, stroke, and other cardiovascular diseases. So, it stands to reason, if dining out means more exposure to sodium, there is no need to altogether avoid the acquisition of FAFH, just be more mindful of your choices:

- When dining out, ask for information on calories, fat, and sodium. Many chains offer the nutritional profiles of their menu options online.
- When possible, ask for meals to be prepared without salt, then add a pinch or two.
- At the market, read nutrition labels and do not buy food that includes a lot of sodium. Processed foods with high sodium tend to be bread, cold cuts and cured meats, frozen meals, and packaged soups. Better yet, remember real food does not have a label, so opt for fresh food that is typically found on the perimeter of the store. Focus less on foods that come in a box, bag, or can.

- Cook at home more and base those meals on fresh and whole foods, not highly processed, heat and serve products that tend to be high in sodium.
- Keep portions in check. To attract customers, most restaurants serve portions that are two to three times larger than sensible dietary guidelines recommend.
- Instead of prepackaged snack foods, opt for these low sodium snacks:
- Organic, air-popped popcorn
  - Low glycemic fruit such as berries.
  - Sprouted or raw, unsalted nuts.
  - Steamed edamame.
  - Homemade kale chips.
  - Homemade roasted chickpeas.
  - Homemade sweet potato chips.
  - Guacamole.
  - Protein smoothie.
  - Vegetables: baby carrots, celery sticks, cherry tomatoes, cucumber slice, red and green peppers, steamed broccoli, cauliflower florets.
  - Coconut milk yogurt with berries (freeze yogurt and blend with berries).

Food prepared with little or no salt should still be delicious and flavorful. Try to load up on fresh herbs and spices such as cumin, paprika, oregano, lemon peel, garlic, onion powder, and rubbed sage to season food. Vinegars, citrus juices, and zests are good, too. Not a fan of salt substitutes or "lite salt" as most of them contain potassium chloride. While these have no sodium, they may cause the body to retain potassium.

And remember, most of the foods we eat regularly today are not the normal foods of our species. Instead, they are foods that have been created to elicit an unnatural, elevated taste response; as a result, these foods are high in processed sugar, fat, and salt. Our taste buds and the pleasure centers in our brain find these unnatural foods very appealing, making whole natural foods less palatable by comparison. But do not despair. Neuroadaptation is a normalizing process, whereby the taste buds will change once you adjust your diet to whole foods.

Based on the patient's need, I recommend somewhere between 1500 and 2300 mg a day for those with cardiovascular disease or high blood pressure. This is the equivalent to about 3/4–1 teaspoon of table salt. Note that the average American takes in about 3400 mg a day.

14.10 RECIPES

1. **Crispy Cauliflower with Gremolata**

   1 head cauliflower, quartered, cored, and cut into bite-size florets

   3–4 tablespoons extra-virgin olive oil, plus extra for drizzling

   Salt and freshly cracked pepper

   1 lemon

   1 large handful fresh parsley (about 1/2 cup/25 g), roughly chopped

   Sea salt, for serving

Preheat the oven to 425°F (220°C). Spread the cauliflower on a baking sheet in a single layer. Drizzle with the oil, season generously with salt and pepper, and toss to coat. Roast the cauliflower, tossing the florets halfway through, until they are deep golden and crispy, 30–35 minutes total.

While the cauliflower is roasting, prepare gremolata. Transfer the roasted cauliflower to a serving bowl and mix with germinate to taste. For some, it is a couple of tablespoons, for others they like more sauce!!!

Gremolata (Italian herb sauce)

1 cup packed Italian parsley (small stems OK)

1–2 garlic cloves

Zest of one small lemon, plus 1–2 teaspoons lemon juice (Meyer lemon is especially nice)

1/2 cup olive oil

1/8 teaspoon kosher salt and pepper, more to taste

Pinch chili flakes – optional

On a cutting board or mat, chop everything very finely and place into a bowl. Stir in olive oil, salt, and pepper.

Add chili flakes for a touch of heat if you like. Store in a jar in the fridge for up to 1 week. An excellent sauce for eggs, fish, or chicken!

2. **Avocado Egg "Toast"**

1/4 medium avocado

1/2 clove garlic, mashed

1/4 ground pepper

1 slice sweet potato toast

1 large egg, poached

1 teaspoon store-bought hot sauce (optional)

1 tablespoon sliced red onion

Combine avocado, pepper, garlic, and hot sauce

Top sweet potato toast with mashed avocado and poached egg. Garnish with red onions.

3. **Salmon with Fresh Herbs**

3 tablespoons olive oil

3/4 teaspoon kosher salt

1/2 teaspoon freshly ground black pepper

4 (6-oz) skin-on salmon fillets

1/4 teaspoon smoked paprika

2 tablespoons chopped fresh tarragon

2 tablespoons chopped fresh dill

2 tablespoons chopped fresh sage

Preheat oven to 450°. Rinse fish, pat dry. Mix herbs together. Spread each salmon fillet olive oil. Sprinkle fillets with salt and pepper. Place prepared salmon fillets skin-side down on baking sheet. Top salmon with herbs. Bake until salmon is firm but still pink in the center 12–14 minutes.

4. **Lemon Asparagus**

1 lb fresh asparagus, trimmed

2 tablespoons olive oil

2 cloves garlic, minced
1 lemon, thinly sliced
2 tablespoons freshly squeezed lemon juice (approximate 1 lemon)
1/2 teaspoon sea salt
1/4 teaspoon ground black pepper
Instructions

Preheat your oven to 400°F and line a rimmed baking sheet with parchment paper.

Add the asparagus, lemon slices, olive oil, freshly squeezed lemon juice, sea salt, ground black pepper, minced garlic, to the baking sheet. Toss to evenly coat. Place in the oven and roast for 8–10 minutes or until the asparagus is crisp on the outside and tender in the center.

5. **Homemade Sweet Potato Chips**

2 medium sweet potatoes
4 tablespoons olive oil
1 teaspoon sea salt
1/2 teaspoon black pepper

Preheat oven to 375°. Use a mandoline to thinly slice potatoes. In a large bowl, toss sweet potatoes with oil, salt, and pepper. Coat a wire rack with cooking spray. Place rack in a shallow baking pan and arrange half of the slices on the rack. Bake 30 minutes until crispy at edges. Repeat with remaining potatoes.

6. **Mexican Cod**

4 4 oz frozen, skinless cod filets
2 tablespoons lime juice
2 teaspoons chili powder
1 teaspoon cumin
1/2 teaspoon sea salt
3 tablespoons avocado oil
Lime wedges

Rinse fish, pat dry. In a small bowl, combine lime juice, chili powder, cumin, and salt. Brush both sides of fish with lime mixture. In a skillet, heat 3 teaspoons avocado oil over medium-high heat. Add fish, cook 4–6 minutes per 1/2 thickness or until fish flakes easily, turning once. Serve with lime wedges.

7. **Cauliflower Tabbouleh**

3 tablespoons extra-virgin olive oil
1 and 1/2 lb (5 cups)head cauliflower, riced, finely chopped or grated
1 and 1/2 teaspoon sea salt
1 lemon, juiced
1/2 cup red onion, chopped
1/2 cup chopped parsley
1/2 cup chopped dill or mint
1 cup cherry tomatoes, halved
1 cup seeded and chopped cucumber
Lemon wedges

Olive oil for drizzle

Heat the olive oil in an extra-large skillet over medium-high heat. Add cauliflower and 1 teaspoon salt to the hot skillet. Cook, stirring occasionally, about 5 minutes or until crisp-tender. Spread cauliflower out on a large baking sheet to cool.

In a large bowl, stir together the remaining salt and lemon. Add cooler cauliflower, red onion, herbs, tomatoes, and cucumber. Cover and let stand at room temperature for 1 hour, stirring occasionally. Drizzle with olive oil, salt, and pepper, if desired.

8. **Thai Cucumber Salad**

2 medium cucumbers, peeled, cut in half lengthwise, seeded, cut into 1/4 in. slices

3 tablespoons seasoned rice vinegar

1 teaspoon red Thai chili pepper

1/2 teaspoon salt

1/2 teaspoon lime zest

1/2 teaspoon freshly grated ginger

3 tablespoons fresh basil, sliced thinly

In a medium bowl, combine vinegar, chili pepper, salt, lime, and ginger. Add cucumbers. Allow to sit for 15 minutes. Add basil. Can store refrigerated for 3 days.

9. **Arugula and Fennel Salad**

1 medium fennel bulb

3 cups baby arugula

3 tablespoons extra-virgin olive oil

3 tablespoons fresh lemon juice

1/2 teaspoon sea salt

1/4 teaspoon freshly ground black pepper

Trim and discard the outer layers and fronds from the fennel. Slice it paper thin using a mandolin and place in a large bowl. In a small bowl, whisk olive oil, lemon juice, salt, and pepper. Pour over the salad and toss to coat evenly.

10. **Avocado Egg Cups**

2 avocados

4 eggs

Salt and pepper to taste

1 tablespoon green onions, chopped

With a knife, cut avocados lengthwise into halves and remove pit. If needed, slightly hollow out the avocados to make room for the eggs.

Arrange avocados in a single layer on a baking dish. Break an egg into each avocado half and season with salt and pepper to taste. Bake in a 425°F oven for about 10–15 minutes or until eggs are cooked to your liking. Remove from oven and garnish with green onions. Serve hot.

11. **Green Beans with Walnuts**

3 cups French green beans, trimmed

1 cup yellow or red onion, halved, sliced thin

1/2 cup walnuts or pecans, chopped
1/2 teaspoon salt
1/4 teaspoon black pepper
2 tablespoons extra-virgin olive oil

In a skillet, add olive oil and over medium-heat, saute green beans, onions, salt, and pepper.

Heat 15 minutes or until green beans are crisp-tender, stirring occasionally. Add walnuts.

12. **Black Cod with Miso**

1 lb black cod, cut into four filets
1/2 white miso paste
1/8 cup Mirin
1/8 cup sake, or other sweet wine
1 tablespoon allulose or erythritol

Combine last four ingredients into a blender until smooth

Pat the black cod fillets thoroughly dry with paper towels and discard. Slather the fish with the miso marinade and place in a nonreactive dish or bowl and cover tightly with plastic wrap. Leave to marinate in the refrigerator for 2–3 days.

Preheat oven to 400°F. Heat an ovenproof skillet over high heat on the stovetop. Lightly wipe off any excess miso clinging to the fillets, but do not rinse. Film the pan with a little olive oil, then place the fish skin-side up on the pan and cook until the bottom of the fish browns and blackens in spots, about 3 minutes. Flip and continue cooking until the other side is browned, 2–3 minutes. Transfer to the oven and bake for 5–10 minutes, until fish is opaque and flakes easily.

13. **White Bean Dip**

1 cup cooked cannellini beans
1/4 cup extra-virgin olive oil
3 cloves garlic, peeled
6 fresh basil leaves, divided
2 teaspoons lemon zest
1/4 teaspoon ground black pepper
1/4 teaspoon sea salt

Place beans, olive oil, garlic, five basil leaves, lemon zest, pepper, and salt in high-speed food processor. Blend about 45 seconds, until creamy. •Transfer into covered glass dish and refrigerate for at least 30 minutes before serving. Serve with basil leaf and drizzled with additional olive oil. Serve with freshly cut peppers, steamed asparagus, cauliflower, or strips of grilled chicken.

14. **Zucchini Noodles with Garlic and Basil**

4 zucchini, medium
4 cloves fresh garlic, minced
4 tablespoons olive or avocado oil
Lemon zest, optional
Celtic salt and freshly ground pepper

Spiral cut zucchini. Add oil to pan on low/medium heat and salute garlic until soft, about 30 seconds.

Add zucchini to pan and cook just until heated through, not mushy. Add salt and pepper and lemon zest to taste.

*This is a very versatile dish that works well with the addition of tomatoes, spices or chicken, fish, or beef. Add your favorite spices and ingredients for a great side dish or entree.

15. **Shaved Brussels Sprouts with Shiitake**

12 oz organic Brussels sprouts
2 tablespoons fat (coconut oil or olive oil)
1 leek, thinly sliced, green and white
2 cloves garlic, minced
1/2 cups shiitake mushrooms
Sea salt and black pepper to taste

Wash Brussels sprouts and remove stems. Shave sprouts with a food processor or slice thinly. Heat oil in large pan over medium heat. Add onion, and let soften for 1–2 minutes.

Add garlic and cook until onions are translucent. Add Brussels sprouts and cook for about 2 minutes. Add mushrooms and sea salt. Cook until sprouts and mushrooms are soft.

16. **Curried Coconut Carrot Soup**

1 tablespoon olive oil
1 medium onion, chopped
1 large shallot, sliced
2 lb carrots, peeled and sliced
1 tablespoon garlic, chopped
1 heaping tablespoon ginger, minced
1 teaspoon minced serrano or jalapeno chili
1 teaspoon ground coriander
3/4 teaspoon Madras style hot curry powder
1 quart organic vegetable or chicken broth
1/2 tablespoon lime juice
2 tablespoon basil, chiffonade

17. **Egg Drop Soup**

4 cups bone broth, preferably homemade
4 eggs, pasture-raised, whole or whisked
1/2 cup red onion or scallions, sliced thinly
1 cup spinach, chard, collards or kale, sliced
2 teaspoons Tamari, gluten-free
1 tablespoon fresh basil, chiffonade
1/2 teaspoon dark sesame oil
Salt and pepper, to taste
Serves 2
Directions

- Place bone broth and tamari in a medium saucepan on medium heat until close to boil.

- Add onions and chard and cook for 2 minutes.
- Drop eggs into soup until cooked, about 2 minutes, with a lid in place.
- Pour into a bowl and add sesame oil and top with fresh basil.
- Heat oil in soup pot over medium heat. (1) Add onion, shallot, and carrots. (2) Add garlic, ginger, chilies, coriander, and curry powder and continue to saute until fragrant, another minute. (3) Add broth, cover partially, and bring to a boil over high heat. Reduce heat and gently simmer for 20 minutes. Remove from heat. (4) Puree soup in blender, working in batches or blend smooth with immersion blender. (5) Stir in coconut milk and lime juice, season to taste with salt and pepper. If soup is too thick, thin soup with water. (6) To serve, ladle into cups and garnish with basil and pepitas. Can be served warm and chilled.

18. **Pumpkin Pie Spiced Seeds**

    Yield: 2 cups

    2 cups pumpkin seeds, organic preferred
    2 teaspoons pumpkin pie spice (Trader Joe's)
    1 tablespoon real maple syrup

    Preheat oven to 375° and line baking sheet with parchment paper. Mix all three ingredients and spread onto prepared baking pan. Roast for 10–15 minutes, checking every 5 minutes to make sure they do not burn. Let cool.

19. **Middle Eastern Spiced Seeds**

    2 cups pumpkin seeds, organic preferred
    1 teaspoon dried thyme
    1 teaspoon dried marjoram
    2 teaspoon za'atar or sumac
    1 and 1/2 teaspoons Celtic or Himalayan salt
    Zest of 1 lemon
    1 tablespoon olive oil

    Preheat oven to 375° and line baking sheet with parchment paper. Mix all three ingredients and spread onto prepared baking pan. Roast for 10–15 minutes. Let cool.

20. **Instant Pot Garlic Lime Shredded Chicken**

    1/2 c low sodium vegetable or chicken broth
    1/4 c olive oil
    1/4 c lime juice
    4 cloves garlic, peeled and smashed
    1 jalapeno, seeded and chopped; see notes
    1–2 teaspoon sea or kosher salt, see notes
    2 teaspoon cumin
    1 teaspoon paprika
    1 teaspoon cracked black pepper
    2 lb boneless skinless chicken breasts
    1/2 c chopped cilantro
    Instructions

Place the chicken broth, olive oil, lime juice, garlic, jalapeno, salt, cumin, paprika, and pepper into a food processor or blender. Blend until smooth. Place chicken in Instant Pot and set on slow cook mode. Pour the sauce over the chicken. Cover and cook on low for 8 hours for best results (or high for 4 hours).

Using two forks, shred the chicken. Add the cilantro to the chicken, and toss again.

21. **Oven Roasted Vegetables with Chimichurri**

Asparagus
Zucchini
Pear tomatoes, cut in half, lengthwise
Carrots
Fennel
Red onion
Green, red and yellow peppers
1 tablespoon fresh thyme
1/2 cup extra-virgin olive oil
Sea salt
Freshly ground pepper
Fresh basil, cut in chiffonade, to taste

Preheat oven to 350°. Wash the vegetables and cut into the preferred sizes and shapes. Place in a bowl and toss with the olive oil, thyme, salt, and pepper. Place all vegetables on a baking sheet, or two, depending on quantity making sure not to overcrowd. Baking time will depend on the size of the vegetables but expect 15–25 minutes.

Remove from oven and toss with fresh basil and a drizzle more olive oil, if needed.

Feel free to experiment with a variety of seasonal produce.

Serve with or without chimichurri

Chimichurri

1 cup extra-virgin olive oil
1 cup flat leaf, or Italian parsley, de-stemmed and packed
1 cup cilantro, de-stemmed and packed
8 cloves fresh garlic
1/4 small red onion
1/4 cup lime juice, freshly squeezed
1 tablespoon oregano, dried
1 and 1/2 teaspoon Celtic or Himalayan sea salt, or to taste
3/4 teaspoon black pepper
1 tablespoon red pepper flakes, optional

Place ingredients into a blender or food processor and pulse until all ingredients are finely chopped and combined. Serve immediately or store in airtight container in the refrigerator for up to a week Bring to room temperature before serving.

22. **Balsamic Skirt Steak with Cherry Tomatoes with Arugula**

Marinade:

1/2 cup balsamic vinegar
1/4 cup olive oil
3 garlic cloves, minced
2 tablespoons fresh herbs such as dill, rosemary, basil, sage, or a combination
3 lb grass-fed skirt or hanger steak
1 basket small cherry tomatoes
1 red chili pepper, optional
1 tablespoon balsamic vinegar
2 cloves garlic, minced
2 tablespoons extra-virgin olive oil
1 cup fresh basil, roughly chopped
3 cups wild arugula

Add all marinade ingredients to a blender until smooth. Season steaks with salt and pepper, and pour contents of blender over steak in a glass dish and allow to marinate overnight. When ready to grill, season the cherry tomatoes with dusting of salt and chilies, if including. Stir in the vinegar, garlic, and olive oil. Grill steak over high heat for a few minutes per side, let rest. Toss the basil and arugula with the tomatoes and put on platter. Add sliced steak to the top of salad.

23. **Clean Salad Dressings – Four Ways**
    - Avocado Dressing

      1/2 cup filtered water
      1 large avocado, peeled and pitted
      2 tablespoons cilantro, chopped
      2 tablespoons, basil, chopped
      2 cloves garlic, fresh
      Squeeze of lime
      Pinch of salt
      *Add 1/2 small jalapeño if you like spicy
      Add ingredients to blender
      Blend until smooth
      Refrigerate in airtight glass container, but use within 3 days
    - Tahini

      1 cup tahini sesame seed paste – I prefer the paste made from light-colored seeds
      3/4 cup lukewarm water, or more for consistency
      3 cloves garlic, minced
      1/4 cup fresh lemon juice, or more to taste
      1/4 teaspoon salt, or more to taste
      2 teaspoons fresh parsley, minced

      Place all ingredients except for parsley into a food processor and blend until smooth and light colored. Scrape down sides every 30 seconds or so. Add water depending on your desired consistency. Refrigerate in airtight glass container, but use within 3 days.
    - Mustard Vinaigrette

1 rounded tablespoon Dijon mustard
2.5 tablespoons fresh lemon juice
Salt
Freshly ground pepper
ó cup extra-virgin olive oil
1 garlic clove, lightly crushed but intact
1/2 teaspoon fresh thyme (dill works nicely, too)

In a small bowl or measuring cup, combine the mustard, lemon juice, salt, and pepper. Whisk in the oil.

Once blended, add thyme. Place the garlic clove in the dressing and allow to marinate for at least 30 minutes. Remove from dressing before serving. Refrigerate in airtight glass container, but use within 3 days

- Raw Ranch
  1/2 cup raw cashews
  1/4 cup filtered water
  1/4 cup cashew milk, unsweetened
  1 garlic clove, minced
  2 tablespoon fresh dill, chopped finely
  1 teaspoon fresh lemon juice, or to taste
  1/2 teaspoon salt
  Freshly ground pepper

  Blend cashews in food processor to flour consistency. Blend in water and cashew milk. Add herbs, salt, and pepper, and blend. Refrigerate in airtight glass container, but use within 3 days

24. **FOUR Ingredient Banana Bread**

1.5 lb of ripe bananas, approximately 4–5 medium bananas
2 cups sprouted rolled oats
1 cup almond, cashew, or peanut butter, unsweetened. Nuts only.
1 cup mini chocolate chips, sweetened with Erythritol

*Optional: add 1/2 cup chopped crystallized ginger when you add the chocolate chips

Preheat oven to 350°. Lightly grease 9 × 5 in. loaf pan with olive oil or line with parchment paper; set aside. Add oats to blender and blend until fine powder, put in medium mixing bowl. Add 4 of your five bananas to blender with nut butter and blend until smooth. Add to bowl with oat powder and stir just until blended. Do not over mix. Add chocolate chips. Batter will be thick. Place in loaf pan and smooth to fill edges of pan. Garnish with remaining banana and sprinkle chocolate chips. Bake for 30 minutes or until toothpick inserted in the center comes out clean. Let cool completely in loaf pan.

25. **Protein Truffles**

1 cup sprouted rolled oats
1/2 cup unsweetened nut butter
1/3 cup raw honey
1/2 cup dark chocolate
2 tablespoons flax seeds

2 tablespoons chia seeds
1 tablespoon vanilla collagen or whey powder

Stir oats, nut butter, honey, chocolate, flax, chia, and protein powder in a bowl until blended. Cover bowl with lid or plastic wrap and refrigerate for 30 minutes. Scoop chilled mixture into balls. Keep cold until ready to eat.

14.11 TAKEAWAYS

1. Ritual matters and creating wellness-oriented rituals in HIP can transform negative patterns into positive ones.
2. CBT is a key component of this, allowing patients to reframe their thinking around food.
3. One habit that has to become a healthy ritual is food shopping and stocking the cupboards and fridge. A more mindful process results in better eating.
4. HIP is highly individualized but there are key principles to it that anyone can leverage in their own approach to nutrition.
5. While HIP varies from patient to patient, beginning with 2 weeks of detox and elimination before reintroducing some foods to test for food sensitivity is a common approach used.

NOTES

1 JI Macdiarmid and JE Blundell BioPsychology group, Department of Psychology, University of Leeds, Leeds, LS2 9JT, United Kingdom

https://newsroom.ucla.edu/releases/Dieting-Does-Not-Work-UCLA-Researchers-7832#:~:text=People%20on%20diets%20typically%20lose,be%20significantly%20higher%2C%20they%20said.

https://www.hsph.harvard.edu/obesity-prevention-source/obesity-causes/food-environment-and-obesity/.

https://www.ecoandbeyond.co/articles/big-food/.

https://www.ncbi.nlm.nih.gov/pmc/articles/PMC5764193/.

REFERENCES

https://www.apa.org/ptsd-guideline/patients-and-families/cognitive-behavioral.

https://www.ncbi.nlm.nih.gov/pmc/articles/PMC5764193/.

https://www.researchgate.net/publication/14137648_Dietary_under-reporting_What_people_say_about_recording_their_food_intake.

15 Treatment of Hypertension with Nutraceutical (Nutritional) Supplements

Over the past 25 years, Dr. Houston, Director of the Hypertension Institute has performed many clinical studies, reviewed thousands of medical articles, done medical research, and treated over 7000 patients with nutritional supplements to lower blood pressure. These nutritional supplements work in conjunction with other aspects of the Hypertension Institute program to lower blood pressure and reduce the risk of cardiovascular disease (CVD). Here are some of the important data and key points that you should know. (1–15)

1. The proof is in the incredible results with our patients treated in the Hypertension Institute has been published. (15) About 62% of patients with high blood pressure are able to stop or reduce their blood pressure medications in 1 year. Those with mild hypertension had an even greater chance to stop or reduce medications for hypertension.
2. Many patients with high blood pressure have micronutrient or macronutrient deficiencies that may increase their blood pressure. Replacing these deficiencies and also using high doses of many single or combined nutritional supplements will reduce blood pressure. There is an additive or synergistic effect of using nutritional supplements in combination and with drugs.
3. In addition, patients may consume foods that contain unhealthy substances that will increase blood pressure such as sodium, *trans*-fatty acids, some saturated fats, sugars, sweets, and refined carbohydrates.
4. Many foods are high in vitamins, minerals, and antioxidants that will improve blood pressure, but many foods do contain enough of some very important nutrients that lower blood pressure such as coenzyme Q-10 (CoQ-10) and lipoic acid. The combination of whole foods with nutritional supplements is better in order to get the best blood pressure–lowering effects.
5. For the purposes of our discussion, let us define a **nutraceutical supplement or nutritional supplement.** The term "nutraceutical" is similar to the term "pharmaceutical," a term that "pharmaceutical" companies use for their drugs. The term "nutraceutical" combines two words – "**nutrient**"

(a nourishing food component) and "**pharmaceutical**" (a medical drug). **Nutraceutical** is a broad umbrella term that is used to describe any product derived from food sources with extra health benefits in addition to the basic nutritional value found in foods. They can be considered non-specific biological therapies used to promote general well-being, health, and control symptoms. A **dietary or nutritional supplement** represents a product that contains nutrients derived from food products and is often concentrated in liquid, capsule, powder, or pill form. Although **dietary or nutritional supplements** are regulated by the FDA as foods, their regulation differs from drugs and other foods. These terms will be considered the same in this chapter to avoid confusion: **Nutraceutical supplement is the same as a nutritional supplement**. We will use nutraceutical supplements broadly in this chapter to include the following:

a. **Nutraceutical supplement or nutritional supplement** such as CoQ-10 and lipoic acid.
b. **Medical foods** such as pomegranate capsules, powder or seeds, whey protein, and green tea capsules or green tea drink.
c. **Antioxidants** such as glutathione liquid, lycopene, and vitamins A and C.
d. **Vitamins** such as B, D, and E.
e. **Minerals or electrolytes** such as sodium, potassium, calcium, and magnesium.

6. A large number of nutraceutical supplements and natural compounds in food produce physiologic effects that that lower blood pressure. They mimic specific classes of antihypertensive medications; improve vascular biology; improve the function and structure of the arteries and heart; reduce oxidative stress, inflammation, and vascular immune dysfunction; and reduce blood pressure. (1–52) These natural compounds can be classified into the major antihypertensive drug groups such as diuretics (D), beta blockers (BB), central alpha agonists (CAA), calcium channel blockers (CCB), angiotensin-converting enzyme (ACE) inhibitors (ACEI), angiotensin receptor blockers (ARBs), and direct renin inhibitors (DRI). (1–14) (Table 15.1)
7. Numerous clinical studies have demonstrated the efficacy of nutritional supplement interventions for the prevention and treatment of hypertension. These "blood pressure–lowering nutraceutical supplements" (antihypertensive nutraceutical supplements) provide a broad range of cardiovascular effects without side effects. Although their potency may not be as much as a blood pressure–lowering drug, when used in rational combinations in the correct amount, they are very effective as antihypertensive nutraceutical supplements.
8. In addition to the "blood pressure–lowering nutraceutical supplements" (antihypertensive nutraceutical supplements), there have been many published studies on the effect of nutrition and diets on the prevention and treatment of hypertension. These include *Dietary Approaches to Stop Hypertension (DASH 1 and DASH 2), the Mediterranean diet (MedDiet)*

TABLE 15.1
Natural Antihypertensive Compounds Categorized by Antihypertensive Class

Antihypertensive Therapeutic Class (Alphabetical Listing)	Foods and Ingredients Listed by Therapeutic Class	Nutrients and Other Supplements Listed by Therapeutic Class
Angiotensin-converting enzyme inhibitors	Egg yolk Fish (specific): Bonito, Dried salted fish, Fish sauce Sardine muscle/protein Tuna Garlic Gelatin Hawthorn berry Isoflavones/flavonoids Milk products (specific): Casein Sour milk Whey (hydrolyzed) Protein Sake Sea vegetables (kelp) Seaweed (wakame) Sesame (also ET1) Wheat germ (hydrolyzed) Zein (corn protein)	Melatonin Omega-3 fatty acids Pomegranate Probiotics Pycnogenol Quercetin (?) Zinc
Angiotensin receptor blockers	Celery Fiber Garlic MUFA	Coenzyme Q-10 Gamma-linolenic acid NAC Oleic acid Resveratrol Potassium Taurine Vitamin C Vitamin B6 (pyridoxine)
Beta blockers	Hawthorn berry	
Calcium channel blockers	Celery Garlic Hawthorn berry MUFA	Alpha-lipoic acid Calcium Magnesium (PGE, NO) *N*-acetylcysteine Oleic acid Omega-3 fatty acids: Eicosapentaenoic acid Docosahexaenoic acid Taurine Vitamin B6 Vitamin C Vitamin E

(*Continued*)

TABLE 15.1 (*Continued*)
Natural Antihypertensive Compounds Categorized by Antihypertensive Class

Antihypertensive Therapeutic Class (Alphabetical Listing)	Foods and Ingredients Listed by Therapeutic Class	Nutrients and Other Supplements Listed by Therapeutic Class
Central alpha agonists (reduce sympathetic nervous system activity)	Celery Fiber Garlic Protein	Coenzyme Q-10 Gamma-linolenic acid Potassium Probiotics Restriction of sodium Taurine Vitamin C Vitamin B6 Zinc
Direct renin inhibitors		Vitamin D
Direct vasodilators	Beets (NO, ED) Celery Cocoa (NO, ED) Cooking oils with monounsaturated fats Fiber Garlic Orange juice Lycopene food (NO, ED) MUFA Soy Teas: green and black	Alpha-linolenic acid Arginine Calcium Carnitines (eNOS, NO) Flavonoids Grape seed extract Lycopene (NO, ED) Magnesium Melatonin (NO, ED) Omega-3 fatty acids (NO, ED) Potassium (NO, ED) Taurine Vitamin C Vitamin E
Diuretics	Celery Fiber Hawthorn berry Protein	Calcium Coenzyme Q-10 Fiber Gamma-linolenic acid L-Carnitine Magnesium Potassium Taurine Vitamin B6 Vitamin C Vitamin E: high gamma-/delta-tocopherols and tocotrienols.

(Predimed), Trials of Hypertension Prevention (TOHP 1 and TOHP 2), Trial of Nonpharmacologic Intervention in the Elderly (TONE), Treatment of Mild Hypertension (TOMHS), INTERMAP, INTERSALT, Premier, Vanguard, and others. (1–5, 10–14, 51, 52) Some of these have been reviewed in the nutrition Chapters 14 and 15. The combination of these diets with "blood pressure–lowering nutraceutical supplements" (antihypertensive nutraceutical supplements) is a very effective treatment program that will treat the blood vessel, the heart and lower the blood pressure.

9. When you purchase a nutritional supplement, it is vitally important that it be high quality from a reputable nutritional supplement company. There are standards that must be met to ensure that what you buy works and has no adverse effects. There are only a handful of these companies in the United States. These are listed in the **Sources section** in the back of this book.
10. If I know of a high quality, standardized nutritional supplement with good research, I will mention the name of the supplement and the company that you can get it from in this chapter. In the **Sources section**, you will find the contact information for each company where you can purchase all of the nutritional supplements mentioned. Use the information in this book and your doctor's advice when you purchase them.

Now let us take a look at all each of these "blood pressure–lowering nutraceutical supplements" (antihypertensive nutraceutical supplements) and the science that supports their use in the treatment of hypertension.

15.1 SODIUM (NA^+)

Increased dietary sodium intake is associated with hypertension, stroke (CVA), left ventricular hypertrophy (LVH), diastolic dysfunction, coronary heart disease (CHD), heart attack (myocardial infarction), renal insufficiency, protein in the urine (microalbuminuria), higher death rate, arterial stiffness, platelet stickiness, and increased sympathetic nervous system activation (the "fight or flight reaction" with fast heart rate, high blood pressure, and nervousness). A high sodium intake also causes abnormalities in vascular immune function, increases inflammation and oxidative stress in the arteries and the heart. A reduction in dietary sodium intake lowers blood pressure and the risk of all of these problems and diseases. (2–5, 10–15, 18, 19, 53–61) Decreasing dietary sodium intake in hypertensive patients, especially the salt-sensitive patients (African-Americans and Chinese), lowers blood pressure by 4–6/2–3 mm Hg proportional to the amount of sodium restriction (54) and may prevent or delay hypertension in high-risk patients.

Salt sensitivity, defined as ≥10% increase in mean arterial pressure (MAP) with salt loading, increases the blood pressure response to dietary salt intake in 51% of hypertensive patients. (57, 58) Cardiovascular events may be more common in salt-sensitive patients compared to salt-resistant patients, independent of blood pressure level. (57, 58) Decreasing sodium intake to below 1500 mg/day was associated with lower blood pressure and a decrease in death rate. However, increasing the intake to >2300 mg/day was associated with an increase in death rate and CVD. (56) The sodium intake should not be overly aggressive either. You should not go below 500 mg of sodium intake per day, as this may increase insulin resistance, and in some patients, this will counterbalance the blood pressure reduction seen with 1500 mg of sodium intake per day.

Sodium promotes hypertension by increasing the endothelial cell stiffness, reducing the size and elasticity of the endothelial cells, decreasing nitric oxide (NO) production, increasing oxidative stress, and abolishing the ability to vasodilate. (59, 60, 64, 65) High sodium intake damages the glycocalyx, increases constriction of the coronary arteries which increases the risk of heart attack, and induces higher nighttime blood pressure and a non-dipping status that increases the risk of all CVDs, especially stroke. In several studies, a sodium intake of 8 g/day increased cardiovascular death by 53%, heart attack by 34%, stroke by 48%, and congestive heart failure (CHF) by 51%. These complications were independent of the increased blood pressure. (2–5, 10–15, 18, 19, 53–61)

All of these effects are increased in the presence of the adrenal hormone, aldosterone, which mimics these same pathophysiologic changes. (59, 60, 63) Endothelial cells act as **vascular salt sensors** and they become damaged and diseased. (59, 60)

A balance of sodium with potassium and magnesium improves blood pressure control and lowers cardiovascular and cerebrovascular (stroke) events. (2, 63, 66–69). Increasing the **sodium/potassium ratio** increases blood pressure and the risk of CVD, but increasing the **potassium/sodium** ratio lowers blood pressure and cardiovascular risk. (66–69) A potassium/sodium ratio of 4:1 is recommended with a daily dietary sodium intake of 1500 mg and a dietary potassium intake of 6000 mg. (2, 66–69) It is important to read the labels of all foods that you eat to determine the amount of sodium in each.

15.2 POTASSIUM (K^+)

Populations that consume high amounts of dietary potassium (K^+) have lower blood pressures and reduced CVD, especially stroke, compared to those who consume lower amounts of dietary potassium. Potassium is the third most abundant element in the body and has many functions, including the nervous system, cardiovascular system, and the muscles. Increased dietary potassium intake reduces blood pressure and CVD. (66–73) The minimal recommended intake of K^+ is 6000 mg/day with a K^+/Na^+ ratio at least 4:1. (66–73) Dietary supplementation of potassium at 2500 mg/day for 12 weeks significantly reduced the systolic blood pressure (SBP) by 5.0 mm Hg in 150 Chinese subjects. (70) Clinical studies have found that 1.64 g or more per day of potassium intake resulted in a 21% lower risk of stroke ($p = 0.0007$) and significant reductions in blood pressure of 4/.2.5 mm Hg. (72) When potassium intake is increased, the incidence of stroke is reduced proportional to blood pressure reduction, but also potassium reduces stroke even if the blood pressure is not reduced. (2) Studies indicate a dose-related reduction in blood pressure of 4.4/2.5–8/4.1 mm Hg with potassium supplementation with doses between 2500 and 5000 mg/day. (2–14, 66–73) Chronic blood levels of potassium below 4.0 meq/dl increase blood pressure, cardiovascular death, CHF, CHD, heart attack, ventricular tachycardia, and ventricular fibrillation that are fatal rhythms of the heart.

(2–14, 66–73) Red blood cell potassium is a better indication of total body stores than blood potassium. (2–14)

Potassium helps to lower blood pressure in many ways. (2–14, 66–73) It causes the artery to dilate, reduces arterial stiffness, increases the loss of sodium and water in the kidney, like a diuretic, and counteracts the effects of sodium on the artery thickness, on endothelial dysfunction, and on damage to the glycocalyx. Potassium increases NO, reduces inflammation and oxidative stress, lowers the potent arterial constrictor, endothelin, improves dipping status, balances the nervous system, and lowers adrenalin levels. It reduces LVH (enlarged heart), reduces heart muscle stiffness, improves kidney function, and reduces insulin resistance and risk for diabetes mellitus. Numerous genetic abnormalities in the renin-angiotensin-aldosterone system (RAAS) system play an important role in determining an individual's blood pressure response to dietary potassium.

For each 1000 mg increase of daily dietary potassium, the death rate is reduced by 20%. For each 1000 mg decrease of daily dietary sodium intake, the death rate is decreased by 20%. (66) Therefore, small changes in the sodium/potassium ratio and daily intake will have a dramatic effect on cardiovascular death and other complications. The recommended daily dietary intake of potassium is 6 g in hypertensive patients with normal kidney function, those not taking potassium retaining medications or in those with some other contraindications. (2–14, 66–73) Potassium sources include dark green leafy vegetables and fruits (Table 15.2), nutritional supplements such as "No Salt" (KCL) substitutes, pure potassium powders or capsules or combined potassium/magnesium powders or capsules, and prescription potassium chloride (KCL) or potassium bicarbonate. An excellent nutritional supplement for combined potassium and magnesium is **Potassium HP powder** from Biotics Research, which contains 1200 mg of potassium and 120 mg of magnesium per scoop (see Sources section). The red blood cell levels should be monitored. (2–4) Red blood cell potassium and serum potassium should be monitored. (2–14)

15.3 MAGNESIUM (MG^{++})

The lower the dietary magnesium intake, the higher the blood pressure. (67, 74–78) In numerous clinical trials, an increased dietary magnesium of 500–1000 mg/day lowers blood pressure within 2 months by about 6/3 mm Hg documented by 24-hour ambulatory blood pressure monitoring, home and office blood pressure readings. (67, 74–78) Low magnesium is also associated with diabetes mellitus, metabolic syndrome, inflammation, CHD, heart attack, atherosclerosis, platelet aggregation, dyslipidemia, sudden death, and stroke. For each 100 mg increase in dietary magnesium, there was a reduction in ischemic stroke by 8%.

The combination of high dietary potassium and magnesium combined with a low dietary sodium intake potentiates the antihypertensive effects in patients treated with blood pressure–lowering medications and hypertensive patients on no blood pressure–lowering medications. (67, 74–78) Magnesium also increases NO levels and improves endothelial function. When calcium enters the blood vessel wall, it causes the artery to constrict and increases the blood pressure. Magnesium blocks that calcium entry, vasodilates, and reduces the blood pressure, similar to the drug

TABLE 15.2
Potassium: Food Sources Ranked by Amounts of Potassium and Energy per Standard Food Portions and per 100 g of Foods

Food	Standard Portion Size	Calories in Standard Portion[a]	Potassium in Standard Portion (mg)[a]
Potato, baked, flesh, and skin	1 medium	163	941
Prune juice, canned	1 cup	182	707
Carrot juice, canned	1 cup	94	689
Passion-fruit juice, yellow or purple	1 cup	126–148	687
Tomato paste, canned	1/4 cup	54	669
Beet greens, cooked from fresh	1/2 cup	19	654
Adzuki beans, cooked	1/2 cup	147	612
White beans, canned	1/2 cup	149	595
Plain yogurt, nonfat	1 cup	127	579
Tomato puree	1/2 cup	48	549
Sweet potato, baked in skin	1 medium	103	542
Salmon, Atlantic, wild, cooked	3 oz	155	534
Clams, canned	3 oz	121	534
Pomegranate juice	1 cup	134	533
Plain yogurt, low-fat	8 oz	143	531
Tomato juice, canned	1 cup	41	527
Orange juice, fresh	1 cup	112	496
Soybeans, green, cooked	1/2 cup	127	485
Chard, Swiss, cooked	1/2 cup	18	481
Lima beans, cooked	1/2 cup	108	478
Mackerel, various types, cooked	3 oz	114–171	443–474
Vegetable juice, canned	1 cup	48	468
Chili with beans, canned	1/2 cup	144	467
Great northern beans, canned	1/2 cup	150	460
Yam, cooked	1/2 cup	79	456
Halibut, cooked	3 oz	94	449
Tuna, yellowfin, cooked	3 oz	111	448
Acorn squash, cooked	1/2 cup	58	448
Snapper, cooked	3 oz	109	444
Soybeans, mature, cooked	1/2 cup	149	443
Tangerine juice, fresh	1 cup	106	440
Pink beans, cooked	1/2 cup	126	430
Chocolate milk (1%, 2%, and whole)	1 cup	178–208	418–425
Amaranth leaves, cooked	1/2 cup	14	423
Banana	1 medium	105	422

(Continued)

TABLE 15.2 (*Continued*)
Potassium: Food Sources Ranked by Amounts of Potassium and Energy per Standard Food Portions and per 100 g of Foods

Food	Standard Portion Size	Calories in Standard Portion[a]	Potassium in Standard Portion (mg)[a]
Spinach, cooked from fresh or canned	1/2 cup	21–25	370–419
Black turtle beans, cooked	1/2 cup	121	401
Peaches, dried, uncooked	1/4 cup	96	399
Prunes, stewed	1/2 cup	133	398
Rockfish, Pacific, cooked	3 oz	93	397
Rainbow trout, wild or farmed, cooked	3 oz	128–143	381–383
Skim milk (nonfat)	1 cup	83	382
Refried beans, canned, traditional	1/2 cup	106	380
Apricots, dried, uncooked	1/4 cup	78	378
Pinto beans, cooked	1/2 cup	123	373
Lentils, cooked	1/2 cup	115	365
Avocado	1/2 cup	120	364
Tomato sauce, canned	1/2 cup	30	364
Plantains, slices, cooked	1/2 cup	89	358
Kidney beans, cooked	1/2 cup	113	357
Navy beans, cooked	1/2 cup	128	354

Source: US Department of Agriculture, Agricultural Research Service, Nutrient Data Laboratory. 2014. USDA National Nutrient Database for Standard Reference, Release 27. Available at: http://www.ars.usda.gov/nutrientdata.

class, called CCB. (2, 74–78) Most of the magnesium in your body is in your bones, teeth, liver, muscles, and soft tissue. Very little is actually in the blood. Intracellular red blood cell levels of magnesium are a more accurate assessment of total body stores compared to blood levels. (2, 67, 78)

Magnesium is involved in over 300 biochemical pathways in the body. These include the relaxation of vascular and skeletal muscle, nerve function, controlling blood sugar, making protein, keeping the heart beating in a normal and regular fashion. Magnesium is a key mineral in the production of ATP (adenosine triphosphate), the basic energy source for all body cells.

In general, rich sources of magnesium are greens, seeds, dry beans (especially kidney beans and black beans), whole-grain cereal (shredded wheat and bran cereals), avocado, brown rice, nuts such as cashews and peanuts, edamame, oatmeal, peanut butter, potato with the skin, pumpkin, raisins, soymilk, spinach, whole-grain bread, low-fat dairy, and yogurt. Magnesium formulations bound or chelated to an amino acid (a small protein) also provide blood pressure reduction. (2, 67, 78)

Transdermal (skin application) preparations of magnesium and magnesium salt baths such as Epsom salts are also effective. (2, 67, 78) A high magnesium diet or magnesium supplements must be used with caution in patients taking medications that promote magnesium retention, in those with known kidney disease or those with other contraindications to high doses of magnesium intake. (2, 67, 78) The recommended daily intake of magnesium is 1000 mg using a combination of whole foods and magnesium supplements. An excellent nutritional supplement for combined magnesium and potassium is **Potassium HP powder** from Biotics Research, which contains 120 mg of magnesium and 1200 mg of potassium per scoop (see Sources section). The red blood cell levels should be monitored.

15.4 CALCIUM (CA^{++})

Calcium supplementation is not recommended as an effective means to reduce blood pressure until more studies are done on specific populations, specific age groups identification of the proper formulation and dose. (79–82) The only exception to this is that calcium may reduce the risk of preeclampsia and its complications for both mother and fetus. (82)

15.5 ZINC (ZN^{++})

Low serum zinc levels correlate with hypertension and other cardiovascular problems such as diabetes mellitus, insulin resistance, low HDL cholesterol, and CHD. (2, 83, 84) Zinc is important for memory, immune function, wound healing, bone health, and reproduction. Genetic disorders of zinc transport into the vascular system and heart may lead to zinc deficiencies with heart failure and hypertension. (83) Zinc reduces vascular oxidative stress, inflammation, vascular immune dysfunction, balances the nervous system, and reduces the levels of two hormones that increase blood pressure, the RAAS, and adrenalin from the sympathetic nervous system. (1, 2, 57, 58, 83, 84) Good dietary sources of zinc include shellfish, legumes like chickpeas, lentils, and beans, seeds, nuts, dairy, yogurt, eggs, oysters, sardines, wheat germ, and whole grains. Dietary zinc intake should be approximately 50 mg/day from whole food and nutritional supplements and levels should be monitored. (1)

15.6 PROTEIN

Lower blood pressure is associated with an increased intake of all types of protein, including animal (meat) protein, fish protein, dairy protein, plant-based protein in the Intermap study, and other types of protein. (85–114, 416–420) The Framingham study followed 1361 men and women (30–54 years) without hypertension, CVD, or diabetes over 11 years for the development of hypertension. (420) Higher protein intakes were associated with lower mean blood pressure. Both animal and plant proteins lowered blood pressure and led to statistically significant reductions in blood pressure by 32% with animal proteins and 49% with plant proteins. Participants in the highest one-third of total protein intake had 40% less risk of developing hypertension. Beneficial effects of protein were apparent for men and women and for normal-weight and overweight individuals. Higher protein diets also characterized by higher fiber intakes led to a 59% reduction in hypertension risk.

Over 40 trials with 3277 subjects were reviewed and there was a significant decrease in blood pressure with increasing levels of protein intake for both animal and vegetable protein:

- Blood pressure reduction 2.27/1.26 mm Hg for vegetable protein ($p < 0.001$, highly significant)
- Blood pressure reduction of 2.54/.95 mm Hg for animal protein ($p < 0.001$, highly significant)

The PROPRESS study was conducted over 4 weeks in 94 subjects with prehypertension and stage I hypertension that compared 25 versus 15% protein intake in isocaloric diet. (419) The proteins were 20% pea, 20% soy, 30% egg, and 30% milk-protein isolate versus maltodextrin. The office blood pressure was about 5/3 mm Hg lower in the protein group.

All of the proteins have a similar mechanism of action in which they inhibit an enzyme called **ACE**. The ACE converts a substance in the RAAS called angiotensin I to angiotensin II, which is a very strong constrictor of the arteries and elevates blood pressure. There is a drug class called **ACEI (angiotensin-converting enzyme inhibitors)** that have this same mechanism of action as protein. Other mechanisms include improved endothelial dysfunction, decrease in adrenalin and sympathetic nervous system activity, diuretic effect, decrease in oxidative stress, lower inflammation, and lower aldosterone levels. (85–114)

Animal protein varies in its ability to lower blood pressure depending on the type of fat present. (2, 6, 85–115) Lean or wild animal protein, with a higher content of omega-3 fatty acids and reduced saturated fat, is more effective in reducing blood pressure. (86–89, 115) In the Intersalt Study, a dietary protein intake 30% above the average US intake (81 g of protein) showed a 3.0/2.5-mm Hg lower blood pressure compared to those that were 30% below the average daily protein intake (44 g of protein). (2, 85, 88) Soy protein intake of 25 g/day significantly lowers blood pressure about 6/3 mm Hg. (89, 101–103, 105, 106, 108) The recommended daily intake of fermented soy is 25 g/day. (2)

Whey protein, milk peptides, and fermented milk lower blood pressure. (2, 6, 90–95, 104, 110–115) Administration of 20–30 g/day of whey protein per day lowered blood pressure within 6–8 weeks by 8.0/5.5 mm Hg but as much as 11/7 mm Hg depending on the dose given per day. (91, 92, 95, 110) In some patients, **Whey Cool** is an excellent nutritional supplement for whey protein from Designs for Health (see Sources section).

Milk peptides (the proteins found in milk) are also rich in ACEI peptides (similar to the drugs called ACEI) that lower blood pressure approximately 4.8/2.2 mm Hg with doses of 5–60 mg/day. (2, 6, 90–95, 104) Powdered fermented milk containing *Lactobacillus helveticus (a probiotic bacteria with active ACEI peptides)* dosed at 12 g daily significantly reduced blood pressure by 11.2/6.5 mm Hg in 1 month. (92)

Marine collagen peptides derived from deep-sea fish have antihypertensive activity. (96–98) Bonito protein (*Sarda orientalis*), from the tuna and mackerel family, have natural ACEI peptides and lower blood pressure by 10/7 mm Hg with a dose of 1.5 g daily. (97) The best source of Bonito protein is **Vasotensin** from Metagenics (see Sources section).

Sardine muscle protein lowered blood pressure by 9.7//5.3 mm Hg over 4 weeks at a dose of 3 mg (sardine muscle concentrated extract). (99) Sardine protein also decreases the adverse effects of fructose on glucose metabolism and oxidative stress that may improve insulin resistance, diabetes mellitus, and metabolic syndrome. A vegetable drink with sardine protein also reduced blood pressure by 8/5 mm Hg over 13 weeks. (100)

Processed and cured meats should be avoided as they increase blood pressure, increase the risk for all CVDs, including heart attack, CHD, CHF, stroke, and increase the death rate. (416–418) Red meat does not increase blood pressure or CHD. Several meta-analysis reports, including a large number of studies, showed no association between red meat consumption and CHD, but processed red meat increased CHD and diabetes mellitus risk and DM risk. Processed meat increased total mortality by 46%. (416–418)

The daily recommended intake of protein from all sources is 1.0–1.5 g/kg (1 kg = 2.2 lb) of body weight depending on kidney function, age, and exercise level.

15.7 L-ARGININE

L-Arginine lowers blood pressure due to its ability to increase NO levels. L-Arginine and endogenous methylarginines produce NO through the important enzyme eNOS. (116–128) Oral L-arginine administration in hypertensive and normotensive patients lowers blood pressure significantly at doses of 10–12 g/day in food or as a supplement by about 6.2/6.8 mm Hg documented in both office and 24-hour ambulatory blood pressure monitor readings. (116, 117, 123, 125, 126) Arginine administered at 4 g daily significantly lowered blood pressure in gestational hypertension, reduced concomitant antihypertensive therapy, and improved maternal and neonatal outcomes with normal delivery time. (123, 124) The combination of arginine (1200 mg/day) and *N*-acetyl cysteine (600 mg twice per day) administered over 6 months to hypertensive patients with type II diabetes, lowered blood pressure about 6/5 mm Hg. (125) Arginine may have a pro-oxidative effect and increase in the death rate in patients with advanced atherosclerosis, CHD, severe unstable angina, or during a heart attack. (127) Pending more studies, arginine is best avoided in these cardiac situations. Arginine has fallen out of favor as a supplement for blood pressure.

15.8 TAURINE

Taurine is a sulfur-based amino acid (protein) that is highly concentrated in the heart, brain, and the retina. (2–5, 14, 129–136) Taurine is one of the most efficacious nutritional supplements for the treatment of hypertension as well as a variety of other CVDs such as CHF and abnormal rhythms of the heart. Taurine dilates the arteries, decreases calcium movement into the artery wall, reduces sympathetic nervous system activity and adrenalin levels (norepinephrine and epinephrine), promotes urinary sodium and water excretion, increases atrial natriuretic factor, elevates NO bioavailability that reduces endothelial dysfunction, and lowers inflammation and oxidative stress. (2–5, 14, 129–136) In addition, taurine increases endothelial progenitor cells, while it decreases the activity of the renin-angiotensin-aldosterone system or RAAS with reductions in plasma renin activity (PRA), angiotensin II and aldosterone, hormones that constrict the arteries and elevate the blood pressure. (2–5, 14, 129–136) In a study of 19 hypertensive patients administered 6 g of taurine per day, the blood pressure was reduced by 9/4.1 mm Hg over 7 days. (130) In another study of 120 prehypertensive individuals, taurine supplementation, even in lower doses of 1.6 g/day, significantly improved endothelial function and decreased 24-hour ambulatory blood pressure readings by 7.2/2.6 mm Hg and the office blood pressure by 4.7/1.3 mm Hg in 12 weeks. (136) In a 4-month study of 97 prehypertensive individuals, 1.6 /day of taurine significantly decreased the clinic and 24-hour ambulatory blood pressure, improved endothelium-vasodilation, and reduced the carotid IMT. (134)

In a placebo-controlled study conducted over 1 month at the Hypertension Institute in Nashville, TN, 42 hypertensive subjects were treated with a combination nutritional supplement in powder form given once daily with highly significant reductions in blood pressure in the treated group of 16/11.5 mm Hg within 4 weeks. (135) The supplement included 6 g of taurine, vitamin C (as magnesium ascorbate) at 1000 mg, grape seed extract (GSE) at 150 mg, magnesium ascorbate at 87 mg, vitamin B6 (pyridoxine HCl) at 100 mg, vitamin D3 at 2000 IU (international units), and biotin at 2 mg. This proprietary product was **CardioSirt BP** from Biotics Research (see Sources section). The recommended dose of taurine if administered alone is 1.5–6 g/day in as a single dose or as divided doses depending on the desired blood pressure reduction. If you want to take only taurine, then there is a good **taurine powder or capsule** nutritional supplement available from Designs for Health (see Sources section). (2, 129–136)

15.9 OMEGA-3 FATS AND SELECTED OMEGA-6 FATS

Omega-3 fatty acids derived from food or nutritional supplements produce a dose-related reduction in blood pressure and CVD in published studies. (2–14, 115, 137–152) Before we discuss all of the data on omega-3 fatty acids, let us review some definitions and their structure.

15.10 DEFINITIONS AND STRUCTURE

1. Omega-3 fatty acids are not the same as fish oil, although they are related. Omega-3 fatty acids are a concentrated form of fish oil, but there are also non-fish sources of omega-3 fatty acid such as algae, green soybeans, butternuts, green leafy vegetables, flaxseed oil, walnuts, and Brazil nuts.
2. A fatty acid is the major component of the fat molecule, just like amino acids are the building blocks of protein. A fatty acid is built around a line of carbon atoms that are attached by various types of bonds to one another and to hydrogen atoms (Figures 15.1–15.3). These bonds are called single or double bonds and the number of carbon atoms and the type and number

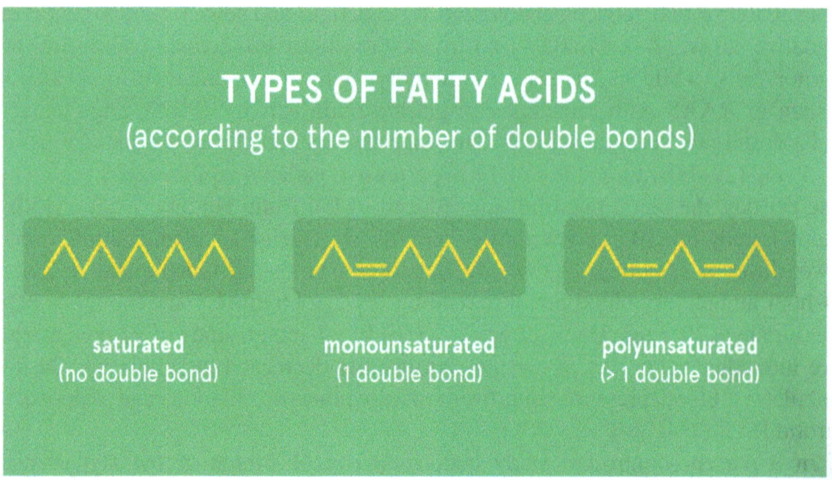

FIGURE 15.1 The three types of fatty acids. Saturated fatty acids have no double bonds. Monounsaturated fatty acids (MUFA) (olive oil) have only one double bond. Polyunsaturated fatty acids (PUFA) have numerous double bonds. Omega-3 fatty acids are a type of PUFA.

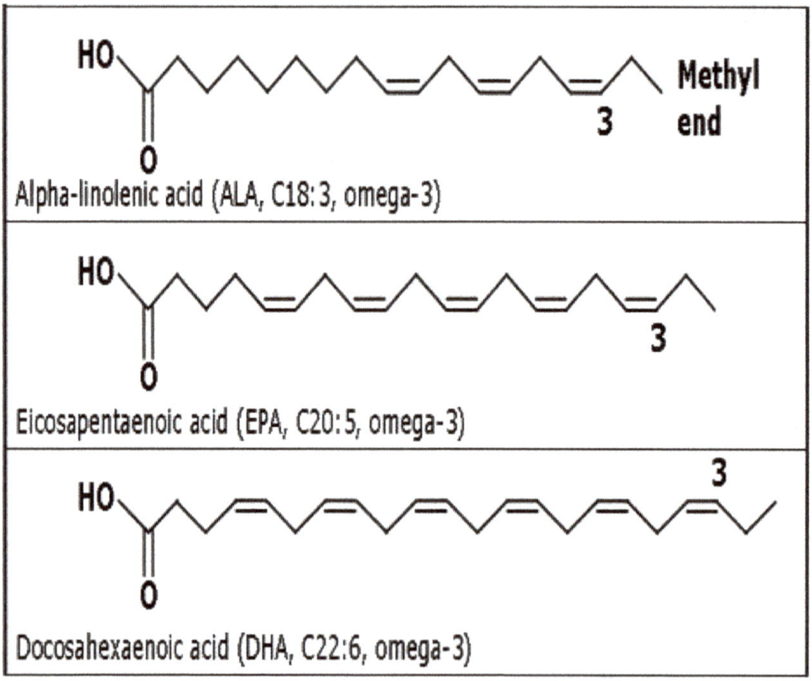

HO
O
3
Methyl end
Alpha-linolenic acid (ALA, C18:3, omega-3)

HO
O
3
Eicosapentaenoic acid (EPA, C20:5, omega-3)

HO
O
3
Docosahexaenoic acid (DHA, C22:6, omega-3)

FIGURE 15.2 The three types of omega-3 fatty acids have different lengths related to the number of carbon atoms: ALA = 18 carbon atoms, EPA has 20 carbon atoms, and DHA has 22 carbon atoms shown below as C18:3 or C20:3 or C22:3. The number 3 indicates the position of the first double bond from the methyl end of the carbon chain.

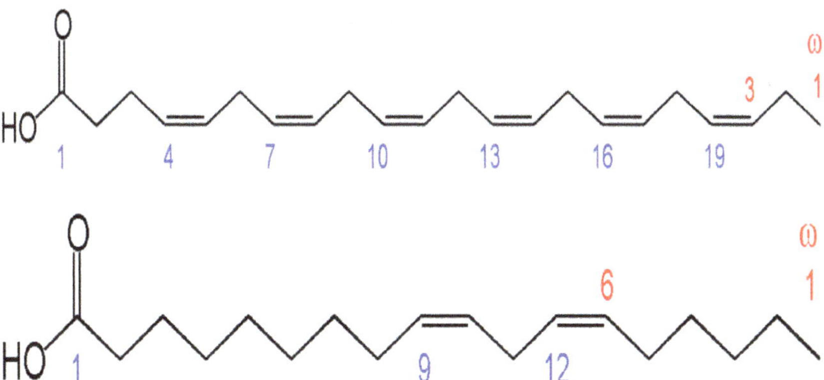

FIGURE 15.3 The location of the first double bond from the methyl end of the carbon chain determines the name of the fatty acid as an omega-3, or 6 or 9 fatty acid.

of bonds determine the function of the fatty acid and the name of the fatty acid, such as saturated fatty acid **(SFA)** (all single bonds) or unsaturated fatty acid (some double bonds). Therefore, an omega-3 fatty acid is a type of polyunsaturated fatty acid **(PUFA)** due to the large number of double bonds, but a saturated fat **(SFA)** has only single bonds and monounsaturated fatty acids **(MUFA),** like olive oil, have only one double bond (Figure 15.1). These structural changes have a major influence on the effects of these fatty acids on our overall health, blood pressure and CVD. The location of the first double bond from the methyl end (CH_3) of the carbon chain determines the name of the fatty acid as a 3 or 6 or 9: omega-3, omega-6, or omega-9 fatty acid (Figure 15.3).

There are three types of omega-3 fatty acids that we will discuss that are defined by the number of carbon atoms in the chain. These are **alpha-linolenic acid (ALA), eicosapentaenoic acid** (**EPA**), and **docosahexaenoic acid (DHA)** (Figure 15.2).

3. Linoleic acid, an omega-6 fatty acid, and ALA, an omega-3 fatty acid, are considered essential fatty acids because they cannot be synthesized by humans.
4. The long-chain omega-3 fatty acids, **EPA** and **DHA,** can be synthesized from **ALA**, but due to low conversion efficiency, it is recommended to take nutritional supplements and consume foods rich in EPA and DHA.
5. Both omega-6 and omega-3 fatty acids are important structural components of cell membranes, serve as precursors to bioactive lipid mediators, and provide a source of energy. Long-chain omega-3 PUFA in particular exert anti-inflammatory effects.
6. Both dietary intake and endogenous metabolism influence whole-body status of essential fatty acids. Genetic abnormalities in fatty acid synthesizing enzymes can have a significant impact on fatty acid concentrations in the body.

A meta-analysis of 70 clinical studies found that, compared with placebo, the consumption of omega-3 fatty acids (0.3–5 g/day) for 4–26 weeks significantly reduced blood pressure by 1.5/1.0 mm Hg. (146) The largest blood pressure reductions were in untreated hypertensive subjects 4.5/3.0 mm Hg. (146) A second meta-analysis found that omega-3 fatty acid supplementation for 6–105 weeks at 900–3000 mg/day improved arterial elasticity and health. (147) DHA is more effective than EPA in reducing the blood pressure with an average reduction of 8/5 mm Hg and it lowers the resting heart rate by 6 beats per minute. (2–14, 137–139, 142–144) Administration of EPA and DHA is preferred to ALA due to minimal conversion to these longer chain omega-3 fatty acids. (2–14, 138, 140) The consumption of cold-water fish three times per week reduces blood pressure due to the combination of protein and omega-3 fatty acids. (2–14, 109, 138) In patients with chronic kidney disease, 4 g of omega-3 fatty acids significantly lowered 24-hour ambulatory blood pressure by 3.3/3 mm Hg compared to placebo. (139) The omega-6 fatty acids, gamma-linolenic acid (GLA), and dihomo-GLA (DGLA) reduce blood pressure and prevent elevations in blood pressure induced by saturated fats. (143) GLA blocks stress-induced hypertension, lowers aldosterone levels, and increases the vasodilating prostaglandins E1 (PGE1) and PGI2. (2–14, 143)

The omega-3 fatty acids reduce CHD and heart attack, (152) reduce inflammation, decrease platelet stickiness, increase NO, improve endothelial function, reduce arterial stiffness, decrease insulin resistance, lower plasma norepinephrine, suppress ACE activity, and increase parasympathetic tone at doses of 900–3000 mg daily. (2–14, 137, 145, 148) The recommended daily dose is 3000–5000 mg/day of combined DHA and EPA in a ratio of three parts EPA to two parts DHA with 50% of this total dose as GLA combined with gamma-/delta-tocopherol (a form of vitamin E) at 100 mg/g of DHA and EPA. The optimal dose is defined by an omega-3 index at 8%. The most effective and balanced omega-3 nutritional supplement that contains all of these components is **EFA-SIRT SUPREME** form Biotics Research (see Sources section). (2–5) There are no adverse effects or safety concerns at these recommended doses. (2–14)

15.11 MONOUNSATURATED FATTY ACIDS (MUFA): OLIVE OIL, MEDITERRANEAN DIET, OMEGA-9 FATS, OLEIC ACID, AND OLIVE LEAF EXTRACT

The MedDiet, which is rich in olive oil, olive leaf extracts (OLEs), extra-virgin olive oil (EVOO), and polyphenols, reduces blood pressure and CVD in published clinical trials. (2–14, 153–176) In a study done over 2 months, 40 borderline hypertensive twins given either 500 or 1000 mg/day of OLE had significant reductions in blood pressure of 6/5 mm Hg (500 mg of OLE) and 13/5 mm Hg reduction (1000 of OLE) compared to controls. (176) Many other studies with OLE have shown reductions in the blood pressure range of 8/6–11/5 mm Hg both in office and with 24-hour ambulatory blood pressure monitoring. There was a decrease in antihypertensive medications by 48% in the MUFA-treated patients. (153, 167–169, 173) The recommended dose of **oleic acid** is 500 mg twice per day from Designs for Health (see Sources section).

EVOO lowered the SBP by 14 mm Hg in elderly hypertensive patients. (154, 155) In the European Prospective Investigation into Cancer and Nutrition study (20,343 subjects), the intake of EVOO and polyphenols documented an inverse relationship with blood pressure. (171) In the prevention with MedDiet (PREDIMED) trial that included 7447 patients at high risk for CVD, the participants on the MedDiet supplemented with EVOO had a significantly lower diastolic blood pressure by 1.5 mm Hg than those in the control group. (172)

EVOO contains lipid-soluble phytonutrients such as nitrates and polyphenols that lower blood pressure by reducing oxidative stress, blocking a receptor on the artery, and improving various hormones that increase vasoconstriction and blood pressure, increasing NO levels and blocking specific areas on the arteries called calcium channels, similar to a calcium channel blocking drug that causes the artery to dilate. (150, 153, 157, 164–166) EVOO with a total phenol content of at least 300 mg/kg at 20–40 g (2–4 tablespoons) per day will significantly lower the blood pressure about 8/6 mm Hg. (2–5, 170) The best source is the organic EVOO from California.

15.12 VITAMIN C

Higher dietary intake of vitamin C and vitamin C blood levels are associated with lower blood pressure. (2–14, 177–199) The administration of vitamin C orally and intravenously reduces blood pressure in clinical studies. (2–14, 177–199) In a clinical trial of 31 patients who were given several doses of vitamin C at 500, 1000, or 2000 mg daily had a decrease in blood pressure by 4.5/2.8 mm Hg. (194) There was no difference between the three vitamin C doses indicating that 500 mg daily or 250 mg twice per day is sufficient to reduce blood pressure in most patients. (194) In a meta-analysis that combined over 29 clinical studies that had given an average dose of vitamin C at 500 mg/day for an average of 2 months, there was a significant reduction in blood pressure of about 4/1.5 mm Hg. (199) Published clinical trials show that vitamin C at a dose of 250 mg twice daily reduces blood pressure by an average of 7/4 mm Hg. (2–14, 177–199) Vitamin C is a potent water-soluble antioxidant, which recycles vitamin E and other antioxidants and enhances the body's total antioxidant ability. (177) In elderly patients with refractory hypertension already on maximum drug therapy, 600 mg of vitamin C daily lowered the blood by an additional 20/16 mm Hg. (186) Vitamin C potentiates the effects of the drugs called CCB. Plasma vitamin C is inversely correlated with blood pressure in healthy patients with normal blood pressure and those with the lowest initial vitamin C blood levels have the largest blood pressure reduction. (2–5, 187, 193) The SBP and the 24-hour ambulatory blood pressure show the most significant reductions with chronic oral administration of vitamin C. (2, 181–186) In a classic clinical study, patients were given no vitamin C in their diet until they were severely deficient and then they had the vitamin replaced in their diet. In this depletion-repletion study of vitamin C, as the vitamin C in the diet and blood level of vitamin C fell, the blood pressure increased, but as the vitamin C in the diet was replaced and blood levels of vitamin C returned to normal the blood pressure normalized. (187) In another meta-analysis of 13 clinical trials with 284 patients, vitamin C at 500 mg/day over 6 weeks reduced blood pressure

3.9/2.1 mm Hg. (188) People who have high blood pressure have significantly lower vitamin C levels compared to those with normal vitamin C levels (40 μmol/l versus 57 μmol/l, respectively). (190, 199) The recommended daily dose of vitamin C is at least 250 mg twice per day. A good source in capsule form is **Stellar C** or in powdered **Buffered vitamin C** from Designs for Health (see Sources section). A serum level of 100 μmol/l is recommended for optimal blood pressure lowering. (2–5)

15.13 VITAMIN E

Very few clinical studies have demonstrated improved blood pressure with the eight different forms of vitamin E (four tocopherols and four tocotrienols called alpha, beta, gamma, and delta forms). (2, 200–204) Patients with type II diabetes mellitus on prescription medications with controlled blood pressure (average blood pressure of 136/76 mm Hg) were administered mixed tocopherols containing 60% gamma, 25% delta, and 15% alpha-tocopherols. (200) The blood pressure increased by 6.8/3.6 mm Hg in the study patients on the mixed tocopherols and increased even more in those patients taking alpha-tocopherol (blood increased 7/5 mm Hg. (200) The blood pressure increase was likely due to drug interactions with tocopherols and their metabolism in the liver by the system that breaks down blood pressure drugs called the cytochrome P450 system. This means that the vitamin E decreased the effective blood levels of the blood pressure–lowering medications and the blood pressure actually increased. (200) Gamma-tocopherol has a diuretic and blood pressure–lowering effect through the inhibition of a potassium channel in the kidney called the thick ascending limb of the loop of Henle. (201) Both alpha- and gamma-tocopherol improve insulin sensitivity with the potential to lower blood pressure and serum glucose. (202)

In a retrospective analysis and data from the National Health and Nutrition Services, the medium and high thirds of vitamin E intake were associated with a significantly lower risk for hypertension, 27% reduction and 19% reduction, respectively. (203) Fifty-eight individuals with type II diabetes given 500 mg/day of alpha-tocopherol, 500 mg/day of mixed tocopherols, or placebo for 6 weeks did not significantly alter the level of daytime or nighttime blood pressure compared to placebo. (204) If vitamin E has a blood pressure–lowering effect, it is probably small and may be limited to untreated hypertensive patients not taking any blood pressure–lowering drugs, those with vitamin E deficiency, known CVD, mild blood volume overload, diabetes mellitus, or high cholesterol. (2–5, 200–204) The recommended dose is a mixed tocopherol at a dose of 1/day from AC Grace called **Unique E** or from Designs for Health called **Ultra Gamma E.** Tocotrienols are also available from these same companies and the dose is 150–200 mg/day of the **Annatto gamma-/delta-tocotrienol** (see Sources section).

15.14 VITAMIN D3

Vitamin D3 has variable blood pressure–lowering effects. (2–5, 205–223) Vitamin D may have an independent and direct role in the regulation of blood pressure, insulin metabolism, and blood glucose, but the results have not been consistent in studies. (205–219, 221, 223) If the vitamin D level is below 30 ng/ml, the circulating PRA levels are higher that increase the potent constrictor of the arteries, angiotensin II, and elevate blood pressure. (215) The lowest fourth quartile of blood vitamin D levels has a 52% incidence of hypertension versus the highest fourth quartile that has a 20% incidence. (215) Compared with a 25-hydroxyvitamin D3 of >30 ng/ml, a 25-hydroxyvitamin D3 of <20 ng/ml was associated with a greater hypertension risk of 122%. (215, 217) A recent analysis from eight trials in which patients were treated with vitamin D for more than 3 months showed that vitamin D supplementation slightly decreased the SBP by 2 mm Hg but the diastolic blood pressure did not change. (219) Vitamin D3 markedly suppresses renin release from the kidney that alters electrolyte balance, volume, and blood pressure. (2, 207) Vitamin D suppresses inflammation, increases NO, improves endothelial function and arterial elasticity, and decreases vascular smooth muscle hypertrophy. (208–215)

The hypotensive effect of vitamin D was inversely related to the pretreatment serum levels of vitamin D_3 and has additive blood pressure reduction when used concurrently with antihypertensive medications. (216) Blacks have significantly higher rates of hypertension than whites and lower circulating levels of 25-hydroxyvitamin D. (222) In a 3-month study of placebo, 1000, 2000, or 4000 IU of vitamin D per day, the difference in SBP between baseline and 3 months was +1.7 mm Hg for those receiving placebo, –0.66 mm Hg for 1000 U/day, –3.4 mm Hg for 2000 U/day, and –4.0 mm Hg for 4000 U/day. This resulted in a –1.4 mm Hg reduction in blood pressure for each additional 1000 U/day of vitamin D. For each 1-ng/ml increase in plasma 25-hydroxyvitamin D, there was a significant 0.2-mm Hg reduction in SBP. (222) There was no effect of vitamin D supplementation on diastolic blood pressure. Vitamin D levels are lower in patients with non-dipping hypertension. (220) A vitamin D level of 80 ng/ml is recommended for optimal blood pressure reduction and cardiovascular risk reduction. (2–5) The recommended dose of vitamin D3 is 2000–4000 IU/day in a liquid form that is combined with some fatty acids to improve absorption. It is important to measure the blood levels and adjust the dose. The best sources are from Designs for Health and Biotics Research and are called **Emulsified Vitamin D3** (see Sources section).

15.15 VITAMIN B6 (PYRIDOXINE)

Low blood vitamin B6 (pyridoxine) levels are associated with hypertension. (2–5, 224–228) High-dose vitamin B6 significantly lowered blood pressure by 14/10 mm Hg and blood adrenalin levels in a study of 20 hypertensive subjects who were administered vitamin B6 at 5 mg/kg/day for 4 weeks. (225) In another trial over 12 weeks, 800 mg of lipoic acid and 80 mg of pyridoxine, the urinary albumin, oxidative stress, and SBP decreased significantly in the supplement group compared to the placebo group. (228) Serum NO increased in the supplement group compared to the placebo group.

Vitamin B6 has similar action to CAA, diuretics, and CCB. (2–5) The recommended dose of vitamin B6 is 200 mg/day orally. (2–5) A good source of vitamin B6 is **B Supreme,** that is balanced with other B vitamins from Designs for Health (see Sources section).

15.16 FLAVONOIDS: RESVERATROL AND POMEGRANATE

Flavonoids (flavonols, flavones, and isoflavones) are potent antioxidants that prevent atherosclerosis, promote vascular relaxation, and have antihypertensive properties. (229–239) There are over 4000 of these in our foods such as fruits, vegetables, tea, grains, wine, olives, onions, and lettuce. Here are two specific ones that have dramatic effects on blood pressure and cardiovascular health.

Resveratrol improves arterial compliance and elasticity and lowers central arterial pressure when administered as 250 ml of either regular or dealcoholized red wine. (231–235) The central arterial pressure was reduced with dealcoholized red wine by 7.4 and 5.4 mm Hg by regular red wine. Resveratrol increases vasodilation in a dose-related manner, improves endothelial dysfunction, increases NO, and blocks the effects of angiotensin II. (231–235) The recommended dose is 250 mg/day of *trans*-resveratrol. (2–5, 233) The best source of resveratrol is **Resveratol HP** from Biotics Research (see Sources section).

Pomegranate (*Punica granatum* L.) reduces serum ACE activity by 36%, improves endothelial function, lowers blood pressure, and reduces carotid IMT. (2–4, 236–239) An analysis of eight studies showed significant reductions in blood pressure of about 5/4 mm Hg after 6 oz of pomegranate juice consumption. (236) Pomegranate may be obtained as the juice or the seeds (fresh or frozen) from most grocery stores. If you use the seeds, then consume about 1/4 cup per day.

15.17 LYCOPENE

Lycopene produces a significant reduction in blood pressure, blood cholesterol levels, inflammation, and oxidative stress. (2–14, 240–246) Dietary sources of lycopene include grapefruit, watermelon, tomatoes, guava, pink apricots, and papaya. (2–14, 240–246) Patients with grade I hypertension given a tomato lycopene extract (10 mg lycopene/day) for 2 months lowered blood pressure by 9/7 mm Hg. (240, 242) Tomato extract administered to 31 hypertensive subjects over 3 months lowered blood pressure by 10/4 mm Hg. (241) Patients on blood pressure medications had an additional significant blood pressure reduction of 5.4/3 mm Hg over 6 weeks when administered a standardized tomato extract. (242) Analysis of multiple studies demonstrates a 6/5 mm Hg average reduction in blood pressure. (245) The doses ranged from 10 to 25 mg/day of lycopene in these trials. (245) Other studies have not shown changes in blood pressure with lycopene. (243) The response to lycopene may be related to the level of blood lycopene before the patient takes it. The recommended daily intake of lycopene is 10–25 mg in food or in a supplement form but it is not clear which has the best effect on blood pressure or cardiovascular risk. (246) However, present data suggest that supplemental forms of lycopene are superior for blood pressure reduction. (246)

15.18 COENZYME Q-10 (COQ-10) (UBIQUINONE AND UBIQUINOL)

CoQ-10 (ubiquinone and ubiquinol) has consistent and significant blood pressure–lowering effects in hypertensive patients. (2–14, 247–264) CoQ-10 increases NO, improves endothelial function and vascular elasticity. (2–14, 256, 257) CoQ-10 serum levels decrease with age, chronic disease, oxidative stress, high cholesterol, CHD, hypertension, diabetes, statin and BB drug use, exercise, and atherosclerosis. (2–14, 256, 257, 262) Compared to normotensive patients, essential hypertensive patients have a higher incidence of CoQ-10 serum deficiency (39 vs 6% of controls) (2–5, 250, 259, 262) In a 12-week study of patients with isolated systolic hypertension (165/81–82 mm Hg), CoQ-10 administered orally at 60 mg twice daily reduced the SBP by 18 mm Hg and the diastolic blood pressure by 2.6 mm Hg. (249) The blood level of CoQ-10 increased by 2.2 μg/dl. There was a 55% response rate defined as a reduction in SBP of over 4 mm Hg. The responders had an average reduction in SBP of 26 mm Hg. (249) The therapeutic serum level of CoQ-10 should be 3 μg/dl. (2, 214, 247, 250, 258, 259) This dose is usually 3–5 mg/kg/day of CoQ-10. (1–5, 247, 252, 258, 259) Combining a targeted intracellular cardiac CoQ-10 (**MitoQ-10**) and low-dose losartan (an angiotensin receptor blocking drug) provides additive therapeutic benefit, significantly attenuating development of hypertension, increasing NO levels, and reducing LVH. (263)

Patients with the lowest CoQ-10 serum levels may have the best blood pressure reduction response to supplementation with CoQ-10. (2–5, 249) The average reduction in blood pressure in all of the clinical studies is about 15/10 mm Hg with office readings (range of 11–17/8–10 mm Hg) (2–5, 247–264) and 18/10 mm Hg with 24-hour ambulatory blood pressure monitoring. (250, 264) The blood pressure–lowering effect peaks at 4 weeks, then the blood pressure remains stable during long-term treatment. (2–5, 249) However, within 2 weeks after discontinuation of CoQ-10, the blood pressure–lowering effect disappears. (2–5, 249) The reduction in blood pressure and arterial constriction are correlated with the pretreatment and posttreatment levels of CoQ-10 and the percent increase in blood levels. (2–5, 249, 250) About 50% of patients respond to oral supplemental CoQ-10. (2–5, 249) Patients administered CoQ-10 with enalapril (an ACEI drug) have better 24-hour ambulatory blood pressure control compared to enalapril monotherapy and better endothelial function. (255) Approximately, 50% of patients on blood pressure–lowering drugs may be able to stop between one and three of these drugs. The literature is supportive of significant reductions in blood pressure in human clinical trials. (2–5, 247–252, 254–262, 264) The recommended starting dose is 100 mg of CoQ-10 and then measures the blood levels. Continue to increase the dose of CoQ-10 by 100 mg increments until the blood level is 3 μg/dl. Good sources of CoQ-10 include Designs for Health, Biotics, Metagenics, MitoQ, and Ortho Molecular (see Sources section). Adverse effects have not been seen in patients in the literature. (2–5, 247–252, 254–262, 264)

15.19 ALPHA LIPOIC ACID (LIPOIC ACID)

Recent research has evaluated the role of ALA or lipoic acid in the treatment of hypertension, especially as part of the metabolic syndrome. (2–5, 265–271) Lipoic acid reduces oxidative stress, inflammation, closes calcium channels in arteries which lead to vasodilation, improves endothelial function, and lowers blood pressure. (2–5, 265–271) Urinary albumin excretion is stabilized in diabetes mellitus patients given 600 mg of lipoic acid compared to placebo for 18 months. (270) In a study of 36 patients with CHD given 200 mg of lipoic acid with 500 mg of acetyl-L-carnitine twice daily for 8 weeks, there was an increase in arterial dilation and a decrease of 11 mg Hg in SBP with no change in diastolic blood pressure. (269) However, patients with metabolic syndrome had a reduction in blood pressure of 7/3 mm Hg. (269) In a 2-month study of 40 patients with diabetes and stage 1 hypertension, quinapril (an ACEI drug) 40 mg daily versus quinapril 40 mg with lipoic acid 600 mg daily reduced urinary albumin excretion by 30% with quinapril and 53% with quinapril with lipoic acid in combination. The blood pressure was reduced significantly by 10% in both groups and the arterial dilation increased 58% with quinapril and 116% with the combination. (268) The blood glucose improved with quinapril and with quinapril plus lipoic acid. The combined administration of lipoic acid and vitamin B6 improves the loss of albumin in the urine in patients with diabetic nephropathy. (271) The recommended daily dose is 100–200 mg/day of lipoic acid. *R*-lipoic acid is recommended instead of the L-lipoic acid form (isomer) because of its preferred use by the mitochondria. (2–5) A good source is **Stabilized *R*-Lipoic Acid** from Designs for Health (see Sources section).

15.20 PYCNOGENOL

Pycnogenol is a bark extract from the French maritime pine that significantly reduces blood pressure and decreases the need for blood pressure–lowering drugs. (2–14, 272–280, 421) Pycnogenol given to patients at a dose of 200 mg/day lowers blood pressure about 3.2/3.1 mm Hg. (271, 421) The antihypertensive effect is mediated by an ACEI effect (similar to this class of drugs) and it reduces endothelin (a strong constrictor of arteries), lowers inflammation and oxidative stress. Pycnogenol improves endothelial function, increases levels of NO and prostaglandins that help to dilate the artery and lower blood pressure. (2–14, 272–280, 421) The recommended dose is 200 mg/day.

15.21 GARLIC

Numerous and clinical studies of garlic administration have shown consistent reductions in blood pressure in hypertensive patients both on antihypertensive medications and those not antihypertensive medications with an average reduction in BP of 7–16/5–9 mm Hg depending on the dose and type of garlic given. (281–291) Garlic is a vasodilator with ACEI activity, calcium channel blocking activity and it increases NO. (2–14, 286)

In a very well-designed clinical trial of 81 prehypertensive and mild hypertensive patients given 300 mg of garlic homogenate for 12 weeks, the blood pressure reduction averaged 7/5 mm Hg. (284) Aged garlic extract at 480 mg/day had the best blood pressure reduction of 12/5 mm Hg. (285) Garlic improves central blood pressure, central pulse pressure, and arterial stiffness. (289) The best garlic supplement with the most studies is **Kyolic Garlic Dried Extract CV formulation** from Japan. This is available in most health food stores. The recommended dose is 600 mg twice a day.

15.22 SEAWEED

Wakame seaweed (*Undaria pinnatifida*) is the most popular, edible seaweed in Japan. (292) It is a type of marine algae and a sea vegetable. It has subtly sweet, but with a distinctive and excellent flavor and texture. It is most often served in soups and salads. Sea farmers in Japan have grown wakame for centuries. A daily dose of 3.3 g of dried wakame for 4 weeks significantly reduced blood pressure by 14/5 mm Hg. (293, 294) The MAP fell 11.2 mm Hg ($p < 0.001$) in the sodium-sensitive subjects and 5.7 mm Hg ($p < 0.05$) in the sodium-insensitive subjects, correlating with PRA. Seaweed and sea vegetables contain 77I minerals and rare-earth elements, and fiber that is well absorbed. (292–294) Wakame has ACEI activity similar to the drug class. (292, 295, 296) Its long-term use in Japan has demonstrated its safety. You can find wakame seaweed in a Japanese health food store or order from many whole food companies on the Internet such as HYPERLINK "https://www.amazon.com/Emerald-Cove-Silver-Wakame-Seaweed/dp/B001BKNFSC" Emerald Cove Silver Grade Wakame (Dried Seaweed). The recommended daily amount is 3–4 g served in a soup or salad.

15.23 COCOA: DARK CHOCOLATE

Dark chocolate (100 g) and cocoa with a high content of polyphenols (30 mg or more) significantly reduce blood pressure in various clinical prospective trials and other analyses. (2–14, 297–308) A meta-analysis of 173 hypertensive patients given cocoa for 2 weeks lowered blood pressure 5/3 mm Hg. (297) Fifteen patients given 100 g of dark chocolate with 500 mg of polyphenols for 15 days had a 6.4 mm Hg reduction in SBP. (298) Cocoa at a dose of 30 mg of polyphenols lowered blood pressure in prehypertensive and stage 1 hypertensive patients by 3/2 mm Hg at 18 weeks. (299) Two meta-analyses, one with 13 trials and the other with 10 trials with a total of 297 patients, found a significant reduction in blood pressure of 3/2 and 4.5/3 mm Hg, respectively, over 2–18 weeks. (301, 304) The blood pressure reduction is the greatest in those with the highest baseline blood pressure and those with a least 50–70% cocoa in dark chocolate at about 100 g/day. (2–5, 297–301, 304) Cocoa improves insulin resistance, NO production, and endothelial function. (298, 304–307) Hershey dark chocolate is a good choice.

15.24 MELATONIN

Melatonin is a natural hormone made in the brain that helps us to sleep. Melatonin lowers blood pressure in many clinical trials as single therapy or in conjunction with antihypertensive medications. (309–336) Melatonin levels are reduced by shortened sleep cycle of less than 6 hours, shift work, age, brief light exposure after darkness, BB (medication used for blood pressure and various types of heart problems), and benzodiazepines (anxiety medications). (328) Melatonin lowers nighttime blood pressure in diabetic and nondiabetic hypertensive patients and improves the dipping pattern in patients with nocturnal non-dipping status. (310–316, 318, 320)

In one study, chronic administration for 3 weeks of melatonin at 2.5 mg before bedtime in hypertensive men, not taking any antihypertensive medications, lowered nocturnal blood pressure by 6/4 mm Hg, reduced day-night and daytime blood pressure by 25% systolic and 15% diastolic, improved sleep, and reduced cortisol levels. (309) In meta-analysis that included 221 participants treated with controlled-release melatonin 2–5 mg/night for 7–90 days, there was a significant decrease in night blood pressure of 6/3.5 mm Hg. (6, 333) Melatonin lowers angiotensin II levels in the brain and stimulates melatonin receptors that lower blood pressure. (322–324, 328) The recommended dose is 3–6 mg/night. A good source is **Melatonin SR 6 mg/night** from Designs for Health (see Sources section).

15.25 GRAPE SEED EXTRACT

GSE produces a significant reduction in blood pressure in many in clinical trials and meta-analyses. (2–5, 337–341) GSE in variable doses and variable amounts of resveratrol was administered to subjects in 9 randomized trials, meta-analysis of 390 subjects, and demonstrated a significant reduction in SBP. (337) A significant reduction in blood pressure of 11/8 mm Hg occurs with 300 mg/day in 1 month. (338) A meta-analysis in 2016 reviewed 16 clinical trials with 810 subjects. (340) There were significant reductions in blood pressure with GSE of 6/3 mm Hg especially in young patients and those with obesity or metabolic syndrome. (340) A 12-week study in 36 patients who consumed a juice containing placebo or 300 mg/day of GSE showed a reduction in SBP by 5.6% and diastolic blood pressure by 4.7%. (341) The blood pressure returned to baseline after the 4-week discontinuation period of GSE beverage. The higher the initial BP, the greater the response. The recommended dose is 300 mg/day. A good source is **Grape Seed Supreme 2 capsules/day** from Designs for Health (see Sources section).

15.26 DIETARY NITRATES AND NITRITES: BEETROOT JUICE AND EXTRACT

The Mediterranean and DASH diets with the ingestion of fruits and vegetables rich in inorganic nitrate (NO_3^-) are effective methods for elevating vascular NO levels through the formation of a nitrite intermediate (NO_2^-) that reduces blood pressure and improves arterial compliance and endothelial function. (6, 342–353) The pathway for NO generation involves the activity of mouth bacteria and the stomach acid and salivary gland cycle to make the conversion of nitrate ingested in the diet, to nitrite. This nitrite eventually enters the circulation where, through the activity of numerous enzymes in the body, it is chemically changed to NO. (6, 342, 343)

Dietary consumption of raw or cooked beets, beet juice or extract, or dark green leafy vegetables (kale and spinach) is a great source of inorganic nitrates. Beet juice at a dose of 250 ml/day reduces blood pressure within 30–60 minutes in normotensive, prehypertensive, or mild hypertensive subjects. (344–345) Meta-analysis shows that daily beetroot juice consumption of 5.1–45 mmol (321–2790 mg) over a period of 2 hours to 15 days is associated with dose-dependent changes in blood pressure. (346) In a recent study, the acute effects of an orally disintegrating lozenge that generates NO in the oral cavity evaluated the effects on blood pressure endothelial function and vascular compliance in 30 unmedicated hypertensive patients with average baseline BP of 144/91 mm Hg. (347) Nitrate supplementation versus placebo resulted in a significant decrease of 4/5 mm Hg from baseline after 20 minutes. In addition, there was a further significant reduction of 6 mm Hg in both systolic and diastolic pressure after 60 minutes. After a half-hour of a single dose, there was a significant improvement in vascular compliance and, after 4 hours, a statistically significant improvement in endothelial function. (347)

Another study of 68 drug-naive and treated patients with hypertension a daily dietary supplementation was given for 4 weeks with either dietary nitrate (250 ml daily, as beetroot juice) or a placebo (250 ml daily, as nitrate-free beetroot juice). (348) Daily supplementation with dietary nitrate was associated with a reduction in blood pressure measured by three different methods.

The clinic BP was decreased by 7.7/2.4 mm Hg, the 24-hour ambulatory blood pressure was reduced by 7.7/5.2 mm Hg and the home blood pressure was reduced by 8.1/3.8 mm Hg. (348) The supplement continued to work as long as the patient continued to take it and it was well tolerated. Endothelial function improved by ≈20% and arterial stiffness was reduced after dietary nitrate consumption with no change after placebo. (348)

In a whole food study of 24 hypertensive subjects, raw beet juice was administered for 2 weeks followed by cooked beets. (351) After 2 weeks, both groups had a washout for 2 weeks then switched to the alternative treatment. Each participant consumed 250 ml/day of beet juice or 250 g/day of cooked beets. The artery dilated significantly and systolic and diastolic blood pressure decreased with beet juice and cooked beet. (351) Based on these studies, there is a dose-related response to blood pressure, endothelial function, and other vascular parameters with beet juice, beet extract, raw, and cooked beets. (342–353)

The consumption of dietary nitrate at 0.1 mmol/kg of body weight per day (high intake of F and V at 4–6 servings a day) reduces blood pressure about 5/4 mm Hg and this effect is potentiated by vitamin C and polyphenols. (342–353)

Vegetables are the primary source of nitrates (80–85%). (352, 353) About 500 mg of beetroot juice with 45 mmol/l or 2.79 g/l of inorganic nitrate lowers blood pressure 10/8 mm Hg and increases artery dilation by 30%. (352, 353) Beetroot tends to be dosed based on the **nitrate** content, with around 0.1–0.2 mmol/kg (6.4–12.8 mg/kg) being the target for nitrate consumption. This is about 436 mg for a 150-lb person, which is comparable to half a kilogram (500 g) of the beetroots themselves (wet weight). (352, 353) We recommend at healthy diet with all of these foods mentioned and a supplement with **NEO 40** one waver twice per day from Human N (see Sources section).

15.27 TEAS

Green tea, black tea, and their respective extracts of active components have demonstrated reduction in blood pressure in many clinical trials and meta-analyses. (354–365) In a study of 379 hypertensive subjects given green tea extract (GTE) 370 mg/day for 3 months, blood pressure was reduced significantly at 4/4 mm Hg. (358)

A meta-analysis of regular consumption of either green or black tea for 4–24 weeks (2–6 cups/day) reduced blood pressure significantly. Green tea lowered blood pressure by 2/2 mm Hg, while black tea reduced blood pressure by 1.4/1.1 mm Hg. (354) A small 4-week study of 21 women administered 1500 mg of GTE (containing 780 mg of polyphenols) or a matching placebo showed significant reductions in blood pressure. (362) The 24-hour ambulatory blood pressure showed an overall decrease in SBP of 3.6 mm Hg, and a daytime reduction of 3.61 mm Hg, and nighttime reduction of 3.9 mm Hg. (362) There was no reduction in diastolic blood pressure. A meta-analysis of 10 trials with 834 subjects noted a reduction in blood pressure of 2.4/1.8 mm Hg with green and black tea in 3 months. The best results were with non-caffeinated tea. Green tea improves endothelial function and induces vasodilation. (363, 364) The required amount is about 500 mg flavonoid content (2 cups of tea/day without caffeine) or a **green tea extract** one twice per day from Designs for Health. (365) (see Sources section).

15.28 L-CARNITINE AND ACETYL-L-CARNITINE

Carnitine has mild blood pressure–lowering effects by increasing NO levels and inhibiting the RAAS. (2–5, 366–376) This results in improved endothelial function and oxidative defense and oxidative stress. (366–370)

Human studies on the effects of L-carnitine and acetyl-L-carnitine are limited, with minimal to no change in blood pressure. (2–5, 371–376) In patients with metabolic syndrome, acetyl-L-carnitine at 1 g twice a day over 8 weeks improved blood sugar and reduced SBP by 8 mm Hg, but diastolic blood pressure was significantly decreased only in those with higher glucose levels. (377) Low carnitine levels are associated with a non-dipping blood pressure pattern in type II diabetes. (376) Doses of 2–3 g twice per day are recommended if carnitine is used. (2–5)

15.29 FIBER

The clinical trials with various types of fiber to reduce blood pressure have been inconsistent. (2–5, 378–383) Soluble fiber, guar gum, guava, psyllium, flaxseed, and oat bran may reduce blood pressure and decrease the need for antihypertensive medications in hypertensive subjects, diabetic subjects, and hypertensive-diabetic subjects especially when incorporated into the MedDiet. (2–5, 378–383) In a meta-analysis, dietary fiber intake was associated with a significant 2 mm Hg reduction in diastolic blood pressure but there was no change in SBP. (378) However, a significant reduction in blood pressure of 6/4 mm Hg was observed in trials conducted among patients with hypertension and in trials with a duration of greater than 8 weeks. (378) A recent meta-analysis of 14 trials, flaxseed, which is a rich dietary source of ALA, lignans, and fiber, lowered BP by 1.8/1.6 mm Hg. (383) You should get about 50 g of mixed fiber in your diet per day.

15.30 SESAME

Sesame has been shown to reduce blood pressure in a several small studies over 30–60 days. (384–392) Sesame lowers blood pressure given alone (185–189) or in combination with nifedipine (a CCB), (184, 188) diuretics, or BB. (185, 189) In a group of 13 mild hypertensive patients, 60 mg of sesamin for 4 weeks lowered SBP 3.5/2 mm Hg. (186) Black sesame meal at 2.52 g/day over 4 weeks in 15 subjects reduced SBP by 8.3/4.2 mm Hg. (187) Sesame oil at 35 g/day significantly lowered central blood pressure within 1 hour and also maintained blood pressure reduction chronically in 30 hypertensive patients. In addition, sesame oil reduced heart rate, arterial stiffness, and inflammation. (392) Also, sesame oil improved NO and antioxidant levels. (392) Finally, sesame lowers serum glucose, HgbA1C, cholesterol, and reduces oxidative stress markers and oxidative defenses. (184, 185, 187–189) The active ingredients are natural ACEIs such as sesamin, sesamolin, and sesaminol compounds that also reduce inflammation. (190, 191)

15.31 *N*-ACETYLCYSTEINE (NAC)

The combination of *N*-acetylcysteine (NAC) and L-arginine (ARG) improves endothelial function and lowers blood pressure in hypertensive patients with and without type II diabetes. (394–397) In 24 subjects with type II diabetes and hypertension treated for 6 months with placebo or NAC with ARG, blood pressure was reduced significantly and NO levels increased. (394) NAC mimics the effects of the CCB and the ARBs. (394–397) The recommended dose of NAC is 500–1000 mg twice a day from Designs for Health (see Sources section).

15.32 HAWTHORN

Hawthorn extract has been used for centuries for the treatment of hypertension, CHF, and other CVDs but the studies are limited and are not convincing of any significant clinical reduction in blood pressure at any dose. (398–402) More studies are needed to determine the efficacy, long-term effects, and dose of hawthorn for the treatment of hypertension. It is not recommended at this time.

15.33 QUERCETIN

Quercetin is an antioxidant flavonoid found in apples, berries, and onions, which reduces blood pressure in hypertensive individuals. (403–405) Quercetin is metabolized by the liver enzyme system called cytochrome 3A4 and should be used with caution in patients on drugs metabolized by this cytochrome system. (403–405) Quercetin was administered to 12 hypertensive men at an oral dose of 1095 mg with reduction in blood pressure of 7/3 mm Hg. (403) Forty-one prehypertensive and stage 1 hypertensive subjects were enrolled in a study with 500 mg of quercetin per day versus placebo. (404) In the stage 1 hypertensive patients, the blood pressure was reduced by 7/5 mm Hg. (404) Quercetin administered to 93 overweight or obese subjects at 150 mg/day over 6 weeks lowered SBP about 3–4 mm Hg. (405) The recommended dose of quercetin is 500 mg twice daily. A good source is **quercetin with nettles** from Designs for Health (see Sources section).

15.34 PROBIOTICS

Gut dysbiosis or dysfunction in hypertension is characterized by a gut microbiome (bacteria) that are less diverse with an increased ratio of bacteria called Firmicutes to Bacteroidetes, a decrease in acetate- and butyrate-producing bacteria and an increase in lactate-producing bacterial populations. There are several meta-analyses that support the role of probiotic supplementation to reduce blood pressure. (111, 406, 408, 409)

One meta-analysis of many studies suggested that consuming probiotics results in a modest lowering of blood pressure with a potentially greater effect with an elevated baseline blood pressure, when multiple species of probiotics are consumed, the duration of the treatment is at least 8 weeks and the daily dose is $\geq 10^{11}$ colony-forming units (CFU). (406) Another meta-analysis of 14 studies, involving 702 participants, showed that, compared with placebo, probiotic fermented milk produced a slight but significant reduction of 3.1/1.1 mm Hg in blood pressure. In a meta-analysis of 11 trials with 641 patients, probiotic consumption significantly decreased blood pressure 3.2/2 mm Hg. (408)

15.35 PUTTING YOUR NUTRITIONAL SUPPLEMENT PROGRAM ALL TOGETHER

I know that you must be a bit overwhelmed with all of the possible nutritional supplements that lower blood pressure which have been discussed in this chapter. I am going to give you my suggestions based on the science and published medical articles but also what has worked the best for the patients in my medical practice in the Hypertension Institute to lower their blood pressure. First of all, remember that the nutritional supplements that I am going to list in the following must be part of the entire Hypertension Institute Program to be the most effective. This includes the nutrition program and the lifestyle programs discussed in those chapters. Second, all of the supplements that are recommended must be from high quality and reputable companies. Do not use any supplement or company that is not recommended or listed in Sources section. Third, go in a stepwise fashion from **Step 1 to Step 3** based on your blood pressure readings. Once you have consistent blood pressure readings at 120/80 mm Hg, then you do not need to keep adding more supplements or more steps. These are my recommendations:

Step 1

1. **CardioSirt BP (from Biotics Research) (see Sources section):** One scoop of the powder in water in the morning on an empty stomach. This supplement has been studied and results published. It will lower the blood pressure about 16/11.5 mm Hg within 4 weeks.

2. **VasculoSirt (from Biotics Research) (see Sources section)**: Take two capsules twice per day with food to start. You can increase up to five capsules twice per day depending on the blood pressure response. VasculoSirt supplies 27 of the nutrients that have been reviewed in this chapter. This will provide a broad spectrum of compounds that lower blood pressure and improve the blood vessel health. VasculoSirt also limits the number of pills that you would need to take if you got all of them separately.

Step 2

1. **Bonito Protein: Vasotension from Metagenics) (see Sources section)**
2. **CoQnol (ubiquinol) (from Designs for Health (see Sources section):** One capsule once or twice per day. This will provide additional coenzyme Q-10 that may be needed in some patients who have higher blood pressures.
3. **Kyolic Garlic extract from Japan:** You can order this online or get in a health food store. Take one capsule twice per day of the cardiovascular formulation.

Step 3

1. **Neo 40 from Human N (see Sources section):** One wafer chewed twice per day then drink 4 oz of water.
2. **Pomegranate seeds** at a dose of 1/4 cup once or twice per day. Get this at a grocery store or health food store as fresh or frozen seeds and make a smoothie.

Other supplements that can be added as needed are discussed in this chapter.

15.36 CLINICAL CONSIDERATIONS

A comprehensive clinical approach to the categories and clinical use of nutraceutical supplements is detailed in Table 15.3.

Several of the strategic combinations of nutraceutical supplements with antihypertensive drugs have been shown to lower blood pressure more than the medication alone. (2–5) These are as follows:

- Pycnogenol with ACEI.
- Lycopene with various antihypertensive medications.
- *R*-lipoic acid with ACEI.
- Vitamin C with CCB.
- *N*-acetylcysteine with arginine.
- Garlic with ACEI, diuretics, and BB.
- CoQ-10 with ACEI and CCB.

Many antihypertensive drugs may cause nutrient depletions that can actually interfere with their antihypertensive action or cause other metabolic adverse effects

TABLE 15.3
An Integrative Approach to the Treatment of Hypertension

Intervention Category	Therapeutic Intervention	Daily Intake
Diet characteristics	DASH I, DASH II-Na^+, or PREMIER diet	Diet type
	Sodium restriction	1500 mg
	Potassium	5000–10,000 mg
	Potassium/sodium ratio	>4:1
	Magnesium	1000 mg
	Zinc	50 mg
Macronutrients	*Protein* Total intake from non-animal sources, organic lean or wild animal protein, or cold-water fish	30% of total calories, which 1.5–1.8 g/kg body weight
	Whey protein	30 g
	Soy protein (fermented sources are preferred)	30 g
	Sardine muscle concentrate extract	3 g
	Milk peptides (VPP and IPP)	30–60 mg
	Fat	30% of total calories
	Omega-3 fatty acids	2–3 g
	Omega-6 fatty acids	1 g
	Omega-9 fatty acids(MUFA)	4 tablespoons (40 g) of EVOO or nuts
	Saturated fatty acids from wild game, bison, or other lean meat	<10% total calories
	Polyunsaturated to saturated fat ratio	>2.0
	Omega-3 to omega-6 ratio	1.1–1.2
	Synthetic *trans*-fatty acids	None (completely remove from diet)
	Nuts in variety	*2–3 servings*
	Carbohydrates as primarily complex carbohydrates and fiber	40% of total calories
	Oatmeal or	60 g
	Oat bran or	40 g
	Beta-glucan or	3 g
	Psyllium	7 g
Specific foods	Garlic as fresh cloves or aged Kyolic garlic	4 fresh cloves (4 g) or 600 mg aged garlic taken twice daily
	Sea vegetables, specifically dried wakame	3.0–3.5 g
	Lycopene as tomato products, guava, watermelon, apricots, pink grapefruit, papaya, or supplements	10–20 mg

(*Continued*)

TABLE 15.3 (*Continued*)
An Integrative Approach to the Treatment of Hypertension

Intervention Category	Therapeutic Intervention	Daily Intake
	Dark chocolate	100 g
	Pomegranate juice or seeds	8 oz or one cup
	Sesame	60 mg sesamin or 2.5 g sesame meal
	Beet juice	500 g
		60 oz of 500 mg bid
	Green tea or EGCG extract	2–6 g/day
	Carnitine	
Exercise	Aerobic	20 minutes daily at 4200 kJ/week
	Resistance	40 minutes/day
Weight reduction	Body mass index <25 Waist circumference: <35 in. for women <40 in. for men Total body fat: <22% for women <16% for men	Lose 1–2 lb/week and increasing the proportion of lean muscle
Other lifestyle recommendations	Alcohol restriction: For men Among the choice of alcohol red wine is preferred due to its vasoactive phytonutrients. Women is 50% of amount listed	<20 g/day Wine 6 oz Beer 12–24 oz Liquor 1–2 oz
	Caffeine restriction or elimination depending on CYP 1A2 450 SNP	<100 mg/day
	Tobacco and smoking	Stop
Medical considerations	Medications which may increase blood pressure.	Minimize use when possible, such as by using disease-specific nutritional interventions
Supplemental foods and nutrients	Alpha-lipoic acid with biotin	100–200 mg twice daily
	Amino acids:	
	Arginine	2 g twice daily
	Carnitine	1–2 g twice daily
	Taurine	1–3 g twice daily
	Chlorogenic acids	150–200 mg
	Coenzyme Q-10	100 mg once to twice daily
	Grape seed extract	300 mg
	Hawthorn extract	500 mg twice a day

(*Continued*)

TABLE 15.3 (*Continued*)
An Integrative Approach to the Treatment of Hypertension

Intervention Category	Therapeutic Intervention	Daily Intake
	Melatonin (long acting)	3 mg
	N-Acetylcysteine (NAC)	500 mg twice a day
	Olive leaf extract (oleuropein)	500 mg twice a day
	Pycnogenol	200 mg
	Quercetin	500 mg twice a day
	Probiotics	10^{11} CFU
	Resveratrol (*trans*)	250 mg
	Vitamin B6	100 mg once to twice daily
	Vitamin C	250–500 mg twice daily
	Vitamin D3	Dose to raise 25-hydroxyvitamin D serum level to 80 ng/ml
	Vitamin E as mixed tocopherols	400 IU

to manifest through the laboratory results or with clinical symptoms. (411, 412) Diuretics decrease potassium, magnesium, phosphorous, sodium, chloride, folate, vitamin B6, zinc, iodine, and CoQ-10. The diuretics increase homocysteine, calcium and blood creatinine levels (kidney function) and elevate serum glucose by inducing insulin resistance. BB reduces CoQ-10. ACEI and ARBs reduce zinc. (411, 412)

Clinical monitoring of blood pressure is required, as well as patient awareness that nutritional supplement interventions need to be taken as consistently as medications. Additional laboratory tests can inform clinical decision-making such as the measurement of intracellular micronutrients, antioxidant capacity, oxidative stress, inflammation biomarkers such as hsCRP, PRA, and serum aldosterone. Blood pressure is improved following the repletion of all micronutrient depletions and with the use of selected higher doses of nutritional supplements based on the clinical studies that have been reviewed. (413)

15.37 SUMMARY AND KEY TAKEAWAY POINTS

- Vascular biology such as endothelial, vascular, and cardiac muscle dysfunction plays a primary and pivotal role in the beginning and continuation of hypertension.
- Nutrient-gene interactions and epigenetics are predominant factors in promoting beneficial or detrimental effects in cardiovascular health and hypertension.
- Oxidative stress, inflammation, and vascular immune dysfunction initiate and promote hypertension and CVD.

- Nutrition, natural whole food, nutraceutical supplements, antioxidants, vitamins, and minerals can prevent, control, and treat hypertension through numerous vascular biology mechanisms and may mimic the effects of the various antihypertensive drug classes.
- There is a role for the selected use of single and combined nutraceutical supplements, vitamins, antioxidants, and minerals in the treatment of hypertension based on prospective randomized placebo-controlled studies and meta-analysis as a complement to optimal nutrition and other lifestyle modifications.
- Only high-quality nutritional supplements from reputable nutritional supplement companies should be used. See the Sources section at the end of this book.
- A clinical approach that incorporates optimal nutrition with scientifically proven nutraceutical supplements, exercise, weight reduction, smoking cessation, alcohol and caffeine restriction, and other lifestyle strategies can be systematically and successfully incorporated into clinical practice for the prevention and treatment of hypertension. Many of the nutritional supplements have a mechanism of activity similar to the various drug classes (Table 15.3). This may allow for a more selective use of the supplement when tapering or stopping a blood pressure medication to mimic that same effect.

REFERENCES

1. Wesa KM, Grimm RH Jr. Recommendations and guidelines regarding the preferred research protocol for investigating the impact of an optimal healing environment on patients with hypertension. J Altern Complement Med. 2004;10(Suppl 1):S245–S250.
2. Houston M. The role of nutrition and nutraceutical supplements in the treatment of hypertension. World J Cardiol. 2014;6(2):38–66.
3. Houston M. Nutrition and nutraceutical supplements for the treatment of hypertension: Part 1. J Clin Hypertens. 2013;15:752–757.
4. Houston M. Nutrition and nutraceutical supplements for the treatment of hypertension: Part II. J Clin Hypertens. 2013;15:845–851.
5. Houston M. Nutrition and nutraceutical supplements for the treatment of hypertension: Part III. J Clin Hypertens. 2013;15:931–937.
6. Borghi C, Cicero AF. Nutraceuticals with a clinically detectable blood pressure-lowering effect: a review of available randomized clinical trials and their meta-analyses. Br J Clin Pharmacol. 2017;83(1):163–171.
7. Sirtori CR, Arnoldi A, Cicero AF. Nutraceuticals for blood pressure control. Rev Ann Med. 2015;47(6):447–456.
8. Cicero AF, Colletti A. Nutraceuticals and blood pressure control: results from clinical trials and meta-analyses. High Blood Press Cardiovasc Prev. 2015;22(3):203–213.
9. Turner JM, Spatz ES. Nutritional supplements for the treatment of hypertension: a practical guide for clinicians. Curr Cardiol Rep. 2016;18(12):126.
10. Caligiuri SP, Pierce GN. A review of the relative efficacy of dietary, nutritional supplements, lifestyle and drug therapies in the management of hypertension. Crit Rev Food Sci Nutr. 2017;57(16):3508–3527.
11. Houston MC, Fox B, Taylor N. What Your Doctor May Not Tell You About Hypertension: The Revolutionary Nutrition and Lifestyle Program to Help Fight High Blood Pressure. AOL Time Warner, Warner Books, New York, NY, 2003.

12. Houston Mark C. Handbook of Hypertension. Wiley-Blackwell, Oxford, UK, 2009.
13. Houston Mark C. What Your Doctor May Not Tell You About Heart Disease. Grand Central Press, New York, NY, 2012.
14. Sinatra S, Houston M, Editors. Nutrition and Integrative Strategies in Cardiovascular Medicine. CRC Press, 2015.
15. Houston MC. The role of cellular micronutrient analysis and minerals in the prevention and treatment of hypertension and cardiovascular disease. Ther Adv Cardiovasc Dis. 2010;4:165–183.
16. Thomopoulos C, Parati G, Zanchetti A. Effects of blood pressure lowering on outcome incidence in hypertension: 7. Effects of more vs. less intensive blood pressure lowering and different achieved blood pressure levels-updated overview and meta-analyses of randomized trials. J Hypertens. 2016;34(4):613–622.
17. Ettehad D, Emdin CA, Kiran A, Anderson SG, Callender T, Emberson J, Chalmers J, Rodgers A, Rahimi K. Blood pressure lowering for prevention of cardiovascular disease and death: a systematic review and meta-analysis. Lancet. 2016;387(10022):957–967.
18. ESH/ESC Task Force for the Management of Arterial Hypertension. 2013 Practice guidelines for the management of arterial hypertension of the European Society of Hypertension (ESH) and the European Society of Cardiology (ESC): ESH/ESC Task Force for the Management of Arterial Hypertension. J Hypertens. 2013;31:1925–1938.
19. Flack JM, Calhoun D, Schiffrin EL. The new ACC/AHA hypertension guidelines for the prevention, detection, evaluation, and management of high blood pressure in adults. Am J Hypertens. 2018;31(2):133–135.
20. Appel LJ, American Society of Hypertension Writing Group. ASH position paper: dietary approaches to lower blood pressure. J Am Soc Hypertens. 2009;3:321–331.
21. Eaton SB, Eaton SB III, Konner MJ. Paleolithic nutrition revisited: a twelve-year retrospective on its nature and implications. Eur J Clin Nutr. 1997;51:207–216.
22. Layne J, Majkova Z, Smart EJ, Toborek M, Hennig B. Caveolae: a regulatory platform for nutritional modulation of inflammatory diseases. J Nutr Biochem. 2011;22:807–811.
23. Dandona P, Ghanim H, Chaudhuri A, Dhindsa S, Kim SS. Macronutrient intake induces oxidative and inflammatory stress: potential relevance to atherosclerosis and insulin resistance. Exp Mol Med. 2010;42(4):245–253.
24. Kizhakekuttu TJ, Widlansky ME. Natural antioxidants and hypertension: promise and challenges. Cardiovasc Ther.2010;28(4):e20–e32.
25. Houston MC. New insights and approaches to reduce end organ damage in the treatment of hypertension: subsets of hypertension approach. Am Heart J. 1992;123:1337–1367.
26. Nayak DU, Karmen C, Frishman WH, Vakili BA. Antioxidant vitamins and enzymatic and synthetic oxygen-derived free radical scavengers in the prevention and treatment of cardiovascular disease. Heart Dis. 2001;3:28–45.
27. Ritchie RH, Drummond GR, Sobey CG, De Silva TM, Kemp-Harper BK. The opposing roles of NO and oxidative stress in cardiovascular disease. Pharmacol Res. 2017;116:57–69.
28. Russo C, Olivieri O, Girelli D, Faccini G, Zenari ML, Lombardi S, Corrocher R. Antioxidant status and lipid peroxidation in patients with essential hypertension. J Hypertens. 1998;16:1267–1271.
29. Tse WY, Maxwell SR, Thomason H, Blann A, Thorpe GH, Waite M, Holder R. Antioxidant status in controlled and uncontrolled hypertension and its relationship to endothelial damage. J Hum Hypertens. 1994;8:843–849.
30. Galley HF, Thornton J, Howdle PD, Walker BE, Webster NR. Combination oral antioxidant supplementation reduces blood pressure. Clin Sci. 1997;92:361–365.
31. Dhalla NS, Temsah RM, Netticadam T. The role of oxidative stress in cardiovascular diseases. J Hypertens. 2000;18:655–673.

32. Loperena R, Harrison DG. Oxidative stress and hypertensive diseases. Med Clin North Am. 2017;101(1):169–193.
33. Pietri P, Vlachopoulos C. Tousoulis D inflammation and arterial hypertension: from pathophysiological links to risk prediction. Curr Med Chem. 2015;22(23):2754–2761.
34. Amer MS, Elawam AE, Khater MS, Omar OH, Mabrouk RA, Taha HM. Association of high-sensitivity C reactive protein with carotid artery intimamedia thickness in hypertensive older adults. J Am Soc Hypertens. 2011;5(5):395–400.
35. Kvakan H, Luft FC, Muller DN. Role of the immune system in hypertensive target organ damage. Trends Cardiovasc Med. 2009;19(7):242–246.
36. Rodriquez-Iturbe B, Franco M, Tapia E, Quiroz Y, Johnson RJ. Renal inflammation, autoimmunity and salt-sensitive hypertension. Clin Exp Pharmacol Physiol. 2012;39(1):96–103.
37. Mansego ML, Solar Gde M, Alonso MP, Martinez F, Saez GT, Escudero JC, Redon J, Chaves FJ. Polymorphisms of antioxidant enzymes, blood pressure and risk of hypertension. J Hypertens. 2011;29(3):492–500.
38. Vongpatanasin W, Thomas GD, Schwartz R, Cassis LA, Osborne-Lawrence S, Hahner L, Gibson LL, Black S, Samois D, Shaul PW. C-reactive protein causes downregulation of vascular angiotensin subtype 2 receptors and systolic hypertension in mice. Circulation. 2007;115(8):1020–1028.
39. Razzouk, Munter P, Bansilal S, Kini AS, Aneja A, Mozes J, Ivan O, Jakkula M, Sharma S, Farkouh ME. C reactive protein predicts long-term mortality independently of low-density lipoprotein cholesterol in patients undergoing percutaneous coronary intervention. Am Heart J. 2009;158(2):277–283.
40. Tian N, Penman AD, Mawson AR, Manning RD Jr, Flessner MF. Association between circulating specific leukocyte types and blood pressure. The atherosclerosis risk in communities (ARIC) study. J Am Soc Hypertens. 2010;4(6):272–283.
41. Muller DN, Kvakan H, Luft FC. Immune-related effects in hypertension and target-organ damage. Curr Opin Nephrol Hypertens. 2011;20(2):113–117.
42. Leibowitz A, Schiffin EL. Immune mechanisms in hypertension. Curr Hypertens Rep. 2011;13(6):465–472.
43. Xiong S, Li Q, Liu D, Zhu Z. Gastrointestinal tract: a promising target for the management of hypertension. Curr Hypertens Rep. 2017;19:(4):31.
44. Caillon A, Mian MO, Fraulob-Aquino JC, Huo KG, Barhoumi T, Ouerd S, Sinnaeve PR, Paradis P, Schiffrin EL. Gamma delta T cells mediate angiotensin II-induced hypertension and vascular injury. Circulation. 2017;135(22):2155–2162. doi: 10.1161/CIRCULATIONAHA.116.027058.
45. Rudemiller NP, Crowley SD. The role of chemokines in hypertension and consequent target organ damage. Pharmacol Res. 2017;119:404–411.
46. De Ciuceis C, Agabiti-Rosei C, Rossini C, Airò P, Scarsi M, Tincani A, Tiberio GA, Piantoni S, Porteri E, Solaini L, Duse S, Semeraro F, Petroboni B, Mori L, Castellano M, Gavazzi A, Agabiti-Rosei E, Rizzoni D. Relationship between different subpopulations of circulating CD4+ T lymphocytes and microvascular or systemic oxidative stress in humans. Blood Press. 2017;6(4):237–245.
47. Caillon A, Schiffrin EL. Role of inflammation and immunity in hypertension: recent epidemiological, laboratory, and clinical evidence. Curr Hypertens Rep. 2016 Mar;18(3):21.
48. Abais-Battad JM, Dasinger JH, Fehrenbach DJ, Mattson DL. Novel adaptive and innate immunity targets in hypertension. Pharmacol Res. 2017;120:109–115. doi: 10.1016/j.phrs.2017.03.015.
49. Biancardi VC, Bomfim GF, Reis WL, Al-Gassimi S, Nunes KP. The interplay between angiotensin II, TLR4 and hypertension. Pharmacol Res. 2017;120:88–96. doi: 10.1016/j.phrs.2017.03.017.

50. Justin Rucker A, Crowley SD. The role of macrophages in hypertension and its complications. Pflugers Arch. 2017;469(3–4):419–430.
51. Miller ER 3rd, Erlinger TP, Appel LJ. The effects of macronutrients on blood pressure and lipids: an overview of the DASH and OmniHeart trials. Curr Atheroscler Rep. 2006;8:460–465.
52. Pérez-López FR, Chedraui P, Quadro JL. Effects of the Mediterranean diet on longevity and age-related morbid conditions. Maturitas. 2009;64:67–79.
53. Cutler JA, Follmann, Allender PS. Randomized trials of sodium reduction: an overview. Am J Clin Nutr. 1997;65:643S–651S.
54. Sacks FM, Svetkey LP, Vollmer WM, Appel LJ, Bray GA, Harsha D, Obarzanek E, Conlin PR, Miller ER 3rd, Simons-Morton DG, Karanja N, Lin PH, DASH-Sodium Collaborative Research Group. Effects on blood pressure of reduced dietary sodium and the Dietary Approaches to Stop Hypertension (DASH) diet. DASH-Sodium Collaborative Research Group. N Engl J Med. 2001;4;344(1):3–10.
55. Messerli FH, Schmieder RE, Weir MR. Salt: a perpetrator of hypertensive target organ disease? Arch Intern Med. 1997;157:2449–2452.
56. Merino J, Guasch-Ferré M, Martínez-González MA, Corella D, Estruch R, Fitó M, Ros E, Arós F, Bulló M, Gómez-Gracia E, Moñino M, Lapetra J, Serra-Majem L, Razquin C, Buil-Cosiales P, Sorlí JV, Muñoz MA, Pintó X, Masana L, Salas-Salvadó J. Is complying with the recommendations of sodium intake beneficial for health in individuals at high cardiovascular risk? Findings from the PREDIMED study. Am J Clin Nutr. 2015;101(3):440–448.
57. Weinberger MH. Salt sensitivity of blood pressure in humans. Hypertension. 1996;27:481–490.
58. Morimoto A, Usu T, Fujii T, et al. Sodium sensitivity and cardiovascular events in patients with essential hypertension. Lancet. 1997;350:1734–1737.
59. Kanbay M, Chen Y, Solak Y, Sanders PW. Mechanisms and consequences of salt sensitivity and dietary salt intake. Curr Opin Nephrol Hypertens. 2011;20(1):37–43.
60. Toda N, Arakawa K. Salt-induced hemodynamic regulation mediated by nitric oxide. J Hypertens. 2011;29(3):415–424.
61. Rust P, Ekmekcioglu C. Impact of salt intake on the pathogenesis and treatment of hypertension. Adv Exp Med Biol. 2017;956:61–84.
62. Oberleithner H, Callies C, Kusche-Vihrog K, Schillers H, Shahin V, Riethmuller C, Macgregor GA, deWardener HE. Potassium softens vascular endothelium and increases nitric oxide release. Proc Natl Acad Sci USA. 2009;106(8):2829–2834.
63. Feis J, Oberleithner H, Kusche-Vihrog K. Menage a trios: aldosterone, sodium and nitric oxide in vascular endothelium. Biochim Biophys Acta. 2010;1802(12):1193–1202.
64. Toda N, Arakawa K. Salt-induced hemodynamic regulation mediated by nitric oxide. J Hypertens. 2011;29(3):415–424.
65. Foulquier S, Dupuis F, Perrin-Sarrado C, Maquin Gate K, Merhi-Soussi F, Liminana P, Kwan YW, Capdeville-Atkinson C, Lartaud I, Atkinson J. High salt intake abolishes AT (2)-mediated vasodilation of pial arterioes in rats. J Hypertens. 2011;29(7):1392–1399.
66. Yang Q, Liu T, Kuklina EV, Glanders WD, Hong Y, Gillespie C, Chang MH, Gwinn M, Dowling N, Khoury MJ, Hu FB. Sodium and Potassium intake and mortality among US adults: prospective data from the third national health and nutrition examination survey. Arch Int Med. 2011;171(13):1183–1191.
67. Houston MC, Harper KJ. Potassium, magnesium, and calcium: their role in both the cause and treatment of hypertension. J Clin Hypertens. 2008;10(7 supp 2):3–11.
68. Perez V, Chang ET. Sodium-to-potassium ratio and blood pressure, hypertension, and related factors. Adv Nutr. 2014;5:712–741.

69. Filippini T, Violi F, D'Amico R, Vinceti M. The effect of potassium supplementation on blood pressure in hypertensive subjects: a systematic review and metaanalysis. Int J Cardiol. 2017;230:127–135.
70. Gu D, He J, Xigui W, Duan X, Whelton PK. Effect of potassium supplementation on blood pressure in Chinese: a randomized, placebo-controlled trial. J Hypertens. 2001;19:1325–1331.
71. D'Elia L, Barba G, Cappuccio FP, Strazzullo P. Potassium intake, stroke, and cardiovascular disease a meta-analysis of prospective studies. J Am Coll Cardiol. 2011;57:1210–1219.
72. Poorolajal J, Zeraati F, Soltanian AR, Sheikh V, Hooshmand E. Maleki oral potassium supplementation for management of essential hypertension: a meta-analysis of randomized controlled trials. PLOS ONE. 2017;12(4):e0174967. doi: 10.1371/journal.pone.0174967.
73. Houston MC. The importance of potassium in managing hypertension. Curr Hypertens Rep. 2011;13(4):309–317.
74. Widman L, Wester PO, Stegmayr BG, Wirell MP. The dose dependent reduction in blood pressure through administration of magnesium: a double-blind placebo controlled cross-over trial. Am J Hypertens. 1993;6:41–45.
75. Laurant P, Touyz RM. Physiological and pathophysiological role of magnesium in the cardiovascular system: implications in hypertension. J Hypertens. 2000;18:1177–1191.
76. Zhang X, Li Y, Del Gobbo LC, Rosanoff A, Wang J, Zhang W, Song Y. Effects of magnesium supplementation on blood pressure: a meta-analysis of randomized double-blind placebo-controlled trials. Hypertension. 2016 Aug;68(2):324–333.
77. Kass L, Weekes J, Carpenter L. Effect of magnesium supplementation on blood pressure: a meta-analysis. Eur J Clin Nutr. 2012;66:411–418.
78. Houston MC. The role of magnesium in hypertension and cardiovascular disease. J Clin Hyperten. 2011;13:843–847.
79. Cormick G, Ciapponi A, Cafferata ML, Belizán JM. Calcium supplementation for prevention of primary hypertension. Cochrane Database Syst Rev. 2015 Jun;30(6):CD010037. doi: 10.1002/14651858.CD010037.
80. Resnick LM. Calcium metabolism in hypertension and allied metabolic disorders. Diabetes Care. 1991;14:505–520.
81. Garcia Zozaya JL, Padilla Viloria M. Alterations of calcium, magnesium, and zinc in essential hypertension: their relation to the renin-angiotensin-aldosterone system. Invest Clin. 1997;38:27–40.
82. Hofmeyr GJ, Lawrie TA, Atallah AN, Duley L. Calcium supplementation during pregnancy for preventing hypertensive disorders and related problems. Cochrane Database Syst Rev. 2010;8: CD001059.
83. Shahbaz AU, Sun Y, Bhattacharya SK, Ahokas RA, Gerling IC, McGee JE, Weber KT. Fibrosis in hypertensive heart disease: molecular pathways and cardioprotective strategies. J Hypetens. 2010;28: S25–S32.
84. Bergomi M, Rovesti S, Vinceti M, Vivoli R, Caselgrandi E, Vivoli G. Zinc and copper status and blood pressure. J Trace Elem Med Biol. 1997;11:166–169.
85. Stamler J, Elliott P, Kesteloot H, Nichols R, Claeys G, Dyer AR, Stamler R. Inverse relation of dietary protein markers with blood pressure. Findings for 10,020 men and women in the Intersalt Study. Intersalt Cooperative Research Group. International study of salt and blood pressure. Circulation. 1996;94:1629–1634.
86. Altorf-van der Kuil W, Engberink MF, Brink EJ, van Baak MA, Bakker SJ, Navis G, van t'Veer P, Geleijnse JM. Dietary protein and blood pressure: a systematic review. PLOS ONE. 2010;5(8);e12102–e12117.
87. Jenkins, DJ, Kendall CW, Faulkner DA, Kemp T, Marchie A, Nquyen TH, Wong JM, de Souza R. Emam A, Vidgen E, Trautwein EA, Lapsley KG, Josse RG, Leiter LA,

Singer W. Long-term effects of a plant-based dietary portfolio of cholesterol-lowering foods on blood pressure. Eur J Clin Nutr. 2008;62(6):781–788.
88. Rebholz CM, Friedman EE, Powers LJ, Arroyave WD, He J, Kelly TN. Dietary protein intake and blood pressure: a meta-analysis of randomized controlled trials. Am J Epidemiol. 2012;176(S7):S27–S43.
89. He J, Wofford MR, Reynolds K, Chen J, Chen CS, Myers L, Minor DL, Elmer PJ, Jones DW, Whelton PK. Effect of dietary protein supplementation on blood pressure: a randomized controlled trial. Circulation. 2011;124(5);589–595.
90. FitzGerald RJ, Murray BA, Walsh DJ. Hypotensive peptides from milk proteins. J Nutr. 2004;134(4):980S–988S.
91. Pins JJ, Keenan JM. Effects of whey peptides on cardiovascular disease risk factors. J Clin Hypertens. 2006;8(11):775–782.
92. Aihara K, Kajimoto O, Takahashi R, Nakamura Y. Effect of powdered fermented milk with *Lactobacillus helveticus* on subjects with high-normal blood pressure or mild hypertension. J Am Coll Nutr. 2005;24(4):257–265.
93. Gemino FW, Neutel J, Nonaka M, Hendler SS. The impact of lactotripeptides on blood pressure response in stage 1 and stage 2 hypertensives. J Clin Hypertens. 2010;12(3):153–159.
94. Geleijnse JM, Engberink MF. Lactopeptides and human blood pressure. Curr Opin Lipidol. 2010;21(1):58–63.
95. Pins J, Keenan J. The antihypertensive effects of a hydrolyzed whey protein supplement. Cardiovasc Drugs Ther. 2002;16(Suppl):68.
96. Zhu CF, Li GZ, Peng HB, Zhang F, Chen Y, Li Y. Therapeutic effects of marine collagen peptides on Chinese patients with type 2 diabetes mellitus and primary hypertension. Am J Med Sci. 2010;340(5):360–366.
97. De Leo F, Panarese S, Gallerani R, Ceci LR. Angiotensin converting enzyme (ACE) inhibitoroy peptides: production and implementation of functional food. Curr Pharm Des. 2009;15(31):3622–3643.
98. Lordan S, Ross P, Stanton C. Marine bioactives as functional food ingredients: potential to reduce the incidence of chronic disease. Mar Drugs. 2011;9(6):1056–1100.
99. Kawasaki T, Seki E, Osajima K, Yoshida M, Asada K, Matsui T, Osajima Y. Antihypertensive effect of valyl-tyrosine, a short chain peptide derived from sardine muscle hydrolyzate, on mild hypertensive subjects. J Hum Hypertens. 2000;14:519–523.
100. Kawasaki T, Jun CJ, Fukushima Y, Seki E. Antihypertensive effect and safety evaluation of vegetable drink with peptides derived from sardine protein hydrolysates on mild hypertensive, high-normal and normal blood pressure subjects. Fukuoka Igaku Zasshi. 2002;93(10):208–218.
101. Yang G, Shu XO, Jin F, Zhang X, Li HL, Li Q, Gao YT, Zheng W. Longitudinal study of soy food intake and blood pressure among middle-aged and elderly Chinese women. Am J Clin Nutr. 2005;81(5):1012–1017.
102. Teede HJ, Giannopoulos D, Dalais FS, Hodgson J, McGrath BP. Randomised, controlled, cross-over trial of soy protein with isoflavones on blood pressure and arterial function in hypertensive patients. J Am Coll Nutr. 2006;25(6):533–540.
103. Welty FK, Lee KS, Lew NS, Zhou JR. Effect of soy nuts on blood pressure and lipid levels in hypertensive, prehypertensive and normotensive postmenopausal women. Arch Inter Med. 2007;167(10):1060–1067.
104. Mohanty DP, Mohapatra S, Misra S, Sahu PS. Milk derived bioactive peptides and their impact on human health. A review. J Biol Sci. 2016;23(5):577–583.
105. Nasca MM, Zhou JR, Welty FK. Effect of soy nuts on adhesion molecules and markers of inflammation in hypertensive and normotensive postmenopausal women. Am J Cardiol. 30008;102(1):84–86.

106. He J, Gu D, Wu X, Chen J, Duan X, Chen J, Whelton PK. Effect of soybean protein on blood pressure: a randomized, controlled trial. Ann Intern Med. 2005;143(1):1–9.
107. Hasler CM, Kundrat S, Wool D. Functional foods and cardiovascular disease. Curr Atheroscler Rep. 2000;2(6):467–475.
108. Liu XX, Li SH, Chen JZ, Sun K, Wang XJ, Wang XG, Hui RT. Effect of soy isoflavones on blood pressure: a meta-analysis of randomized controlled trials. Nutr Metab Cardiovasc Dis. 2012;22:463–470.
109. Begg DP, Sinclari AJ, Stahl LA, Garg ML, Jois M, Weisinger RS. Dietary proteins level interacts with omega-3 polyunsaturated fatty acid deficiency to induce hypertension. Am J Hyperten. 2010;23(2):125–128.
110. Fekete ÁA, Giromini C, Chatzidiakou Y, Givens DI, Lovegrove JA. Whey protein lowers blood pressure and improves endothelial function and lipid biomarkers in adults with prehypertension and mild hypertension: results from the chronic Whey2Go randomized controlled trial. Am J Clin Nutr. 2016;104(6):1534–1544.
111. Dong JY, Szeto IM, Makinen K, Gao Q, Wang J, Qin LQ, Zhao Y. Effect of probiotic fermented milk on blood pressure: a meta-analysis of randomised controlled trials. Br J Nutr. 2013;110:1188–1194.
112. Cicero AF, Gerocarni B, Laghi L, Borghi C. Blood pressure lowering effect of lactotripeptides assumed as functional foods: a meta-analysis of current available clinical trials. J Hum Hypertens. 2011;25:425–436.
113. Cicero AF, Aubin F, Azais-Braesco V, Borghi C. Do the lactotripeptides isoleucine-proline-proline and valine-proline-proline reduce systolic blood pressure in European subjects? A meta-analysis of randomized controlled trials. Am J Hypertens. 2013;26:442–449.
114. Cicero AF, Rosticci M, Gerocarni B, Bacchelli S, Veronesi M, Strocchi E, Borghi C. Lactotripeptides effect on office and 24-h ambulatory blood pressure, blood pressure stress response, pulse wave velocity and cardiac output in patients with high-normal blood pressure or first-degree hypertension: a randomized double-blind clinical trial. Hypertens Res. 2011;34:1035–1040.
115. Morris MC. Dietary fats and blood pressure. J Cardiovasc Risk. 1994;1:21–30.
116. Siani A, Pagano E, Iacone R, Iacoviell L, Scopacasa F, Strazzullo P. Blood pressure and metabolic changes during dietary L-arginine supplementation in humans. Am J Hypertens. 2000;13:547–551.
117. Vallance P, Leone A, Calver A, Collier J, Moncada S. Endogenous dimethylarginine as an inhibitor of nitric oxide synthesis. J Cardiovasc Pharmacol. 1992;20:S60–S62.
118. Ruiz-Hurtado, G, Delgado C. Nitric oxide pathway in hypertrophied heart: new therapeutic uses of nitric oxide donors. J Hypertens. 2010;28(Suppl1):56–61.
119. Sonmez A, Celebi G, Erdem G, Tapan S, Genc H, Tasci K, Ercin CN, Dogru T, Kilic S, Uckaya G, Yilmaz MI, Erbil MK, Kutlu M. Plasma apelin and ADMA levels in patients with essential hypertension. Clin Exp Hypertens. 2010;32(3):179–183.
120. Michell DL, Andrews KL, Chin-Dusting JP. Endothelial dysfunction in hypertension: the role of arginase. Front Biosci (Schol Ed). 2011;3:946–960.
121. Rajapakse NW, Mattson DL. Role of L-arginine in nitric oxide production in health and hypertension. Clin Exp Pharmacol Physiol. 2009;36(3):249–255.
122. Tsioufis C, Dimitriadis K, Andrikou E, Thomopoulos C, Tsiachris D, Stefanadi E, Mihas C, Miliou A, Papademetriou V, Stefanadis C. ADMA, C-reactive protein and albuminuria in untreated essential hypertension: a cross-sectional study. Am J Kidney Dis. 2010;55(6):1050–1059.
123. Facchinetti F, Saade GR, Neri I, Pizzi C, Longo M, Volpe A. L-Arginine supplementation in patients with gestational hypertension: a pilot study. Hypertens Pregnancy. 2007;26(1):121–130.

124. Neri I, Monari F, Sqarbi L, Berardi A, Masellis G, Facchinetti F. L-Arginine supplementation in women with chronic hypertension: impact on blood pressure and maternal and neonatal complications. J Matern Fetal Neonatal Med. 2010;23(12):1456–1460.
125. Martina V, Masha A, Gigliardi VR, Brocato L, Manzato E, Berchio A, Massarenti P, Settanni F, Della Casa L, Bergamini S, Iannone A. Long-term *N*-acetylcysteine and L-arginine administration reduces endothelial activation and systolic blood pressure in hypertensive patients with type 2 diabetes. Diabetes Care. 2008;31(5):940–944.
126. Ast J, Jablecka A, Bogdanski I, Krauss H, Chmara E. Evaluation of the antihypertensive effect of L-arginine supplementation in patients with mild hypertension assessed with ambulatory blood pressure monitoring. Med Sci Monit. 2010;16(5):CR266–CR271.
127. Schulman SP, Becker LC, Kass DA, Champion HC, Terrin ML, Forman S. Ernst KV, Kelemen MD, Townsend SN, Capriotti A, Hare JM, Gerstenblith G. L-Arginine therapy in acute myocardial infraction: the vascular interaction with age in myocardial infarction (VINTAGE MI) randomized clinical trial. JAMA. 2006;295(1):58–64.
128. Dong JY, Qin JQ, Zhang ZL, Zhao Y, Wang J, Arigoni F, Zhang W. Effect of oral L-arginine supplementation on blood pressure: a meta-analysis of randomized, double-blind, placebo-controlled trials. Am Heart J. 2011;162:959–965.
129. Huxtable RJ. Physiologic actions of taurine. Physiol Rev. 1992;72:101–163.
130. Fujita T, Ando K, Noda H, Ito Y, Sato Y. Effects of increased adrenomedullary activity and taurine in young patients with borderline hypertension. Circulation. 1987;75:525–532.
131. Huxtable RJ, Sebring LA. Cardiovascular actions of taurine. Prog Clin Biol Res. 1983;125:5–37.
132. Tanabe Y, Urata H, Kiyonaga A, Ikede M, Tanake H, Shindo M, Arakawa K. Changes in serum concentrations of taurine and other amino acids in clinical antihypertensive exercise therapy. Clin Exp Hypertens. 1989;11:149–165.
133. Yamori Y, Taguchi T, Mori H, Mori M. Low cardiovascular risks in the middle age males and females excreting greater 24-hour urinary taurine and magnesium in 41 WHO-CARDIAC study populations in the world. J Biomed Sci. 2010;17(Suppl 1):s21–s26.
134. Wang B, Li Y, Sun F, Li P, Xia W, Zhou X, Li Q, Wang X, Chen J, Zeng X, Zhao Z, He H, Liu D, Zhu Z. Taurine supplementation lowers blood pressure and improves vascular function in prehypertension: randomized, double-blind, placebo-controlled study. Hypertension. 2016;67(3):541–549.
135. Houston Mark C. Combination nutraceutical supplement lowers blood pressure in hypertensive individuals. Integr Med. 2013;12(3):22–28.
136. Sun Q, Wang B, Li Y, Sun F, Li P, Xia W, Zhou X, Li Q, Wang X, Chen J, Zeng X, Zhao Z, He H, Liu D, Zhu Z. Taurine supplementation lowers blood pressure and improves vascular function in prehypertension: randomized, double-blind, placebo-controlled study. Hypertension. 2016;67(3):541–549.
137. Mori TA, Bao DQ, Burke V, Puddey IB, Beilin LJ. Docosahexaenoic acid but not eicosapentaenoic acid lowers ambulatory blood pressure and heart rate in humans. Hypertension. 1999;34:253–260.
138. Bønaa KH, Bjerve KS, Straume B, Gram IT, Thelle D. Effect of eicosapentaenoic and docosahexanoic acids on blood pressure in hypertension: a population-based intervention trial from the Tromso study. N Engl J Med. 1990;322:795–801.
139. Mori TA, Burke V, Puddey I, Irish A. The effects of omega 3 fatty acids and coenzyme Q 10 on blood pressure and heart rate in chronic kidney disease: a randomized controlled trial. J Hypertens. 2009;27(9):1863–1872.
140. Ueshima H, Stamler J, Elliot B, Brown, CQ. Food omega 3 fatty acid intake of individuals (total, linolenic acid, long chain) and their blood pressure: INTERMAP study. Hypertension. 2007;50(20):313–319.

141. Mon TA. Omega 3 fatty acids and hypertension in humans. Clin Exp Pharmacol Physiol. 2006;33(9):842–846.
142. Liu JC, Conkin SM, Manuch SB, Yao JK, Muldoon MF. Long-chain omega-3 fatty acids and blood pressure. Am J Hypertens. 2011;24(10):1121–1126.
143. Engler MM, Schambelan M, Engler MB, Goodfriend TL. Effects of dietary gamma-linolenic acid on blood pressure and adrenal angiotensin receptors in hypertensive rats. Proc Soc Exp Biol Med. 1998;218(3):234–237.
144. Sagara M, Njelekela M, Teramoto T, Taquchi T, Mori M, Armitage L, Birt N, Birt C, Yamori Y. Effects of docoahexaenoic acid supplementation on blood pressure, heart rate, and serum lipid in Scottish men with hypertension and hypercholesterolemia. Int J Hypertens. 2011;8:8091–8098.
145. Colussi G, Catena C, Novello M, Bertin N, Sechi LA. Impact of omega-3 polyunsaturated fatty acids on vascular function and blood pressure: relevance for cardiovascular outcomes. Nutr Metab Cardiovasc Dis. 2017;27(3):191–200.
146. Miller PE, Van Elswyk M, Alexander DD. Long-chain omega-3 fatty acids eicosapentaenoic acid and docosahexaenoic acid and blood pressure: a meta-analysis of randomized controlled trials. Am J Hypertens. 2014;27:885–896.
147. Pase MP, Grima NA, Sarris J. Do long-chain n-3 fatty acids reduce arterial stiffness? A meta-analysis of randomised controlled trials. Br J Nutr. 2011;106:974–980.
148. Cicero AF, Ertek S, Borghi C. Omega-3 polyunsaturated fatty acids: their potential role in blood pressure prevention and management. Curr Vasc Pharmacol. 2009;7:330–337.
149. Minihane AM, Armah CK, Miles EA, Madden JM, Clark AB, Caslake MJ, Packard CJ, Kofler BM, Lietz G, Curtis PJ, Mathers JC, Williams CM, Calder PC. Consumption of fish oil providing amounts of eicosapentaenoic acid and docosahexaenoic acid that can be obtained from the diet reduces blood pressure in adults with systolic hypertension: a retrospective analysis. J Nutr. 2016;146(3):516–523.
150. Rodriguez-Leyva D, Weighell W, Edel AL, LaVallee R, Dibrov E, Pinneker R, Maddaford TG, Ramjiawan B, Aliani M, Guzman R, Pierce GN. Potent antihypertensive action of dietary flaxseed in hypertensive patients. Hypertension. 2013 Dec;62(6):1081–1089.
151. Saravanan P, Davidson NC, Schmidt EB, Calder PC. Cardiovascular effects of marine omega-3 fatty acids. Lancet. 2010;376(9740):540–550.
152. Alexander DD, Miller PE, Van Elswyk ME, Kuratko CN, Bylsma LC. A meta-analysis of randomized controlled trials and prospective cohort studies of eicosapentaenoic and docosahexaenoic long-chain omega-3 fatty acids and coronary heart disease risk. Mayo Clin Proc. 2017 Jan;92(1):15–29.
153. Ferrara LA, Raimondi S, d'Episcopa I. Olive oil and reduced need for antihypertensive medications. Arch Intern Med. 2000;160:837–842.
154. Perona JS, Canizares J, Montero E, Sanchez-Dominquez JM, Catala A, Ruiz Gutierrez V. Virgin olive oil reduces blood pressure in hypertensive elderly patients. Clin Nutr. 2004;23(5):1113–1121.
155. Perona JS, Montero E, Sanchez-Dominquez JM, Canizares J, Garcia M, Ruiz-Gutierrez V. Evaluation of the effect of dietary virgin olive oil on blood pressure and lipid composition of serum and low-density lipoprotein in elderly type 2 subjects. J Agric Food Chem. 2009;57(23):11427–11433.
156. Lopez-Miranda J, Perez-Jimenez F, Ros E, De Caterina F, Badimon L, Cocas MI, Escrich E, Ordovas JM, et al. Olive oil and health: summary of the II international conference on olive oil and health consensus report, Jaen and Cordoba (Spain) 2008. Nutr Metab Cardiovasc Dis. 2010;20(4):284–294.
157. Thomsen C, Rasmussen OW, Hansen KW, Vesterlund M, Hermansen K. Comparison of the effects on the diurnal blood pressure, glucose, and lipid levels of a diet rich in

monounsaturated fatty acids with a diet rich in polyunsaturated fatty acids in type 2 diabetic subjects. Diabet Med. 1995;12:600–606.
158. Sofi F, Abbate R, Gensini GF, Casini A. Accruing evidence on benefits of adherence to the Mediterranean diet on health: an updated systematic review and meta-analysis. Am J Clin Nutr. 2010;92(5):1189–1196.
159. Estruch R, Ros E, Salas-Salvadó J, Covas MI, Corella D, Arós F, Gómez-Gracia E, Ruiz-Gutiérrez V, Fiol M, Lapetra J, Lamuela-Raventos RM, Serra-Majem L, Pintó X, Basora J, Muñoz MA, Sorlí JV, Martínez JA, Martínez-González MA, PREDIMED Study Investigators. Primary prevention of cardiovascular disease with a Mediterranean diet. N Engl J Med. 2013;368(14):1279–1290.
160. Nadtochiy SM, Redman EK. Mediterranean diet and cardioprotection: the role of nitrite, polyunsaturated fatty acids, and polyphenols. Nutrition. 2011;27(7–8):733–744.
161. Salas-Salvadó J, Bulló M, Estruch R, Ros E, Covas MI, Ibarrola-Jurado N, Corella D, Arós F, Gómez-Gracia E, Ruiz-Gutiérrez V, Romaguera D, Lapetra J, Lamuela-Raventós RM, Serra-Majem L, Pintó X, Basora J, Muñoz MA, Sorlí JV, Martínez-González MA. Prevention of diabetes with Mediterranean diets: a subgroup analysis of a randomized trial. Ann Intern Med. 2014;160(1):1–10.
162. Lopez S, Bermudez B, Montserrat-de la Paz S, Jaramillo S, Abia R, Muriana FJ. Virgin olive oil and hypertension. Curr Vasc Pharmacol. 2016;14(4):323–329.
163. Martín-Peláez S, Castañer O, Konstantinidou V, Subirana I, Muñoz-Aguayo D, Blanchart G, Gaixas S, de la Torre R, Farré M, Sáez GT, Nyyssönen K, Zunft HJ, Covas MI, Fitó M. Effect of olive oil phenolic compounds on the expression of blood pressure-related genes in healthy individuals. Eur J Nutr. 2017;56(2):663–670.
164. Storniolo CE, Casillas R, Bulló M, Castañer O, Ros E, Sáez GT, Toledo E, Estruch R, Ruiz-Gutiérrez V, Fitó M, Martínez-González MA, Salas-Salvadó J, Mitjavila MT, Moreno JJ. A Mediterranean diet supplemented with extra virgin olive oil or nuts improves endothelial markers involved in blood pressure control in hypertensive women. Eur J Nutr. 2017;56(1):89–97.
165. Hohmann CD, Cramer H, Michalsen A, Kessler C, Steckhan N, Choi K, Dobos G. Effects of high. phenolic olive oil on cardiovascular risk factors: a systematic review and meta-analysis. Phytomedicine. 2015;22(6):631–640.
166. Doménech M, Roman P, Lapetra J, García de la Corte FJ, Sala-Vila A, de la Torre R, Corella D, Salas-Salvadó J, Ruiz-Gutiérrez V, Lamuela-Raventós RM, Toledo E, Estruch R, Coca A, Ros E. Mediterranean diet reduces 24-hour ambulatory blood pressure, blood glucose, and lipids: one-year randomized, clinical trial. Hypertension. 2014;64(1):69–76.
167. Lockyer S, Rowland I, Spencer JP, Yaqoob P, Stonehouse W. Impact of phenolic-rich olive leaf extract on blood pressure, plasma lipids and inflammatory markers: a randomized controlled trial. Eur J Nutr. 2017;56(4):1421–1432.
168. Cabrera-Vique C, Navarro-Alarcón M, Rodríguez Martínez C, Fonollá-Joya J. Hypertensive effect of an extract of bioactive compounds olive leaves preliminary clinical study. Nutr Hosp. 2015;32(1):242–249.
169. Susalit E, Agus N, Effendi I, Tjandrawinata RR, Nofiarny D, Perrinjaquet-Moccetti T, Verbruggen M. Olive (*Olea europaea*) leaf extract effective in patients with stage-1 hypertension: comparison with captopril. Phytomedicine. 2011;18(4):251–258.
170. Flynn, M, Wang S. Olive Oil as Medicine: The Effect on Blood Pressure. The Report of UCD Olive Center, December 2015.
171. Psaltopoulou T, Naska A, Orfanos P, Trichopoulos D, Mountokalakis T, Trichopoulou A. Olive oil, the Mediterranean diet, and arterial blood pressure: the Greek European Prospective Investigation into Cancer and Nutrition (EPIC) study. Am J Clin Nutr. 2004;80:1012–1018.
172. Toledo E, Hu FB, Estruch R, Buil-Cosiales P, Corella D, Salas-Salvadó J, Covas MI, Arós F, Gómez-Gracia E, Fiol M, Lapetra J, Serra-Majem L, Pinto X, Lamuela-Raventós

RM, Saez G, Bulló M, Ruiz-Gutiérrez V, Ros E, Sorli JV, Martinez-Gonzalez MA. Effect of the Mediterranean diet on blood pressure in the PREDIMED trial: results from a randomized controlled trial. BMC Med. 2013;11:207.

173. Perrinjaquet-Moccetti T, Busjahn A, Schmidlin C, Schmidt A, Bradl B, Aydogan C. Food supplementation with an olive (*Olea uropaea* L.) leaf extract reduces blood pressure in borderline hypertensive monozygotic twins. Phytother Res. 2008;22:1239–1242.
174. Hodgson JM, Woodman R Bryan J, Wilson C, Murphy KJ. A Mediterranean diet lowers blood pressure and improves endothelial function: results from the MedLey randomized intervention trial. Am J Clin Nutr. 2017;105(6):1305–1313.
175. Miura K, Stamler J, Brown IJ, Ueshima H, Nakagawa H, Sakurai M, Chan Q, Appel LJ, Okayama A, Okuda N, Curb JD, Rodriguez BL, Robertson C, Zhao L, Elliott P, INTERMAP Research Group. Relationship of dietary monounsaturated fatty acids to blood pressure: the international study of macro/micronutrients and blood pressure. J Hypertens. 2013 Jun;31(6):1144–1150.
176. Perrinjaquet-Moccetti T, Busjahn A, Schmidlin C, Schmidt A, Bradl B, Aydogan C. Food supplementation with an olive (*Olea europaea* L.) leaf extract reduces blood pressure in borderline hypertensive monozygotic twins. Phytother Res. 2008;22(9):1239–1242.
177. Sherman DL, Keaney JF, Biegelsen ES, et al. Pharmacological concentrations of ascorbic acid are required for the beneficial effect on endothelial vasomotor function in hypertension. Hypertension. 2000;35:936–941.
178. Ness AR, Khaw K-T, Bingham S, Day NE. Vitamin C status and blood pressure. J Hypertens. 1996;14:503–508.
179. Duffy SJ, Bokce N, Holbrook. Treatment of hypertension with ascorbic acid. Lancet. 1999;354:2048–2049.
180. Enstrom JE, Kanim LE, Klein M. Vitamin C intake and mortality among a sample of the United States population. Epidemiology. 1992;3:194–202.
181. Block G, Jensen, CD, Norkus EP, Hudes M, Crawford PB. Vitamin C in plasma is inversely related to blood pressure and change in blood pressure during the previous year in young black and white women. Nutr J. 2008;17(7):35–46.
182. Hatzitolios A, Iliadis F, KatsikiN, Baltatzi M. Is the antihypertensive effect of dietary supplements via aldehydes reduction evidence based: a systemic review. Clin Exp Hypertens. 2008;30(7):628–639.
183. Mahajan AS, Babbar R, Kansai N, Agarwai, SK, Ray PC. Antihypertensive and antioxidant action of amlodipine and Vitamin C in patients of essential hypertension. J Clin Biochem Nutr. 2007;40(2):141–147.
184. Ledlerc PC, Proulx, CD, Arquin G, Belanger S. Ascorbic acid decreases the binding affinity of the AT1 receptor for angiotensin II. Am J Hypertens. 2008;21(1):67–71.
185. Plantinga Y, Ghiadone L, Magagna, A, Biannarelli C. Supplementation with vitamins C and E improves arterial stiffness and endothelial function in essential hypertensive patients. Am J Hypertens. 2007;20(4):392–397.
186. Sato K, Dohi Y, Kojima, M, Miyagawa K. Effects of ascorbic acid on ambulatory blood pressure in elderly patients with refractory hypertension. Arzneimittelforschung. 2006;56(7):535–540.
187. Block G, Mangels AR, Norkus EP, Patterson BH, Levander OA, Taylor PR. Ascorbic acid status and subsequent diastolic and systolic blood pressure. Hypertension. 2001;37:261–267.
188. McRae MP. Is vitamin C an effective antihypertensive supplement? A review and analysis of the literature. J Chiropr Med. 2006;5(2):60–64.
189. Simon JA. Vitamin C and cardiovascular disease: a review. J Am Coll Nutr. 1992;11(2):107–125.
190. Ness AR, Chee D, Elliott P. Vitamin C and blood pressure—an overview. J Hum Hypertens. 1997;11(6):343–350.

191. Trout DL. Vitamin C and cardiovascular risk factors. Am J Clin Nutr. 1991;53(1 Suppl):322S–325S.
192. Ried K, Travica N, Sali A. The acute effect of high-dose intravenous vitamin C and other nutrients on blood pressure: a cohort study. Blood Press Monit. 2016 Jun;21(3):160–167.
193. Buijsse B, Jacobs DR Jr, Steffen LM, Kromhout D, Gross MD. Plasma ascorbic acid, a priori diet quality score, and incident hypertension: a prospective cohort study. PLOS ONE. 2015;10(12).
194. Hajjar IM, George V, Sasse EA, Kochar MS. A randomized, double-blind, controlled trial of vitamin C in the management of hypertension and lipids. Am J Ther. 2002 Jul-Aug;9(4):289–293.
195. National Center for Health Statistics, Fulwood R, Johnson CL, Bryner JD. Hematological and Nutritional Biochemistry Reference Data for Persons 6 Months-74 Years of Age: United States, 1976-80. US Public Health Service, Washington, DC, 1982. Vital and Health Statistics Series 11, No. 232, DHHS Publication No. (PHS) 83-1682.
196. McCartney DM, Byrne DG, Turner MJ. Dietary contributors to hypertension in adults reviewed. Ir J Med Sci. 2015;184:81–90.
197. Enstrom JE, Kanim LE, Klein M. Vitamin C intake and mortality among a sample of the United States population. Epidemiology. 1992;3:194–202.
198. Block G, Jensen CD, Norkus EP, Hudes M, Crawford PB. Vitamin C in plasma is inversely related to blood pressure and change in blood pressure during the previous year in young black and white women. Nutr J. 2008;17:35–46.
199. Juraschek SP, Guallar E, Appel LJ, Miller ER 3rd. Effects of vitamin C supplementation on blood pressure: a meta-analysis of randomized controlled trials. Am J Clin Nutr. 2012;95:1079–1088.
200. Ward NC, Wu JH, Clarke MW, Buddy IB. Vitamin E effects on the treatment of hypertension in type 2 diabetics. J Hypertens. 2007;227:227–234.
201. Murray ED, Wechter WJ, Kantoci D, Wang WH, Pham T, Quiggle DD, Gibson KM, Leipold D, Anner BM. Endogenous natriuretic factors 7: biospecificity of a natriuetic gamma-tocopherol metabolite LLU alpha. J Pharmacol Exp Ther. 1997;282(2):657–662.
202. Gray B, Swick J, Ronnenberg AG. Vitamin E and adiponectin: proposed mechanism for vitamin E-induced improvement in insulin sensitivity. Nutr Rev. 2011;69(3):155–161.
203. Kuwabara A, Nakade M, Tamai H, Tsuboyama-Kasaoka N, Tanaka K. The association between vitamin E intake and hypertension: results from the re-analysis of the National Health and Nutrition Survey. J Nutr Sci Vitaminol (Tokyo). 2014;60(4):239–245.
204. Hodgson JM, Croft KD, Woodman RJ, Puddey IB, Bondonno CP, Wu JH, Bilin LJ, Lukoshkova EV, Head GA, Ward NC. Effects of vitamin E, vitamin C and polyphenols on the rate of blood pressure variation: results of two randomised controlled trials. Br J Nutr. 2014;112(9):1551–1561.
205. Hanni LL, Huarfner LH, Sorensen OH, Ljunghall S. Vitamin D is related to blood pressure and other cardiovascular risk factors in middle-aged men. Am J Hypertens. 1995;8:894–901.
206. Bednarski R, Donderski R, Manitius L. Role of vitamin D in arterial blood pressure control. Pol Merkur Lekarski. 2007;136:307–310.
207. Li YC, Kong H, Wei M, Chen ZF. 1,25-Dihydroxyvitamin D(3) is a negative endocrine regulator of the renin–angiotensin system. J Clin Invest. 2002;110(2):229–238.
208. Ngo DT, Sverdlov AL, McNeil JJ, Horowitz JD. Does vitamin D modulate asymmetric dimethylargine and C-reactive protein concentrations? Am J Med. 2010;123(4):335–341.
209. Rosen CJ. Clinical practice. Vitamin D insufficiency. N Engl J Med. 2011;364(3):248–254.
210. Boldo A, Campbell P, Luthra P, White WB. Should the concentration of vitamin D be measured in all patients with hypertension? J Clin Hypertens. 2010;12(3):149–152.

211. Pittas AG, Chung M, Trikalinos T, Mitri J, Brendel M, Patel K, Lichtenstein HA, Lau J, Balk EM. Systematic review: vitamin D and cardiometabolic outcomes. Ann Intern Med. 2010;152(5):307–314.
212. Movano Peregrin C, Lopez Rodriguez R, Castilla Castellano MD. Vitamin D and hypertension. Med Clin (Barc). 2012;138(9):397–401.
213. Motiwala Sr, Want TJ. Vitamin D and cardiovascular disease. Curr Opin Nephrol Hypertens. 2011;20(4):345–353.
214. Cosenso-Martin LN, Vitela-Martin JF. Is there an association between vitamin D and hypertension. Recent Pat Cardiovasc Drug Discov. 2011;6(2):140–147.
215. Bhandari SK, Pashayan S, Liu IL, Rasgon SA, Kujubu DA, Tom TY, Sim JJ. 25-hydroxyvitamin D levels and hypertension rates. J Clin Hypertens. 2011;13(3):170–177.
216. Pfeifer M, Begerow B, Minne HW, Nachtigall D, Hansen C. Effects of a short-term vitamin D (3) and calcium supplementation on blood pressure and parathyroid hormone levels in elderly women. J Clin Endocrinol Metab. 2001;86:1633–1637.
217. Qi D, Nie XL, Wu S, Cai J. Vitamin D and hypertension: prospective study and meta-analysis. PLOS ONE. 2017;12(3):e0174298.
218. McMullan CJ, Borgi L, Curhan GC, Fisher N, Forman JP. The effect of vitamin D on renin-angiotensin system activation and blood pressure: a randomized control trial. J Hypertens. 2017;35(4):822–829.
219. Qi D, Nie X, Cai J. The effect of vitamin D supplementation on hypertension in non-CKD populations: a systemic review and meta-analysis. Int J Cardiol. 2017;227:177–186.
220. Yilmaz S, Sen F, Ozeke O, Temizhan A, Topaloglu S, Aras D, Aydogdu S. The relationship between vitamin D levels and nondipper hypertension. Blood Press Monit. 2015;20(6):330–334.
221. Beveridge LA, Struthers AD, Khan F, Jorde R, Scragg R, Macdonald HM, Alvarez JA, Boxer RS, Dalbeni A, Gepner AD, Isbel NM, Larsen T, NagpalJ, Petchey WG, Stricker H, Strobel F, Tangpricha V, Toxqui L, Vaquero MP, Wamberg L, Zittermann A, Witham MD, D-PRESSURE Collaboration. Effect of vitamin D supplementation on blood pressure: a systematic review and meta-analysis incorporating individual patient data. JAMA Intern Med. 2015;175(5):745–754.
222. Forman JP, Scott JB, Ng K, Drake BF, Suarez EG, Hayden DL, Bennett GG, Chandler PD, Hollis BW, Emmons KM, Giovannucci EL, Fuchs CS, Chan AT. Effect of vitamin D supplementation on blood pressure in blacks. Hypertension. 2013;61(4):779–785.
223. McMullan CJ, Borgi L, Curhan GC, Fisher N, Forman JP. The effect of vitamin D on renin-angiotensin system activation and blood pressure: a randomized control trial. J Hypertens. 2017;35(4):822–829.
224. Keniston R, Enriquez JI Sr. Relationship between blood pressure and plasma vitamin B_6 levels in healthy middle-aged adults. Ann NY Acad Sci. 1990;585:499–501.
225. Aybak M, Sermet A, Ayyildiz MO, Karakilcik AZ. Effect of oral pyridoxine hydrochloride supplementation on arterial blood pressure in patients with essential hypertension. Arzneimittelforschung. 1995;45:1271–1273.
226. Paulose CS, Dakshinamurti K, Packer S, Stephens NL. Sympathetic stimulation and hypertension in the pyridoxine-deficient adult rat. Hypertension. 1988;11(4):387–391.
227. Dakshinamurti K, Lal KJ, Ganguly PK. Hypertension, calcium channel and pyridoxine (vitamin B6). Mol Cell Biochem. 1998;188(1–2):137–148.
228. Noori N, Tabibi H, Hosseinpanah F, Hedayati M, Nafar M. Effects of combined lipoic acid and pyridoxine on albuminuria, advanced glycation end-products, and blood pressure in diabetic nephropathy. Int J Vitam Nutr Res. 2013;83(2):77–85.
229. Moline J, Bukharovich IF, Wolff MS, Phillips R. Dietary flavonoids and hypertension: is there a link? Med Hypotheses. 2000;55:306–309.

230. Knekt P, Reunanen A, Järvinen R, Seppänen R, Heliövaara M, Aromaa A. Antioxidant vitamin intake and coronary mortality in a longitudinal population study. Am J Epidemiol. 1994;139:1180–1189.
231. Karatzi KN, Papamichael CM, Karatizis EN, Papaioannou TG, Aznaouridis KA, Katsichti PP, Stamatelopuolous KS. Red wine acutely induces favorable effects on wave reflections and central pressures in coronary artery disease patients. Am J Hypertens. 2005;18(9):1161–1167.
232. Biala A, Tauriainen E, Siltanen A, Shi J, Merasto S, Louhelainen M, Martonen E, Finckenberg P, Muller DN, Mervaala E. Resveratrol induces mitochondrial biogenesis and ameliorates Ang II-induced cardiac remodeling in transgenic rats harboring human renin and angiotensinogen genes. Blood Press. 2010;19(3):196–205.
233. Wong RH, Howe PR, Buckley JD, Coates AM, Kunz L, Berry NM. Acute resveratrol supplementation improves flow-mediated dilatation in overweight/obese individuals with mildly elevated blood pressure. Nutr Metab Cardiovasc Dis. 2011;21(11):851–856.
234. Bhatt SR, Lokhandwala MF, Banday AA. Resveratrol prevents endothelial nitric oxide synthase uncoupling and attenuates development of hypertension in spontaneously hypertensive rats. Eur J Pharmacol. 2011;667(1–3):258–264.
235. Rivera L, Moron R, Zarzuelo A, Galisteo M. Long-term resveratrol administration reduces metabolic disturbances and lowers blood pressure in obese Zucker rats. Biochem Pharmacol. 2009;77(6):1053–1063.
236. Sahebkar A, Ferri C, Giorgini P, Bo S, Nachtigal P, Grassi D. Effects of pomegranate juice on blood pressure: a systematic review and meta-analysis of randomized controlled trials. Pharmacol Res. 2017;115:149–161.
237. Tjelle TE, Holtung L, Bøhn SK, Aaby K, Thoresen M, Wiik SÅ, Paur I, Karlsen AS, Retterstøl K, Iversen PO, Blomhoff R. Polyphenol-rich juices reduce blood pressure measures in a randomised controlled trial in high normal and hypertensive volunteers. Br J Nutr. 2015;114(7):1054–1063.
238. de Jesús Romero-Prado MM, Curiel-Beltrán JA, Miramontes-Espino MV, CardonaMuñoz EG, Rios-Arellano A, Balam-Salazar LB. Dietary flavonoids added to pharmacological antihypertensive therapy are effective in improving blood pressure. Basic Clin Pharmacol Toxicol. 2015;117(1):57–64.
239. Asgary S, Sahebkar A, Afshani MR, Keshvari M, Haghjooyjavanmard S, Rafieian-Kopaei M. Clinical evaluation of blood pressure lowering, endothelial function improving, hypolipidemic and anti-inflammatory effects of pomegranate juice in hypertensive subjects. Phytother Res. 2014;28(2):193–199.
240. Paran E, Engelhard YN. Effect of lycopene, an oral natural antioxidant on blood pressure. J Hypertens. 2001;19:S74.
241. Engelhard YN, Gazer B, Paran E. Natural antioxidants from tomato extract reduce blood pressure in patients with grade-1 hypertension: a double blind placebo controlled pilot study. Am Heart J. 2006;151(1):100.
242. Paran E, Novac C, Engelhard YN, Hazan-Halevy I. The effects of natural antioxidants form tomato extract in treated but uncontrolled hypertensive patients. Cardiovasc Durgs Ther. 2009;23(2):145–151.
243. Reid K, Frank OR, Stocks NP. Dark chocolate or tomato extract for prehypertension: a randomized controlled trial. BMC Complement Altern Med. 2009;9:22.
244. Paran E, Engelhard Y. Effect of tomato's lycopene on blood pressure, serum lipoproteins, plasma homocysteine and oxidative stress markers in grade I hypertensive patients. Am J Hypertens. 2001;14:141A.
245. Ried K, Fakler P. Protective effect of lycopene on serum cholesterol and blood pressure: meta-analyses of intervention trials. Maturitas. 2011;68(4):299–310.

246. Burton-Freeman B, Sesso HD. Whole food versus supplement: comparing the clinical evidence of tomato intake and lycopene supplementation on cardiovascular risk factors. Adv Nutr. 2014;5(5):457–485.
247. Langsjoen PH, Langsjoen AM. Overview of the use of CoQ 10 in cardiovascular disease. Biofactors. 1999;9:273–284.
248. Singh RB, Niaz MA, Rastogi SS, Shukla PK, Thakur AS. Effect of hydrosoluble coenzyme Q10 on blood pressure and insulin resistance in hypertensive patients with coronary heart disease. J Hum Hypertens. 1999;12:203–208.
249. Burke BE, Neustenschwander R, Olson RD. Randomized, double-blind, placebo-controlled trial of coenzyme Q10 in isolated systolic hypertension. South Med J. 2001;94:1112–1117.
250. Rosenfeldt FL, Haas SJ, Krum H, Hadu A. Coenzyme Q 10 in the treatment of hypertension: a meta-analysis of the clinical trials. J Hum Hypertens. 2007;21(4):297–306.
251. Singh RB, Niaz MA, Rastogi SS, Shukia PK, Thakur AS. Effect of hydrosoluble coenzyme Q 10 on blood pressures and insulin resistance in hypertensive patients with coronary artery disease. J Hum Hypertens. 1999;13(3):302–308.
252. Ankola DD, Viswanas B, Bhardqaj V, Ramarao P, Kumar MN. Development of potent oral nanoparticulate formulation of coenzyme Q10 for treatment of hypertension: can the simple nutritional supplement be used as first line therapeutic agents for prophylaxis/therapy? Eur J Pharm Biopharm. 2007;67(2):361–369.
253. Ho MJ, Li EC, Wright JM. Blood pressure lowering efficacy of coenzyme Q10 for primary hypertension. Cochrane Database Syst Rev. 2016;3:CD007435.
254. Ho MJ, Bellusci A, Wright JM. Blood pressure lowering efficacy of coenzyme Q10 for primary hypertension. Cochrane Database Syst Rev. 2009 Oct;7(4):CD007435.
255. Mikhin VP, Kharchenko AV, Rosliakova EA, Cherniatina MA. Application of coenzyme Q(10) in combination therapy of arterial hypertension. Kardiologiia. 2011;51(6):26–31.
256. Tsai KL, Huang YH, Kao CL, Yang DM, Lee HC, Chou HY, Chen YC, Chiou GY, Chen LH, Yang YP, Chiu TH, Tsai CS, Ou HC, Chiou SH. A novel mechanism of coenzyme Q10 protects against human endothelial cells from oxidative stress-induced injury by modulating NO-related pathways. J Nutr Biochem. 2012;23(5):458–468.
257. Sohet FM, Delzenne NM. Is there a place for coenzyme Q in the management of metabolic disorders associated with obesity? Nutr Rev. 2012;70(11):631–641.
258. Digiesi V, Cantini F, Oradei A, Bisi G, Guarino GC, Brocchi A, Bellandi F, Mancini M, Littarru GP. Coenzyme Q10 in essential hypertension. Mol Aspects Med. 1994;15(Suppl):s257–s263.
259. Langsjoen P, Langsjoen P, Willis R, Folkers K. Treatment of essential hypertension with coenzyme Q10. Mol Aspects Med. 1994;15(Suppl):S265–S272.
260. Trimarco V, Cimmino CS, Santoro M, Pagnano G, Manzi MV, Piglia A, Giudice CA, De Luca N, Izzo R. Nutraceuticals for blood pressure control in patients with high-normal or grade 1 hypertension. High Blood Press Cardiovasc Prev. 2012;19(3):117–122.
261. Young JM, Florkowski CM, Molyneux SL, McEwan RG, Frampton CM, Nicholls MG, Scott RS, George PM. A randomized, double-blind, placebo-controlled crossover study of coenzyme Q10 therapy in hypertensive patients with the metabolic syndrome. Am J Hypertens. 2012;(2):261–270.
262. Kontush A, Reich A, Baum K, Spranger T, Finckh B, Kohlschütter A, Beisiegel U. Plasma ubiquinol-10 is decreased in patients with hyperlipidaemia. Atherosclerosis. 1997;129(1):119–126.
263. McLachlan J, Beattie E, Murphy MP, Koh-Tan CH, Olson E, Beattie W, Dominiczak AF, Nicklin SA, Graham D. Combined therapeutic benefit of mitochondria-targeted antioxidant, MitoQ10, and angiotensin receptor blocker, losartan, on cardiovascular function. J Hypertens. 2014;32(3):555–564.

264. Rosenfeldt F, Hilton D, Pepe S, Krum H. Systematic review of effect of coenzyme Q10 in physical exercise, hypertension and heart failure. Biofactors. 2003;18(1–4):91–100.
265. McMackin CJ, Widlansky ME, Hambury NM, Haung AL. Effect of combined treatment with alpha lipoic acid and acetyl carnitine on vascular function and blood pressure in patients with coronary artery disease. J Clin Hypertens. 2007;9:249–255.
266. Hatzitolios A, Iliadis F, Katsiki N, Baltazi M. Is the anti-hypertensive effect of dietary supplements via aldehydes reduction evidenced based? A systematic review. Clin Exp Hypertens. 2008;30(7):628–639.
267. Salinthone S, Schillace RV, Tsang C, Regan JW, Burdette DN, Carr DW. Lipoic acid stimulates cAMP production via G protein-coupled receptor-dependent and -independent mechanisms. J Nutr Biochem. 2011;22(7):681–690.
268. Rahman ST, Merchant N, Hague T, Wahi J, Bhaheetharan S, Ferdinand KC, Khan BV. The impact of lipoic acid on endothelial function and proteinuria in quinapril-treated diabetic patients with stage I hypertension: results from the QUALITY study. J Cardiovasc Pharmacol Ther. 2012;17(2):139–145.
269. Huang YD, Li N, Zhang WG, Hu XJ, Wang Q, Wang CC, Xu RW, Uan K, Hou XY, Naer K, Want XL, Yan WL. The effect of oral alpha-lipoic acid in overweight/obese individuals on the brachial-ankle pulse wave velocity and supine blood pressure: a randomized, crossover, double-blind, placebo-controlled trial. Zhonghua Liu Xing Bing Xue Za Zhi. 2011;32(3):290–296.
270. Morcos M, Borcea V, Isermann B, et al. Effect of alpha-lipoic acid on the progression of endothelial cell damage and albuminuria in patients with diabetes mellitus: an exploratory study. Diabetes Res Clin Prac. 2001;52(3):175–183.
271. Noori N, Tabibi H, Hosseinpanah F, Hedayati M, Nafar M. Effects of combined lipoic acid and pyridoxine on albuminuria, advanced glycation end-products, and blood pressure in diabetic nephropathy. Int J Vitam Nutr Res. 2013;83(2):77–85.
272. Hosseini S, Lee J, Sepulveda RT, et al. A randomized, double-blind, placebo-controlled, prospective 16 week crossover study to determine the role of pycnogenol in modifying blood pressure in mildly hypertensive patients. Nutr Res. 2001;21:1251–1260.
273. Zibadi S, Rohdewald PJ, Park D, Watson RR. Reduction of cardiovascular risk factors in subjects with type 2 diabetes by pycnogenol supplementation. Nutr Res. 2008;28(5):315–320.
274. Liu X, Wei J, Tan F, Zhou S, Wurthwein G, Rohdewald P. Pycnogenol French maritime pine bark extract improves endothelial function of hypertensive patients. Lif Sci. 2004;74(7):855–862.
275. Van der Zwan LP, Scheffer PG, Teerlink T. Reduction of myeloperoxidase activity by melatonin and pycnogenol may contribute to their blood pressure lowering effect. Hypertension. 2010;56(3):e35.
276. Cesarone MR, Belcaro G, Stuard S, Schonlau F, Di Renzo A, Grossi MG, Dugall M, Cornelli U, Cacchio M, Gizzi G, Pellegrini L. Kidney flow and function in hypertension: protective effects of pyconogenol in hypertensive particpants – a controlled study. J Cardiovasc Pharmacol Ther. 2010;15(1):41–46.
277. Gulati OP. Pycnogenol in metabolic syndrome and related disorders. Phytother Res. 2015;29(7):949–968.
278. Hu S, Belcaro G, Cornelli U, Luzzi R, Cesarone M, Dugall M, Feragalli B, Errichi B, Ippolito E, Grossi M, Hosoi M, Gizzi G, Trignani M. Effects of pycnogenol on endothelial dysfunction in borderline hypertensive, hyperlipidemic, and hyperglycemic individuals: the borderline study. Int Angiol. 2015;34(1):43–52.
279. Enseleit F, Sudano I, Périat D, Winnik S, Wolfrum M, Flammer AJ, Fröhlich GM, Kaiser P, Hirt A, Haile SR, Krasniqi N, Matter CM, Uhlenhut K, Högger P, Neidhart M, Lüscher TF, Ruschitzka F, Noll G. Effects of pycnogenol on endothelial function in patients with stable coronary artery disease: a double-blind, randomized, placebo-controlled, cross-over study. Eur Heart J. 2012;33(13):1589–1597.

280. Luzzi R, Belcaro G, Hosoi M, Feragalli B, Cornelli U, Dugall M, Ledda A. Normalization of cardiovascular risk factors in peri-menopausal women with Pycnogenol®. Minerva Ginecol. 2017;69(1):29–34.
281. Simons S, Wollersheim H, Thien T. A systematic review on the influence of trial quality on the effects of garlic on blood pressure. Neth J Med. 2009;67(6):212–219.
282. Reinhard KM, Coleman CI, Teevan C, Vacchani P. Effects of garlic on blood pressure in patients with and without systolic hypertension: a meta-analysis. Ann Pharmacother. 2008;42(12):1766–1771.
283. Reid K, Frank OR, Stocks NP. Aged garlic extract lowers blood pressure in patients with treated but uncontrolled hypertension: a randomized controlled trial. Maturitas. 2010;67(2):144–150.
284. Nakasone Y, Nakamura Y, Yamamoto T, Yamaguchi H. Effect of a traditional Japanese garlic preparation on blood pressure in prehypertensive and mildly hypertensive adults. Exp Ther Med. 2013;5(2):399–405.
285. Ried K, Frank OR, Stocks NP. Aged garlic extract reduces blood pressure in hypertensives: a dose-response trial. Eur J Clin Nutr. 2013;67(1):64–70.
286. Shouk R, Abdou A, Shetty K, Sarkar D, Eid AH. Mechanisms underlying the antihypertensive effects of garlic bioactives. Nutr Res. 2014;34(2):106–115.
287. Stabler SN, Tejani AM, Huynh F, Fowkes C. Garlic for the prevention of cardiovascular morbidity and mortality in hypertensive patients. Cochrane Database Syst Rev. 2012 Aug;15(8):CD007653.
288. Mahdavi-Roshan M, Nasrollahzadeh J, Mohammad Zadeh A, Zahedmehr A. Does garlic supplementation control blood pressure in patients with severe coronary artery disease? A clinical trial study. Iran Red Crescent Med J. 2016 Aug;18(11):e23871.
289. Ried K, Travica N, Sali A. The effect of aged garlic extract on blood pressure and other cardiovascular risk factors in uncontrolled hypertensives: the AGE at Heart Trial. Integr Blood Press Control. 2016;9:9–21.
290. Varshney R, Budoff MJ. Garlic and heart disease. J Nutr. 2016;146(2):416S–421S.
291. Xiong XJ, Wang PQ, Li SJ, Li XK, Zhang YQ, Wang J. Garlic for hypertension: a systematic review and meta-analysis of randomized controlled trials. Phytomedicine. 2015;22(3):352–361.
292. Suetsuna K, Nakano T. Identification of an antihypertensive peptide from peptic digest of wakame (*Undaria pinnatifida*). J Nutr Biochem. 2000;11:450–454.
293. Nakano T, Hidaka H, Uchida J, Nakajima K, Hata Y. Hypotensive effects of wakame. J Jpn Soc Clin Nutr. 1998;20:92.
294. Krotkiewski M, Aurell M, Holm G, Grimby G, Szckepanik J. Effects of a sodium-potassium ion-exchanging seaweed preparation in mild hypertension. Am J Hypertens. 1991;4:483–488.
295. Sato M, Oba T, Yamaguchi T, Nakano T, Kahara T, Funayama K, Kobayashi A, Nakano T. Antihypertensive effects of hydrolysates of wakame (*Undaria pinnatifida*) and their angiotnesin-1-converting inhibitory activity. Ann Nutr Metab. 2002;46(6):259–267.
296. Sato M, Hosokawa T, Yamaguchi T, Nakano T, Muramoto K, Kahara T, Funayama K, Kobayashi A, Nakano T. Angiotensin I converting enzyme inhibitory peptide derived from wakame (*Undaria pinnatifida*) and their antihypertensive effect in spontaneously hypertensive rats. J Agric Food Chem. 2002;50(21):6245–6252.
297. Taubert D, Roesen R, Schomig E. Effect of cocoa and tea intake on blood pressure: a meta-analysis. Arch Intern Med. 2007;167(7):626–634.
298. Grassi D, Lippi C, Necozione S, Desideri G, Ferri C. Short-term administration of dark chocolate is followed by a significant increase in insulin sensitivity and a decrease in blood pressure in healthly persons. Am J Clin Nutr. 2005;81(3):611–614.
299. Taubert D, Roesen R, Lehmann C, Jung N, Schomig E. Effects of low habitual cocoa intake on blood pressure and bioactive nitric oxide: arandomized controlled trial. JAMA. 2007;298(1):49–60.

300. Cohen DL, Townsend RR. Cocoa ingestion and hypertension-another cup please? J Clin Hypertens. 2007;9(8):647–648.
301. Reid I, Sullivan T, Fakler P, Frank OR, Stocks NP. Does chocolate reduce blood pressure? A meta-analysis. BMC Med. 2010;8:39–46.
302. Egan BM, Laken MA, Donovan JL, Woolson RF. Does dark chocolate have a role in the prevention and management of hypertension? Commentary on the evidence. Hypertension. 2010;55(6):1289–1295.
303. Desch S, Kobler D, Schmidt J, Sonnabend M, Adams V, Sareben M, Eitel I, Bluher M, Shuler G, Thiele H. Low vs higher-dose dark chocolate and blood pressure in cardiovascular high-risk patients. Am J Hypertens. 2010;23(6):694–700.
304. Desch S, Schmidt J, Sonnabend M, Eitel I, Sareban M, Rahimi K, Schuler G, Thiele H. Effect of cocoa products on blood pressure: systematic review and meta-analysis. Am J Hypertens. 2010;23(1):97–103.
305. Grassi D, Desideri G, Necozione S, Lippi C, Casale R, Properzi G, Blumberg JB, Ferri C. Blood pressure is reduced and insulin sensitivity increased in glucose intolerant hypertensive subjects after 15 days of consuming high-polyphenol dark chocolate. J Nutr. 2008;138(9):1671–1676.
306. Grassi D, Necozione S, Lippi C, Croce G, Valeri L, Pasqualetti P, Desideri G, Blumberg JB, Ferri C. Cocoa reduces blood pressure and insulin resistance and improved endothelium-dependent vasodilation in hypertensives. Hypertension. 2005;46(2):398–405.
307. Grassi D, Desideri G, Necozione S, Ruggieri F, Blumberg JB, Stornello M, Ferri C. Protective effects of flavanol-rich dark chocolate on endothelial function and wave reflection during acute hyperglycemia. Hypertension. 2012;60:827–832.
308. Ried K, Sullivan TR, Fakler P, Frank OR, Stocks NP. Effect of cocoa on blood pressure. Cochrane Database Syst Rev. 2012;8: CD008893.
309. Scheer FA, Van Montfrans GA, van Someren EJ, Mairuhu G, Buijs RM. Daily nighttime melatonin reduces blood pressure in male patients with essential hypertension. Hypertension. 2004;43(2):192–197.
310. Cavallo A, Daniels SR, Dolan LM, Khoury JC, Bean JA. Blood pressure response to melatonin in type I diabetes. Pediatr Diabetes. 2004;5(1):26–31.
311. Cavallo A, Daniels SR, Dolan LM, Bean JA, Khoury JC. Blood pressure-lowering effect of melatonin in type 1 diabetes. J Pineal Res. 2004;36(4):262–266.
312. Cagnacci A, Cannoletta M, Renzi A, Baldassari F, Arangino S, Volpe A. Prolonged melatonin administration decreases nocturnal blood pressure in women. Am J Hypertens. 2005;18(12 Pt 1):1614–1618.
313. Grossman E, Laudon M, Yalcin R, Zengil H, Peleg E, Sharabi Y, Kamari Y, Shen-Orr Z, Zisapel N. Melatonin reduces night blood pressure in patients with nocturnal hypertension. Am J Med. 2006;119(10):898–902.
314. Rechcinski T, Kurpese M, Trzoa E, Krzeminska-Pakula M. The influence of melatonin supplementation on circadian pattern of blood pressure in patients with coronary artery disease-preliminary report. Pol Arch Med Wewn. 2006;115(6):520–528.
315. Merkureva GA, Ryzhak GA. Effect of the pineal gland peptide preparation on the diurnal profile of arterial pressure in middle-aged and elderly women with ischemic heart disease and arterial hypertension. Adv Gerontol. 2008;21(1):132–142.
316. Zaslavskai RM, Scherban EA, Logvinenki SI. Melatonin in combined therapy of patients with stable angina and arterial hypertension. Klin Med (Mosk). 2009;86:64–67.
317. Zamotaev IuN, Enikeev AKh, Kolomets NM. The use of melaxen in combined therapy of arterial hypertension in subjects occupied in assembly line production. Klin Med (Mosk). 2009;87(6):46–49.
318. Rechcinski T, Trzos E, Wierzbowski-Drabik K, Krzeminska-Pakute M, Kurpesea M. Melatonin for nondippers with coronary artery disease: assessment of blood pressure profile and heart rate variability. Hypertens Res. 2002;33(1):56–61.

319. Kozirog M, Poliwczak AR, Duchnowicz P, Koter-Michalak M, Sikora J, Broncel M. Melatonin treatment improves blood pressure, lipid profile and parameters of oxidative stress in patients with metabolic syndrome. J Pineal Res. 2011;50(3):261–266.
320. Zeman M, Dulkova K, Bada V, Herichova I. Plasma melatonin concentrations in hypertensive patients with the dipping and nondipping blood pressure profile. Life Sci. 2005;75(16):1795–1803.
321. Jonas M, Garfinkel, D, Zisapel N, Laudon M, Grossman E. Impaired nocturnal melatonin secretion in non-dipper hypertensive patients. Blood Pressure. 2003;12(1):19–24.
322. Simko, F, Pechanova O. Potential roles of melatonin and chronotherapy among the new trends in hypertension treatment. J Pineal Res. 2009;47(2):127–133.
323. Cui HW, Zhang ZX, Gao MT, Liu Y, Su AH, Wang MY. Circadian rhythm of melatonin and blood pressure changes in patients with essential hypertension. Zhonghua Xin Xue Guan Bing Za Zhi. 2008;36(1):20–23.
324. Ostrowska Z, Kos-Kudla B, Marek B, Kajdaniuk D, Wolkowska K, Swietochowska E, Gorski J, Szapska B. Circadian rhythm of melatonin in patients with hypertension. Pol Merkur Lekarski. 2004;17(97):50–54.
325. Shatilo VB, Bondarenke EV, Amtoniuk-Shcheglova IA. Pineal gland melatonin-producing function in elderly patients with hypertensive disease: age peculiarities. Adv Gerontol. 2010;23(4):530–542.
326. Forman JP, Curhan GC, Schemhammer ES. Urinary melatonin and risk of incident hypertension among young women. J Hypetens. 2010;28(3):336–351.
327. van der Zwan LP, Scheffer PG, Teerlink T. Reduction of myeloperoxidase activity by melatonin and pycnogenol may contribute to their blood pressure lowering effect. Hypertension. 2010;56(3):e35.
328. Li HL, Kang YM, Yu L, Xu HY, Zhao H. Melatonin reduces blood pressure in rats with stress-induced hypertension via GABAA receptors. Clin Exp Pharmacol. 2009;36(4):436–440.
329. Simko F, Paulis L. Melatonin as a potential antihypertensive treatment. J Pineal Res. 2007;42(4):319–322.
330. Irmak MK, Sizlan A. Essential hypertension seems to result from melatonin-induced epigenetic modifications in area postrema. Med Hypthesis. 2006;66(5):1000–1007.
331. De-Leersnyder H, de Biois MC, Vekemans M, Sidi D, Villain E, Kindermans C, Munnich A. Beta (1) adrenergic antagonists improve sleep and behavioural disturbances in a circadian disorder, Smith-Magenis syndrome. J Med Genet. 2010;38(9):586–590.
332. Rodella LF, Favero G, Foglio E, Rossini C, Castrezzati S, Lonati C, Rezzani R. Vascular endothelial cells and dysfunctions: role of melatonin. Front Biosci. 2013;5:119–129.
333. Grossman E, Laudon M, Zisapel N. Effect of melatonin on nocturnal blood pressure: meta-analysis of randomized controlled trials. Vasc Health Risk Manag. 2011;7:577–584.
334. Scheer FA, Morris CJ, Garcia JI, Smales C, Kelly EE, Marks J, Malhotra A, Shea SA. Repeated melatonin supplementation improves sleep in hypertensive patients treated with beta-blockers: a randomized controlled trial. Sleep. 2012;35:1395–1402.
335. Zaslavskaya RM, Lilitsa GV, Dilmagambetova GS, Halberg F, Cornélissen G, Otsuka K, Singh RB, Stoynev A, Ikonomov O, Tarquini R, Perfetto F, Schwartzkopff O, Bakken EE. Melatonin, refractory hypertension, myocardial ischemia and other challenges in nightly blood pressure lowering. Biomed Pharmacother. 2004;58(S1):S129–S134.
336. Sun H, Gusdon AM, Qu S. Effects of melatonin on cardiovascular diseases: progress in the past year. Curr Opin Lipidol. 2016 Aug;27(4):408–413.
337. Feringa HH, Laskey DA, Dickson JE, Coleman CI. The effect of grape seed extract on cardiovascular risk markers: a meta-analysis of randomized controlled trials. J Am Diet Assoc. 2011;111(8):1173–1181.

338. Sivaprakasapillai B, Edirsinghe K, Randolph J, Steinberg F, Kappagoda T. Effect of grape seed extract on blood pressure in subjects with the metabolic syndrome. Metabolism. 2009;58(12):1743–1746.
339. Edirisinghe I, Burton-Freeman B, Tissa Kappagoda C. Mechanism of the endothelium-dependent relaxation evoked by grape seed extract. Clin Sci (Lond). 2008;114(4):331–337.
340. Zhang H, Liu S, Li L, Liu S, Liu S, Mi J, Tian G. The impact of grape seed extract treatment on blood pressure changes: a meta-analysis of 16 randomized controlled trials. Medicine (Baltimore). 2016;95(33):e4247.
341. Park E, Edirisinghe I, Choy YY, Waterhouse A, Burton-Freeman B. Effects of grape seed extract beverage on blood pressure and metabolic indices in individuals with pre-hypertension: a randomised, double-blinded, two-arm, parallel, placebo-controlled trial. Br J Nutr. 2016 Jan;115(2):226–238.
342. Clements WT, Lee SR, Bloomer RJ. Nitrate ingestion: a review of the health and physical performance effects. Nutrients. 2014;6:5224–5264.
343. Kapil V, Milsom AB, Okorie M, Maleki-Toyserkani S, Akram F, Rehman F, Arghandawi S, Pearl V, Benjamin N, Loukogeorgakis S, Macallister R, Hobbs AJ, Webb AJ, Ahluwalia A. Inorganic nitrate supplementation lowers blood pressure in humans: role for nitrite-derived NO. Hypertension. 2010;56:274–281.
344. Kapil V, Khambata RS, Robertson A, Caulfield MJ, Ahluwalia A. Dietary nitrate provides sustained blood pressure lowering in hypertensive patients: a randomized, phase 2, double-blind, placebo-controlled study. Hypertension. 2015;65:320–327.
345. Coles LT, Clifton PM. Effect of beetroot juice on lowering blood pressure in free-living, disease-free adults: a randomized, placebo-controlled trial. Nutr J. 2012;11:106.
346. Siervo M, Lara J, Ogbonmwan I, Mathers JC. Inorganic nitrate and beetroot juice supplementation reduces blood pressure in adults: a systematic review and meta-analysis. J Nutr. 2013;143:818–826.
347. Houston M. Acute effects of an oral nitric oxide supplement on blood pressure, endothelial function, and vascular compliance in hypertensive patients. J Clin Hypertens (Greenwich). 2014;16(7):524–529.
348. Kapil V, Khambata RS, Robertson A, Caulfield MJ, Ahluwalia A. Dietary nitrate provides sustained blood pressure lowering in hypertensive patients: a randomized, phase 2, double-blind, placebo-controlled study. Hypertension. 2015;65(2):320–327.
349. Hobbs DA, Kaffa N, George TW, Methven L, Lovegrove JA. Blood pressure-lowering effects of beetroot juice and novel beetroot-enriched bread products in normotensive male subjects. Br J Nutr. 2012;108(11):2066–2074.
350. Kapil V, Pearl V, Ghosh S, Ahluwalia A. Inorganic nitrate ingestion improves vascular compliance but does not alter flow-mediated dilatation in healthy volunteers. Nitric Oxide. 2012;26(4):197–202.
351. Asgary S, Afshani MR, Sahebkar A, Keshvari M, Taheri M, Jahanian E, Rafieian-Kopaei M, Malekian F, Sarrafzadegan N. Improvement of hypertension, endothelial function and systemic inflammation following short-term supplementation with red beet (*Beta vulgaris* L.) juice: a randomized crossover pilot study. J Hum Hypertens. 2016;30(10):627–632.
352. Bryan NS. Application of nitric oxide in drug discovery and development. Expert Opin Drug Discov. 2011 Nov;6(11):1139–1154.
353. Machha A, Schechter AN. Inorganic nitrate: a major player in the cardiovascular health benefits of vegetables? Nutr Rev. 2012 Jun;70(6):367–372.
354. Liu G, Mi XN, Zheng XX, Xu YL, Lu J, Huang XH. Effects of tea intake on blood pressure: a meta-analysis of randomised controlled trials. Br J Nutr. 2014;112:1043–1054.
355. Hodgson JM, Puddey IB, Burke V, Beilin LJ, Jordan N. Effects on blood pressure of drinking green and black tea. J Hypertens. 1999;17:457–463.

356. Kurita I, Maeda-Yamamoto M, Tachibana H, Kamei M. Anti-hypertensive effect of Benifuuki tea containing *O*-methylated EGCG. J Agric Food Chem. 2010;58(3):1903–1908.
357. McKay DL, Chen CY, Saltzman E, Blumberg JB. *Hibiscus sabdariffa* L. tea (tisane) lowers blood pressure in pre-hypertensive and mildly hypertensive adults. J Nutr. 2010;140(2):298–303.
358. Bogdanski P, Suliburska J, Szulinska M, Stepien M, Pupek-Musialik D, Jablecka A. Green tea extract reduces blood pressure, inflammatory biomarkers, and oxidative stress and improves parameters associated with insulin resistance in obese, hypertensive patients. Nutr Res. 2012 Jun;32(6):421–427.
359. Hodgson JM, Woodman RJ, Puddey IB, Mulder T, Fuchs D, Croft KD. Short-term effects of polyphenol-rich black tea on blood pressure in men and women. Food Funct. 2013 Jan;4(1):111–115.
360. Medina-Remón A, Estruch R, Tresserra-Rimbau A, Vallverdú-Queralt A, Lamuela-Raventos RM. The effect of polyphenol consumption on blood pressure.
361. Jiménez R, Duarte J, Perez-Vizcaino F. Epicatechin: endothelial function and blood pressure. J Agric Food Chem. 2012;60(36):8823–8830.
362. Nogueira LP, Nogueira Neto JF, Klein MR, Sanjuliani AF. Short-term effects of green tea on blood pressure, endothelial function, and metabolic profile in obese prehypertensive women: a crossover randomized clinical trial. J Am Coll Nutr. 2017;36(2):108–115.
363. Wasilewski R, Ubara EO, Klonizakis M. Assessing the effects of a short-term green tea intervention in skin microvascular function and oxygen tension in older and younger adults. Microvasc Res. 2016;107:65–71.
364. Bogdanski P, Suliburska J, Szulinska M, Stepien M, Pupek-Musialik D, Jablecka A. Green tea extract reduces blood pressure, inflammatory biomarkers, and oxidative stress and improves parameters associated with insulin resistance in obese, hypertensive patients. Nutr Res. 2012;32(6):421–427.
365. Yarmolinsky J, Gon G, Edwards P. Effect of tea on blood pressure for secondary prevention of cardiovascular disease: a systematic review and meta-analysis of randomized controlled trials. Nutr Rev. 2015;73(4):236–246.
366. Houston MC. Treatment of hypertension with nutraceuticals, vitamins, antioxidants and minerals. Expert Review of Cardiovascular Therapy. 2007;5:681–691.
367. Miguel-Carrasco JL, Monserrat MT, Mate A, Vázquez CM. Comparative effects of captopril and l-carnitine on blood pressure and antioxidant enzyme gene expression in the heart of spontaneously hypertensive rats. Eur J Pharmacol. 2010;632(1–3):65–72.
368. Zambrano S, Blanca AJ, Ruiz-Armenta MV, Miguel-Carrasco JL, Arévalo M, Vázquez MJ, Mate A, Vázquez CM. L-Carnitine protects against arterial hypertension-related cardiac fibrosis through modulation of PPAR-γ expression. Biochem Pharmacol. 2013;85(7):937–944.
369. Vilskersts R, Kuka J, Svalbe B, Cirule H, Liepinsh E, Grinberga S, Kalvinsh I, Dambrova M. Administration of L-carnitine and mildronate improves endothelial function and decreases mortality in hypertensive Dahl rats. Pharmacol Rep. 2011;63(3):752–762.
370. Mate A, Miguel-Carrasco JL, Monserrat MT, Vázquez CM. Systemic antioxidant properties of L-carnitine in two different models of arterial hypertension. J Physiol Biochem. 2010 Jun;66(2):127–136.
371. Digiesi V, Cantini F, Bisi G, Guarino G, Brodbeck B. L-Carnitine adjuvant therapy in essential hypertension. Clin Ter. 1994;144:391–395.
372. Ghidini O, Azzurro M, Vita G, Sartori G. Evaluation of the therapeutic efficacy of L-carnitine in congestive heart failure. Int J Clin Pharmacol Ther Toxicol. 1988;26(4):217–220.
373. Digiesi V, Palchetti R, Cantini F. The benefits of L-carnitine therapy in essential arterial hypertension with diabetes mellitus type II. Minerva Med. 1989;80(3):227–231.

374. Ruggenenti P, Cattaneo D, Loriga G, Ledda F, Motterlini N, Gherardi G, Orisio S, Remuzzi G. Ameliorating hypertension and insulin resistance in subjects at increased cardiovascular risk: effects of acetyl-L-carnitine therapy. Hypertension. 2009;54(3):567–574.
375. Martina V, Masha A, Gigliardi VR, Brocato L, Manzato E, Berchio A, Mate A, Miguel-Carrasco JL, Vázquez CM. The therapeutic prospects of using L-carnitine to manage hypertension-related organ damage. Drug Discov Today. 2010;15(11–12):484–492.
376. Korkmaz S, Yıldız G, Kılıçlı F, Yılmaz A, Aydın H, Içağasıoğlu S, Candan F. [Low L-carnitine levels: can it be a cause of nocturnal blood pressure changes in patients with type 2 diabetes mellitus?]. Anadolu Kardiyol Derg. 2011;11(1):57–63.
377. Velasquez MT, Ramezani A, Manal A, Raj DS. Trimethylamine N-oxide: the good, the bad and the unknown. Toxins (Basel). 2016;8(11):1–12.
378. He J, Whelton PK. Effect of dietary fiber and protein intake on blood pressure: a review of epidemiologic evidence. Clin Exp Hypertens. 1999;21:785–796.
379. Pruijm M, Wuerzer G, Forni V, Bochud M, Pechere-Bertschi A, Burnier M. Nutrition and hypertension: more than table salt. Rev Med Suisse. 2010;6(282): 1715–1720.
380. Cicero AF, Derosa G, Manca M, Bove M, Borghi C, Gaddi AV. Different effect of psyllium and guar dietary supplementation on blood pressure control in hypertensive overweight patients: a six-month, randomized clinical trial. Clin Exp Hypertens. 2007;29:383–394.
381. Pal S, Khoussousi A, Binns C, Dhaliwal S, Radavelli-Bagatini S. The effects of 12-week psyllium fibre supplementation or healthy diet on blood pressure and arterial stiffness in overweight and obese individuals. Br J Nutr. 2012;107:725–734.
382. Houston MC. Nutrition and nutraceuticals supplements in the treatment of hypertension. Prog Cardiovasc Dis. 2005;47:396–449.
383. Caligiuri SP, Edel AL, Aliani M, Pierce GN. Flaxseed for hypertension: implications for blood pressure regulation. Curr Hypertens Rep. 2014;16:499.
384. Sankar D, Sambandam G, Ramskrishna Rao M, Pugalendi KV. Modulation of blood pressure, lipid profiles and redox status in hypertensive patients taking different edible oils. Clin Chim Acta. 2005;355(1–2):97–104.
385. Sankar D, Rao MR, Sambandam G, Pugalendi KV. Effect of sesame oil on diuretics or beta-blockers in the modulation of blood pressure, athropometry, lipid profile and redox status. Yale J Biol Med. 2006;79(1):19–26.
386. Miyawaki T, Aono H, Toyoda-Ono Y, Maeda H, Kiso Y, Moriyama K. Anti-hypertensive effects of sesamin in humans. J Nutr Sci Vitaminol (Toyko). 2009;55(1):87–91.
387. Wichitsranoi J, Weerapreeyakui N, Boonsiri P, Settasatian N, Komanasin N, Sirjaichingkul S, Teerajetgul Y, Rangkadilok N, Leelayuwat N. Antihypertensive and antioxidant effects of dietary black sesame meal in pre-hypertensive humans. Nutr J. 2011;10(1):82–88.
388. Sudhakar B, Kalaiarasi P, Al-Numair KS, Chandramohan G, Rao RK, Pugalendi KV. Effect of combination of edible oils on blood pressure, lipid profile, lipid peroxidative markers, antioxidant status, and electrolytes in patients with hypertension on nifedipine treatment. Saudi Med J. 2011;32(4):379–385.
389. Sankar D, Rao MR, Sambandam G, Pugalendi KV. A pilot study of open label sesame oil in hypertensive diabetics. J Med Food. 2006;9(3):408–412.
390. Harikumar KB, Sung B, Tharakan ST, Pandey MK, Joy B, Guha S, Krishnan S, Aggarwai BB. Sesamin manifests chemopreventive effects through the suppression of NF-kappa-B-regulated cell survival, proliferation, invasion and angiogenic gene products. Mol Cancer Res. 2010;8(5):751–761.

391. Nakano D, Ogura K, Miyakoshi M, Ishii F, Kawanishi H, Kuramazuka D, Kwak CJ, Ikemura K, Takaoka M, Moriguchi S, Ling T, Kusomoto A, Asami S, ShibataK, Kis Y, Matsumura Y. Antihyptensive effect of angiotensin I-converting enzyme inhibitory peptides from a sesame protein hydrolysate in spontaneously hypertensive rats. Biosci Biotechnol Biochem. 2006;70(5):1118–1126.
392. Karatzi K, Stamatelopoulos K, Lykka M, Mantzouratou P, Skalidi S, Manios E, Georgiopoulos G, Zakopoulos N, Papamichael C, Sidossis LS. Acute and long-term hemodynamic effects of sesame oil consumption in hypertensive men. J Clin Hypertens (Greenwich). 2012;14(9):630–636.
393. Morand C, Dubray C, Milenkovic D, Lioger D, Martin JF, Scalber A, Mazur A. Hesperidin contributes to the vascular protective effects of orange juice: a randomized crossover study in healthy volunteers. Am J Clin Nutr. 2011;93(1):73–80.
394. Massarenti P, Settanni F, Della Casa L, Bergamini S, Iannone A. Long-term *N*-acetylcysteine and L-arginine administration reduces endothelial activation and systolic blood pressure in hypertensive patients with type 2 diabetes. Diabetes Care. 2008;31(5):940–944.
395. Jiang B, Haverty M, Brecher P. *N*-acetyl-L-cysteine enhances interleukin-1beta-induced nitric oxide synthase expression. Hypertension. 1999;34(4 Pt 1):574–579.
396. Vasdev S, Singal P, Gill V. The antihypertensive effect of cysteine. Int J Angiol. 2009;18(1):7–21.
397. Meister A, Anderson ME, Hwang O. Intracellular cysteine and glutathione delivery systems. J Am Coll Nutr. 1986;5(2):137–151.
398. Asher GN, Viera AJ, Weaver MA, Dominik R, Caughey M, Hinderliter AL. Effect of hawthorn standardized extract on flow mediated dilation in prehypertensive and mildly hypertensive adults: a randomized, controlled cross-over trial. BMC Complement Altern Med. 2012;12:26–30.
399. Koçyildiz ZC, Birman H, Olgaç V, Akgün-Dar K, Melikoğlu G, Meriçli AH. Crataegus tanacetifolia leaf extract prevents L-NAME-induced hypertension in rats: a morphological study. Phytother Res. 2006;20(1):66–70.
400. Schröder D, Weiser M, Klein P. Efficacy of a homeopathic *Crataegus* preparation compared with usual therapy for mild (NYHA II) cardiac insufficiency: results of an observational cohort study. Eur J Heart Fail. 2003;5(3):319–326.
401. Walker AF, Marakis G, Simpson E, Hope JL, Robinson PA, Hassanein M, Simpson HC. Hypotensive effects of hawthorn for patients with diabetes taking prescription drugs: a randomised controlled trial. Br J Gen Pract. 2006;56(527):437–443.
402. Walker AF, Marakis G, Morris AP, Robinson PA. Promising hypotensive effect of hawthorn extract: a randomized double-blind pilot study of mild, essential hypertension. Phytother Res. 2002;16(1):48–54.
403. Larson A, Witman MA, Guo Y, Ives S, Richardson RS, Bruno RS, Jalili T, Symons JD. Acute, quercetin-induced reductions in blood pressure in hypertensive individuals are not secondary to lower plasma angiotensin-converting enzyme activity or endothelin-1: nitric oxide. Nutr Res. 2012;32(8):557–564.
404. Edwards RL, Lyon T, Litwin SE, Rabovsky A, Symons JD, Jalili T. Quercetin reduces blood pressure in hypertensive subjects. J Nutr. 2007;137(11):2405–2411.
405. Egert S, Bosy-Westphal A, Seiberl J, Kürbitz C, Settler U, Plachta-Danielzik S, Wagner AE, Frank J, Schrezenmeir J, Rimbach G, Wolffram S, Müller MJ. Quercetin reduces systolic blood pressure and plasma oxidised low-density lipoprotein concentrations in overweight subjects with a high-cardiovascular disease risk phenotype: a double-blinded, placebo-controlled cross-over study. Br J Nutr. 2009;102(7):1065–1074.
406. Khalesi S, Sun J, Buys N, Jayasinghe R. Effect of probiotics on blood pressure: a systematic review and meta-analysis of randomized, controlled trials. Hypertension. 2014;64:897–903.

407. de Sousa VP, Cavalcanti Neto MP, Magnani M, Braga VA, da Costa-Silva JH, Leandro CG, Vidal H, Pirola L. New insights on the use of dietary polyphenols or probiotics for the management of arterial hypertension. Front Physiol. 2016;7:448–460.
408. Hendijani F, Akbari V. Probiotic supplementation for management of cardiovascular risk factors in adults with type II diabetes: a systematic review and meta-analysis. Clin Nutr. 2018;37(2):532–541. doi: 10.1016/j.clnu.2017.02.015.
409. Robles-Vera I, Toral M, Romero M, Jiménez R, Sánchez M, Pérez-Vizcaíno F, Duarte J. Antihypertensive effects of probiotics. Curr Hypertens Rep. 2017;19(4):26.
410. Dairi DB, Lee BH, Oh DH. Current perspectives on antihypertensive probiotics. Probiotics Antimicrob Proteins. 2017;9(2):91–101.
411. Trovato A, Nuhlicek DN, Midtling JE. Drug-nutrient interactions. Am Fam Physician. 1991;44(5):1651–1658.
412. McCabe BJ, Frankel EH, Wolfe JJ, Editors. Handbook of Food-Drug Interactions. CRC Press, Boca Raton, FL, 2003.
413. Houston MC. The role of cellular micronutrient analysis and minerals in the prevention and treatment of hypertension and cardiovascular disease. Ther Adv Cardiovasc Dis. 2010;4:165–183.
414. Zeraatkar D, Johnston BC, Bartoszko J, Cheung K, Bala MM, Valli C, Rabassa M, Sit D, Milio K, Sadeghirad B, Agarwal A, Zea AM, Lee Y, Han MA, Vernooij RWM, Alonso-Coello P, Guyatt GH, El Dib R. Effect of lower versus higher red meat intake on cardiometabolic and cancer outcomes: a systematic review of randomized trials. Ann Intern Med. 2019;171(10):721–731. doi: 10.7326/M19-0622.
415. Vernooij RWM, Zeraatkar D, Han MA, El Dib R, Zworth M, Milio K, Sit D, Lee Y, Gomaa H, Valli C, Swierz MJ, Chang Y, Hanna SE, Brauer PM, Sievenpiper J, de Souza R, Alonso-Coello P, Bala MM, Guyatt GH, Johnston BC. Patterns of red and processed meat consumption and risk for cardiometabolic and cancer outcomes: a systematic review and meta-analysis of cohort studies. Ann Intern Med. 2019;171(10): 732–741. 10.7326/M19-1583.
416. Han MA, Zeraatkar D, Guyatt GH, Vernooij RWM, El Dib R, Zhang Y, Algarni A, Leung G, Storman D, Valli C, Rabassa M, Rehman N, Parvizian MK, Zworth M, Bartoszko JJ, Lopes LC, Sit D, Bala MM, Alonso-Coello P, Johnston BC. Reduction of red and processed meat intake and cancer mortality and incidence: a systematic review and meta-analysis of cohort studies. Ann Intern Med. 2019;171(10):711–720. doi: 10.7326/M19-0699.
417. PTeunissen-Beekman KF. Protein supplementation lowers blood pressure in overweight adults: effect of dietary proteins on blood pressure (PROPRES), a randomized trial. Am J Clin Nutr. 2012 Apr;95(4):966–971.
418. Buendia JR, Bradlee ML, Singer MR, Moore LL. Diets higher in protein predict lower high blood pressure risk in Framingham Offspring Study adults. Am J Hypertens. 2015;28(3):372–379.
419. Zheng Z, Xing T, Yu-Lu W, Lin Z, Jia-Ying X, Li-Qiang Q. Effect of pycnogenol supplementation on blood pressure: a systematic review and meta-analysis. Iran J Public Health. 2018;47(6):779–787.

16 Life Style Changes and Blood Pressure

Non-pharmacologic (Drug) Treatment of High Blood Pressure

1. **Exercise: The ABCT (Aerobics, Build, Contour, and Tone) Exercise Program**
2. **Weight, Body Fat, and Visceral Fat Reduction**
3. **Stop Smoking**
4. **Alcohol Reduction**
5. **Caffeine Reduction or Discontinuation**
6. **Relaxation, Stress Reduction, and Breathing**
7. **Sleep**

Non-pharmacologic or lifestyle therapy should be an initial and adjunctive treatment to all the supplements and drugs and should be continued during therapy to enhance efficacy, reduce the dose and number of drugs, limit adverse effects, and promote cardiovascular health. In a compliant patient, these measures can be an effective means of blood pressure reduction. Let us take a look at each of these in more detail.

16.1 EXERCISE

16.1.1 The ABCT (Aerobics, Build, Contour, and Tone) Exercise Program to Lower Blood Pressure and Reduce Cardiovascular Disease

Exercise has numerous health benefits such as lowering blood pressure (Tables 16.1 and 16.2). Prior to starting any exercise program, it is necessary to consult with your physician for medical clearance with a history, physical exam, and cardiopulmonary exercise testing to be sure that you do not have heart disease, marked elevations in blood pressure with exercise, or other contraindications to an exercise program. Then the exercise should be slowly progressive until training is achieved. You should do a combination of aerobic training (AT) and resistance training (RT) for at least 60 minutes/day at least 6 days/week to lower blood pressure and reduce cardiovascular risk. The aerobic exercises should be for 20 min/day to 60–80% of maximal aerobic capacity (MAC) for age:

$$\text{MAC} = \text{MHR (maximal heart rate)} = (220 - \text{age}).$$

TABLE 16.1
Exercise Activities and Kilocalories Used

Energy Values in Kilocalories per Hour of Selected Activities						
Weight (lb.)	95	125	155	185	215	245
Slow walking	86	114	140	168	196	222
Fast walking	172	228	280	336	392	555
Hiking	285	342	420	504	588	666
Jogging	430	570	700	840	980	1110
Running	480	770	945	1134	1323	1499
Heavy work	194	256	315	378	441	500
Sweeping	108	142	175	210	245	278
Scrubbing	237	313	385	462	539	611
Tennis	301	399	490	588	686	777
Golf (walk)	237	313	385	462	539	611
Golf (in cart)	151	200	245	294	343	389
Swimming (light laps)	344	456	560	672	784	888
Swimming (hard laps)	430	570	700	840	980	1,110

RT should be for 40 minutes/day alternating muscle groups each day such as upper or lower body exercises. RT should be progressive, initially with lighter weights to avoid elevations in blood pressure, if not done under supervision. Progressive RT under supervision will improve lean muscle mass, improve insulin sensitivity, and lower blood pressure. Once the patient has optimal cardiovascular conditioning, the blood pressure will fall about 11/8 mmHg. This is equal to one blood pressure lowering medication. Exercise increases nitric oxide, improves endothelial function, increases coronary artery blood flow, dilates arteries, lowers insulin resistance and reduces inflammation. Table 16.1 shows various exercises that you can do and the number of kilocalories burned (a kilocalorie = 1000 calories).

Skeletal muscle is a secretory/endocrine organ and exercise increases the metabolic and secretory/endocrine capacity of muscle. (1) Specific kinds of exercise can alter the ways genes function and how they interact with cells. (1) By triggering the right exercise-gene interactions, inflammation, oxidative stress and immune dysfunction are improved. (1)

The slow physical deterioration of the cardiovascular system and body in general that is seen with age is not inevitable. It is largely the result of diet and movement – or the lack thereof. Movement is one of the primary keys to overall health and especially cardiovascular health. The movement required is the same kind of natural movement that kept humans in robust physical health for millennia. This is not the kind of exercise that most personal trainers, fitness enthusiasts, or doctors recommend. As a matter of fact, most doctors and trainers recommend the exact opposite approach to movement and exercise, one that may actually accelerate deterioration of health, cardiovascular benefits, and overall aging. There is an optimal type and duration of exercise that is required to improve health. It is important to avoid the overtraining syndrome which actually increases muscle breakdown, elevates cortisol

TABLE 16.2
ABCT Exercise Program Health Benefits Summary of the Aerobics, Build, Contour, and Tone Exercise Program

The ABCT Exercise Program has numerous positive effects on body and mind, much more than the typical aerobic-based programs. Among other things, it:

- Reduces risk of heart disease and heart attack, and lowers risk of recurrent heart attack
- Improves heart function
- Lowers blood pressure and reduces risk of developing hypertension
- Reduces total cholesterol, triglycerides, and LDL
- Increases HDL
- Reduces body weight and body fat
- Reduces clotting tendencies
- Lowers blood sugar and decreases risk of diabetes
- Improves insulin sensitivity
- Improves all abnormalities of metabolic syndrome
- Improves immune function
- Reduces risk of stroke
- Reduces risk of certain cancers, such as colon, breast, and prostate
- Improves memory and focus and reduces risk of Alzheimer's Disease, disease and dementia
- Improves skin tone and, elasticity and decreases wrinkles
- Improves depression, stress, and anxiety, and overall psychological well-being
- Improves sleep
- ABCT stands for Aerobics, Build, Contour, and Tone. It has additional meanings that help define its goals:
    - A = Aerobics, plus action and adaptation. The program focuses on the types of action best suited for muscle and cardiovascular conditioning. You will adapt to new exercises so your muscles do not accommodate or become "used to" to the same daily training.
    - B = Build, plus bulk, burn, and breathe. The program builds and increases muscle strength more than any other exercise regimen you have tried before. (Males will build bulk, while women generally do not increase bulk but will instead tone, firm, and sculpture, due to hormonal differences.) You'll use the muscle burn to best advantage. And with proper breathing, you'll increase oxygen consumption while removing carbon dioxide to improve cardiovascular and muscle conditioning and function, while reducing fatigue.
    - C = Contour, plus core and controlling your genes, and core. Muscular exercise regulates the expression of over more than four hundred 400 genes that mediate the beneficial effects of physical activity. In addition to aerobics and resistance exercise, you will practice core exercises that improve abdominal and back muscular strength while increasing flexibility and balance.
    - T = Tone, plus trim and tight. You will trim away total fat, as well as central or visceral body fat, lose weight, and increase your lean muscle mass. Your muscles, subcutaneous tissue, and skin will become tight and look more youthful.

levels increases sympathetic tone, increases oxidative stress and inflammation, and results in the opposite effects that one desires. The power of exercise relates to the numerous hormones, mediators, and signaling molecules that lower blood pressure, blood sugar and cholesterol that are released with the proper type of exercise that influence genes, inflammation, oxidative stress, and immune function.

The ABCT (Aerobics, Build, Contour, and Tone) exercise program is a modern way of exercising the way our ancestors did. The program is specifically designed to get the muscles and body moving in short burns of intense activity, mixing anaerobic with just enough aerobic exercise to improve cardiovascular health, overall health and conditioning. (1–13) In addition, proper nutrition is emphasized before, during and after exercise training. (14–41) The ABCT exercise program has numerous positive effects on body and mind. The ABCT exercise program is simple, effective, scientifically proven, and adaptable to everyone's exercise needs. It allows for optimal training benefits in a shorter period of time to build and tone muscle, reduce body and visceral fat, lose weight, improve hormone levels, lower inflammation and oxidation, decrease blood sugar, reduce blood pressure, improve the lipid profile, improve one's quality of life, increase life expectancy, and slow the aging process. In addition, this type of exercise avoids overtraining associated with increased cortisol levels, catabolic effects on muscle, or chronic fatigue.

16.2 THE ABCs OF EXERCISE WITH A TWIST

The most efficient and effective means of achieving all the health benefits of exercise is to combine interval aerobic training (AE) with anaerobic or resistance exercise or RT in a way that causes body restoration and proper muscle growth and efficiency. The ABCT exercise program represents ABCT and is designed for both genders and allows for specific outcomes (Table 16.3). It has additional meanings that help define its goals.

- **A = Aerobics**, plus action and adaptation – The program focuses on the types of action best suited for muscle and cardiovascular conditioning to adapt to new exercises so muscles do not accommodate to the same daily training.
- **B = Build**, plus bulk, burn, and breathe – The program builds and increases muscle strength more than any other exercise regimen while learning to use muscle burn to the best advantage with proper breathing to increase oxygen consumption and eliminating carbon dioxide to improve cardiovascular and muscle conditioning and function while reducing fatigue.
- **C = Contour**, plus core and controlling your genes – Muscular exercise regulates the expression of more than four hundred genes that mediate the beneficial effects of physical activity. In addition to aerobics and resistance exercise, this program will combine core exercises that improve abdominal and back muscle strength as well as exercises for flexibility and balance.
- **T = Tone**, plus trim and tight – Total body fat, visceral body fat, and body weight are decreased while lean muscle mass increases.

The ABCT exercise program emphasizes interval aerobic and anaerobic resistance movements. Proper warm up and stretching before beginning every exercise session and of cooling down and stretching again when finished are mandatory to avoid muscle, tendon, and ligament injuries while promoting the flexibility that's necessary for exercising.

TABLE 16.3
Recommended Exercises for ABCT Fitness with Aerobic Intervals and Resistance Training Based on Time Schedule

15 MINUTES: Aerobic intervals for 5 minutes
- Resistance training for 10 minutes
- Two upper body exercises with ABCT 1
- Two lower body exercises
- One core exercise

30 MINUTES: Aerobic intervals for 10 minutes
- Resistance training for 20 minutes
- Three upper body exercises with ABCT 1 and 2
- Two lower body exercises
- One core exercises
- One flexibility exercise

45 MINUTES: Aerobic intervals for 15 minutes
- Resistance training for 30 minutes
- Three upper body exercises with ABCT 1, 2, and 3
- Three lower body exercises
- Two core exercises
- One flexibility exercise

60 MINUTES: Aerobic intervals for 20 minutes
- Resistance training for 40 minutes
- Four upper body exercises with ABCT 1, 2, 3, and 4
- Three lower body exercises
- Two core exercises
- One flexibility exercise

90 MINUTES: Aerobic intervals for 30 minutes
- Resistance training for 60 minutes
- Five upper body exercises with ABCT 1, 2 3, 4, and 5
- Three lower body exercises
- Two core exercises
- One flexibility exercise

120 MINUTES: Aerobic intervals for 40 minutes
- Resistance training for 80 minutes
- Six upper body exercises with ABCT 1, 2, 3, 4, and 5
- Four lower body exercises
- Three core exercises
- Two flexibility exercises

Before embarking on an exercise program of any kind or changing the exercise regimen, you already have a complete history, physical exam, labs, cardiovascular risk factor analysis, and cardiopulmonary exercise test are suggested. Interval training with rapid bursts of activity may precipitate plaque rupture in a coronary artery in some predisposed individuals and result in a myocardial infarction or heart attack.

16.3 THE ELEMENTS OF ABCT

Here are the main elements of ABCT, each of which will later be discussed in more detail.

- RT – Weight lifting modified properly will encourage optimal muscle physiology and release of hormones, mediators, and interleukins. ABCT uses graduated weights and variable repetitions. In brief, initially lift the heaviest weight possible 12 times to get the muscle burn, then decrease the weight with each subsequent set but keep increasing the number of times that weight is lifted. This maximizes post-exercise oxygen consumption, depletes glycogen, and increases the production of lactic acid to achieve all the muscle-, hormone-, cytokine-, and interleukin-stimulating effects that lead to the health benefits of exercise.
- Aerobic Training in Intervals – Jogging, swimming, biking, and other forms of continual movement should be done at specific levels of submaximal and MAC or estimated heart rate for age and level of exercise (maximum heart rate [MHR]). The best technique is aerobic interval training, which consists of short periods ranging from 20 seconds to 2 minutes of "burst" aerobic training of varying intensities, depending on one's present level of exercise conditioning. This more closely mimics the natural activities we evolved to perform and benefit from and strings together several periods of intense and semi-intense activity into a single, longer exercise period that still burns calories and builds endurance.
- Proper Ratio of Aerobic Training to RT – The optimal ratio of resistance to interval aerobic training should be 2:1. For example, during a 60-minute workout, you would perform 40 minutes of RT and 20 minutes of interval aerobics, with the aerobics coming after the RT.
- Core Exercises – Exercises designed to improve abdominal and back strength while increasing flexibility. These exercises are important for the core (abdomen and lower back), which is often neglected.
- Time-Intense Exercise – Rather than methodically working one muscle or muscle group after another, then doing the aerobic exercises – or even saving the aerobics for the next day – ABCT challenges the body by combining exercises as much as possible. For example, instead of doing leg squats followed by shoulder presses, with ABCT they are done at the same time, mimicking the real-life movements,
- Busy Rest Periods – These are used to insert small bursts of aerobic exercises into the RT period.
- Water and the ABCT Energy Shake – Drinking plenty of water while working out is vital. (If you get thirsty during the workout, you have waited too long to drink.) You must drink water before beginning to exercise, at set intervals during exercise, and afterwards. Your water should be of high quality and not from plastic containers, due to the risk of certain chemical compounds like PCBs (polychorobeniprienes and triglycerides) that get into the water from the plastic. In addition, about 10 minutes after

starting your workout, you begin consuming an energy drink consisting of fresh orange juice (4 oz) and water (6 oz), d-ribose (5 g), and whey protein (30 g) to provide ATP and energy as well as nutritional substrates to maximize exercise performance and increase muscle strength and performance as well as lean muscle mass (1, 14–24).

- Exercise in the Morning – Exercising in the morning after a 12-hour fast is best for numerous reasons, including the fact that an empty stomach optimizes fat burning, interleukin 10 (IL-10) which lowers inflammation but increases the myokine surges. This results in an increase in muscle strength, bulk, tone and contour, as well as weight and body fat loss, improved energy level, focus and concentration during the day.
- Exercise on an Empty Stomach – Begin exercising on an empty stomach after a 12-hour fast, except for water and whey protein consumed about 10 minutes before exercise, and have nothing but more water and the energy drink while exercising. This allows for depletion of liver and muscle glycogen while generating maximal surges of IL-10. It also increases fat burning and accelerates weight and fat loss from both inside and outside the skeletal muscle.
- Push and Rest – Exercise to maximal effort during each set until "the burn" is significant. The burn should be severe and last for about 4–5 seconds after you stop the exercise. Then rest for 60 seconds before beginning the next set of exercises. You may take 3-second rest periods between repetitions, if necessary. Also performing supersets with minimal rest between sets of exercises or use the rest period for core exercises or alternative upper or lower body exercises will improve the time intensity of the exercise session.
- Exercise Daily, Utilizing Cross-Training – To achieve the best results, perform interval aerobic and RT at least 6 days/week, or if desired every day but alternate the muscle groups for upper and lower body as well as the type of aerobic exercise performed. It is important to change the exercise routine every few weeks to avoid "muscle accommodation" to the exercise regimen.
- Breathe – Mastering proper breathing techniques will ensure ample oxygenation for the muscle performance, as well as prompt the removal of carbon dioxide.

16.4 THE ABCT ELEMENTS IN DETAIL

16.4.1 Resistance Training

ABCT RT takes a radically different approach, mixing heavier weights and lower repetitions with lower weights and greater repetitions to increase the lactic acid burn as well as to maximize muscle contractions and the release of muscle enzymes (myokines). With ABCT, the real goal is not only to bulk and to contour the muscles but to use muscle movements to improve body biochemistry and improve blood pressure, cardiovascular health, and overall health.

ABCT RT is based on five sets, each with a different number of repetitions in each set. Here's the ABCT Five-Set Schedule that starts with the heaviest weight with low repetitions and advances to lighter weight with increasing repetitions.

- ABCT Set 1: 12 repetitions at maximum weight
- ABCT Set 2: 18 repetitions at 75% of maximum weight
- ABCT Set 3: 24 repetitions at 50% of maximum weight
- ABCT Set 4: 50 repetitions at 25% of maximum weight
- ABCT Set 5: 12 repetitions at maximum weight

ABCT Five-Set schedule should be phased in slowly to avoid injury or excessive fatigue, depending on one's present level of physical conditioning.

- Beginners: ABCT 1, or ABCT 1 and 2.
- Intermediate: ABCT 1, 2, and 3
- Advanced: ABCT 1, 2, 3, and 4
- Professional: ABCT 1, 2, 3, 4, and 5

This burn scale can be used as a guide to the exercise level. The idea is to attempt to score a 5 multiple times during your workouts, stopping only briefly (3 seconds) to clear the burn before continuing again.

1. No burn in the muscle
2. Light burn
3. Moderate burn
4. Strong burn
5. Intense burn; must rest

16.5 WHAT, HOW, AND WHEN TO LIFT

Descriptions of the key ABCT resistance exercises are found at the end of the chapter under the heading "Getting Started with ABCT: Training Session Schedules and Descriptions of the Lifts".

16.6 UPPING THE INTENSITY WITH SUPERSETS, HYBRIDS, AND RAPID SETS

Simply following the ABCT 5-Set Schedule will improve blood pressure, cardiovascular and general health. Incorporating hybrids, supersets, and rapid sets as one gains strength and endurance will improve exercise outcomes.

1. Hybrids are two exercises performed at once; i.e., do a full leg squat while also performing an overhead press. Using more muscles simultaneously increases the burn, lactic acid, release of IL-10, and post-exercise oxygen consumption.
2. Supersets are exercises done back to back, with almost no rest period between (15 seconds maximum). These can be the same exercise, such as

biceps curls back to back, or different exercises, such as a biceps curl followed immediately by a triceps lift. Supersets dramatically increase the burn and other beneficial effects of exercise. Supersets should be done only after one has trained for some time to avoid overuse injury or excessive heart rate.

3. Rapid sets are sets performed faster than normal to compress the workout time, enhance mechanical and metabolic burnout, and improve both resistance and aerobic conditioning. For example, with a biceps curl, increase the speed from 1 every second to 2 every 3 seconds.

16.7 ABCT RESISTANCE TRAINING HINTS

1. Take 3-second breaks along the way, if necessary.
2. Drink water and the ABCT energy drink after each set of exercises.
3. Even if the number of repetitions cannot be done in each set, attempt to push to the limit until the maximum burn occurs.
4. If the percentage reduction in weight is a fraction of a number, round up to the next highest whole number on the weight system you are using. This may be 1 or 5 lb. in most systems.

16.7.1 Aerobic Training in Intervals

Aerobic means "with oxygen" and refers to the use of oxygen in the body's metabolic processes. Aerobic training consists of continuous movements that demand more oxygen consumption and ultimately improve the body's oxygen use. Rapid walking, jogging, running, swimming, bicycling, dancing, and aerobics classes can all be aerobic exercises if they keep the body in moderate-to-intense motion for a moderately long period of time, with an elevated heart rate representing the body's heightened level of activity.

For best results, aerobic training should be broken up into periods of differing intensities or interval training with differing lengths and intensities. In general, the interval would be at 90% of MHR for a period of time followed by 50% of MHR for one to three times that period depending on conditioning. For example, a 30-second sprint would be followed by at 30 to 90-second slow jog.

For best results, an interval aerobic exercise program should consist of a 5-minute warm-up period, followed by moderate to intense interval training involving large

ONE TO THREE

The ideal ratio for aerobic interval training is 1:3. This means for every unit of time spent exercising at 90% of your maximal heart rate, spend an additional three units of time exercising at 50% of MHR. Then you repeat this 1:3 sequence about six times over about 20 minutes. The MHR calculation is shown next.

and multiple muscle groups lasting about 20 minutes, followed by a cooling-down period of about 5 minutes at the end.

Aerobic sessions should utilize cross-training, by rotating through different aerobic activities to improve cardiovascular and muscle performance. For example, jog or run on Monday, Wednesday, and Friday; swim on Tuesday and Thursday; bike on Saturday and Sunday.

16.8 MAXIMUM HEART RATE AND MAXIMUM AEROBIC CAPACITY

- MHR Calculation – 220 minus age gives the MAC, and then multiply by the desired heart rate, which should range between 50 and 90% depending on level of exercise and age.

For example, if you are age 40 the MAC would be 220–40 or 180. If you wanted to push to 80% of MAC then multiply 180 × .80 = 144 beats/min as MHR.

16.8.1 Always Combine Resistance and Aerobic Exercises

The optimal ratio is two parts RT to one part interval aerobic training, with the RT first. Here's how the ratio works out with differing total exercise time frames.

- 15 minutes total = 10 minutes of RT, 5 minutes of aerobic training
- 30 minutes total = 20 minutes of RT, 10 minutes of aerobic training
- 45 minutes total = 30 minutes of RT, 15 minutes of aerobic training
- 60 minutes total = 40 minutes of RT, 20 minutes of aerobic training

16.9 CORE EXERCISES

Exercising body core such as the belly and lower back increases abdominal and back strength while improving flexibility and balance. These can be done in sets of one to four per exercise, with the number of repetitions necessary to create the same burn that one gets with the resistance weight training program. Doing the core exercises during the 60-second break periods while the upper or lower body muscles are resting will improve the time efficiency of the workout. Core exercises include sit-ups, abdominal crunches, leg lifts, and leg scissor crosses.

16.10 TIME-INTENSIVE EXERCISE

Two additional steps are required to efficiently and effectively build muscle strength, tone, and contour while simultaneously improving cardiovascular conditioning and cardiovascular health: time-intensive resistance exercises and combined aerobic and RT.

1. Time-Intensive Resistance Exercises – Performing time-intense exercises requires using multiple and large muscle groups simultaneously, with

minimal rest periods; for example, lifting light weights over the head while doing deep knee bends. This increases the release of IL-10 and other muscle cytokines, reduces inflammation, increases lactic acid "burn," enhances post-exercise oxygen consumption, builds muscle, optimizes metabolic and hormonal responses, and increases fat metabolism and fat and weight loss.

2. Combined Aerobic and RT – Instead of standing or sitting during the 60-second between-set rest periods, another resistance or aerobic exercise should be done to maintain heart rate and respiratory rate. For example, on completing an upper body exercise, immediately start doing a lower body exercise or a core exercise that engages large muscle groups and requires "big" action. This technique maintains heart rate and provides more cardiovascular and muscular conditioning.

16.11 NUTRITION, WATER, AND ABCT ENERGY DRINK

Nutritional macronutrient and micronutrient intake relative to exercise is important to optimize recovery, enhance subsequent performance, synthesize muscle (anabolism > catabolism) and provide optimal metabolic and nutrient-genetic interaction for muscle signaling (17). During exercise, inflammation and oxidative stress are linked via muscle metabolism and muscle damage (18). Consumption of a carbohydrate supplement immediately after exercise will improve insulin action and synthesize muscle glycogen significantly faster than when the same amount of carbohydrate is consumed 2 hours post-exercise (17). Protein intake and exercise have synergistic effects on increasing the rate of muscle protein synthesis leading to a more positive protein balance but vary depending the timing of the protein intake and the exercise session (17). The timing of whole protein may not be as crucial as the timing of specific amino acid supplements and anabolism (17). Most studies suggest that consuming free amino acids immediately prior to exercise or within 10 minutes of the initiation of exercise is more effective to increase muscle protein accretion compared to consumption after exercise (15, 17). In contrast, whey protein ingestion may be consumed before, during or after exercise. The effects on muscle anabolism are enhanced with immediate and simultaneous consumption post-exercise of carbohydrates and fats as long as this occurs within less than 2 hours post-exercise. (17) Hydration before, during, and after the exercise program is vital. Two types of hydration are necessary: plain water and the ABCT energy drink. Begin the exercise program well hydrated, drinking about 6 oz of water.

The amount of fluids and water consumed depends on body size, the ambient temperature, and the length and intensity of the workout. As a rule of thumb, 24–32 oz or more of fluid and water are needed during the typical 60-minute workout

Whey protein supplies glutathione precursors is anabolic with an increase in muscle mass, and reduces oxidative stress and inflammation (1, 17). The ingredients in whey help maximize ATP (adenosine triphosphate) production, improve muscle performance, increase muscle mass, and reduce muscle fatigue (1, 17).

16.12 EXERCISE ON AN EMPTY STOMACH (EXCEPT FOR WATER-WHEY MIX)

The exercising program should begin in the morning on an empty stomach, following an 8–12-hour fast, with the exception of drinking water and whey protein that is followed during exercise by and the ABCT Energy Drink.

Consumption of carbohydrates before exercise decreases fat burning and weight loss. Exercising on an empty stomach burns more than twice as much fat as does exercising after consuming carbohydrates. Exercising in a fasting state may increase the utilization of muscle protein for energy slightly, but this effect is relatively small and is minimized when whey protein is consumed.

Optimal exercise benefits occur when skeletal muscle and liver glycogen are depleted. Glycogen depletion triggers the maximal release of IL-10 from muscle, increases muscle growth and fat burning for energy, accelerates fat loss from inside and outside muscle, and improve weight loss. All of this, in turn, reduces inflammation by increasing the levels of IL-10 while lowering other interleukins such as IL-1, IL-6 and increasing the production of testosterone and growth hormone, improving insulin sensitivity and lowering insulin and glucose levels.

The intramuscular triglycerides are metabolized better during glycogen-depleted exercise. The intramuscular triglycerides are far less responsive to insulin which slows the breakdown of stored fat. Exercising while fasting suppresses insulin levels and but maximizes the hormonal and cytokine effects of the exercise program.

HORMONAL CHANGES

Perform ABCT exercises on an empty stomach, after consuming only water and whey,

- testosterone levels increase, enhancing muscle growth, mass, tone, and contour; improving insulin sensitivity, which lowers blood sugar and reduces the risk of diabetes and heart disease; elevating the energy level and libido; and slowing aging.
- growth hormone levels increase, improving muscle growth, mass, tone, and contour; improving energy; increasing the sense of well-being; and slowing aging.
- insulin levels decrease as a result of the improved insulin sensitivity that develops as lean muscle mass increases. (Lean muscle accounts for about 80% of insulin sensitivity or resistance in humans.) These changes help reduce intramuscular triglycerides and extramuscular fat tissue while reducing the risk of heart disease and inflammation.
- cortisol levels drop, improving muscle growth, lowering cholesterol, and TG, reducing blood sugar, and decreasing visceral fat which is associated with inflammation, diabetes, metabolic syndrome, insulin resistance, high blood pressure, elevated cholesterol, cancer, heart disease, and stroke.

16.13 NUTRITION BEFORE, DURING, AND AFTER THE EXERCISE SESSION

Nutrient availability serves as potent modulator of many acute responses and chronic adaptations to both RT and AE. Changes in the macronutrient intake quickly change the concentration of substrates and hormones with alterations in the storage profile of skeletal muscle and other insulin-sensitive organs. This, in turn, regulates the gene expression and cell signaling. Nutrient-exercise interactions activate or inhibit biochemical pathways during training. Proper nutrition after exercise with a breakfast containing fluids, high-quality protein, complex carbohydrates, omega-3 fatty acids, and monounsaturated fatty acids is essential to increase muscle mass and overall muscle performance and cardiovascular conditioning for each subsequent exercise session (42–56).

- A small bowl whole-grain cereal or steel cut oats with whole milk, rice milk, or almond milk.
- 1/2 cup of one of the following: fresh blueberries, raspberries, blackberries, and strawberries.
- 4 oz fresh orange or vegetable juice or another fresh juice, such as pomegranate, grape, or grapefruit or have an orange, grapefruit, grapes or green vegetable like kale, spinach, or broccoli.
- 4-oz of smoked salmon spiced with lemon juice, capers and perhaps add some hot sauce, and jalapeño peppers.
- Whole-wheat toast with omega-3 margarine and raw honey.
- One egg.
- Instead of salmon, you might try tuna or other cold-water fish, lean organic meat (buffalo, elk, venison, beef), organic chicken, or organic turkey.

16.14 GETTING STARTED WITH ABCT: TRAINING SCHEDULES AND DESCRIPTIONS OF THE LIFTS

This section contains different training schedules, ranging from beginner to professional levels,

- Alternate days with the various resistance programs (numbers 1–4) listed next for each of the week's sessions.
- Vary the type of aerobic exercise; for example, running 1 day, swimming the next, and bicycling the third.
- Do the aerobic exercise after the resistance exercises.
- Always do the correct number of sets with each type of ABCT session for the upper body, lower body, core, flexibility, and balance exercises. For example, if you are doing ABCT 1, do only one set for each exercise. With ABCT 2, do two sets for each exercise, with ABCT 3, do three sets for each exercise, and so on.
- Customize the exercise program depending on your goals and time commitment. If you wish to build more muscle, do ABCT 1, 2, and 5; or ABCT 1, 2, 3, and 5. If your goal is to contour and tone, do ABCT 2, 3, and 4. If you wish to have bulk, contour, and tone, then do ABCT 1–5.

16.14.1 The ABCT Training Schedules

Week 1: Beginning Session #1, with ABCT 1

1. RT for 10 minutes: Pick the maximum weight you can do for 12 repetitions, and do one set for each exercise.
   a. 2 upper body exercises: 1 biceps, 1 triceps
   b. 2 lower body exercises: squat, lunges
   c. 1 core: 25–50 or more sit-ups until maximum burn
2. Aerobic exercise for 5 minutes

Week 1: Beginning Session #2, with ABCT 1

3. RT for 10 minutes: Pick the maximum weight you can do for 12 repetitions, and do 1 set for each exercise.
   a. 2 upper body exercises: one chest, one deltoid
   b. 2 lower body exercises: leg press, hamstring press
   c. 1 core: abdominal crunches until maximum burn
4. Aerobic exercise for 5 minutes

Week 1: Beginning Session #3, with ABCT 1

5. RT for 10 minutes: Pick the maximum weight you can do for 12 repetitions, and do 1 set for each exercise.
   a. 2 upper body exercises: 1 shoulder, 1 forearm
   b. 2 lower body exercises: squat with weights, lunges
   c. 1 core: leg lift
6. Aerobic exercise for 5 minutes

Week 1: Beginning Session #4, with ABCT 1

7. RT for 10 minutes: Pick the maximum weight you can do for 12 repetitions, and do 1 set for each exercise.
   a. 2 upper body exercises: 1 reverse biceps curl, 1 pull-down back exercise
   b. 2 lower body exercises: leg press, hamstring press
   c. 1 core: leg scissor crosses
8. Aerobic exercise for 5 minutes

Week 2: Beginning Session #1, with ABCT 1 and 2

9. RT for 20 minutes: Do 12 repetitions at the maximum weight you can do, then 18 repetitions at 75% of original weight.
   a. 3 upper body exercises: 1 chest press, 1 biceps, 1 triceps
   b. 2 lower body exercises: squats, lunges
   c. 1 core exercise: sit-ups
10. Aerobic exercise for 10 minutes

Week 2: Beginning Session #2, with ABCT 1 and 2

11. RT for 20 minutes: Do 12 repetitions at the maximum weight you can do, then 18 repetitions at 75% of original weight.
    a. 3 upper body exercises: 1 chest press, 1 biceps, 1 deltoid
    b. 2 lower body exercise: lunges, hamstring leg press
    c. 1 core exercise: abdominal crunches
12. Aerobic exercise for 10 minutes

Week 2: Beginning Session #3, with ABCT 1 and 2

13. RT for 20 minutes: Do 12 repetitions at the maximum weight you can do, then 18 repetitions at 75% of weight.
    a. 3 upper body exercises: 1 upper shoulder and trapezius, 1 biceps with reverse curl, 1 forearm
    b. 2 lower body exercises: squat with overhead press, quadriceps leg press
    c. 1 core: leg lifts at variable heights
14. Aerobic exercise for 10 minutes

Week 2: Beginning Session #4, with ABCT 1 and 2

15. RT for 20 minutes: Do 12 repetitions at the maximum weight you can do, then 18 repetitions at 75% of weight.
    a. 3 upper body exercises: 1 reverse bicep, 1 pull-down back exercise, 1 chest
    b. 2 lower body exercises: lunges with weights, squats
    c. 1 core: leg scissor crosses
16. Aerobic exercise for 10 minutes

Week 3: Intermediate Session # 1 with ABCT 1 through 3

17. Resistance exercise for 30 minutes with ABCT 1–3: Use maximum weight for 12 repetitions, 75% weight for 18 repetitions, 50% weight for 24 repetitions.
    a. 3 upper body exercises: 1 biceps, 1 chest, 1 triceps
    b. 3 lower body exercises: squat, lunges, quadriceps leg press
    c. 2 core exercises: sit-ups, leg lifts
18. Aerobic exercise for 15 minutes

Week 3: Intermediate Session #2 with ABCT 1 through 3

19. Resistance exercise for 30 minutes with ABCT 1–3: Use maximum weight for 12 repetitions, 75% weight for 18 repetitions, 50% weight for 24 repetitions.
    a. 3 upper body exercises: 1 deltoid, 1 reverse biceps curl, 1 pull-down back exercise
    b. 3 lower body exercises: squats with weights, lunges, hamstring press
    c. 2 core exercises: leg scissor crosses, abdominal crunches
20. Aerobic exercise for 15 minutes

Week 3: Intermediate Session #3 with ABCT 1 through 3

21. Resistance exercise for 30 minutes with ABCT 1–3: Use maximum weight for 12 repetitions, 75% weight for 18 repetitions, 50% weight for 24 repetitions.
    a. 3 upper body exercises: 1 forearm, 1 upper shoulder and trapezius, 1 chest
    b. 3 lower body exercises: lunges with weights, quadriceps leg press, hamstring press
    c. 2 core exercises: leg lifts to chest with floor extension, supine "bicycle" movement with elbows to opposite knees

22. Aerobic exercise for 15 minutes

Week 3: Intermediate Session #4 with ABCT 1 through 3

23. Resistance exercise for 30 minutes with ABCT 1–3: Use maximum weight for 12 repetitions, 75% weight for 18 repetitions, 50% weight for 24 repetitions.
    a. 3 upper body exercises: 1 biceps, 1 triceps, one forearm
    b. 3 lower body exercises: leg quadriceps press, squats, hamstring press
    c. 2 core exercises: leg lifts, sit-ups
24. Aerobic exercise for 15 minutes

Week 4: Advanced Session #1 with ABCT 1 through 4

25. Resistance exercise for 40 minutes with ABCT 1–4: Use maximum weight for 12 repetitions, 75% weight for 18 repetitions, 50% weight for 24 repetitions, 25% weight for 50 repetitions.
    a. 4 upper body exercises: 1 biceps, 1 triceps, 1 shoulder and trapezius, 1 deltoid
    b. 3 lower body exercises: leg quadriceps press, leg hamstring press, squats
    c. 2 core exercises: sit-ups, leg lifts
26. Aerobic exercise for 20 minutes

Week 4: Advanced Session #2 with ABCT 1 through 4

27. Resistance exercise for 40 minutes with ABCT 1–4: Use maximum weight for 12 repetitions, 75% weight for 18 repetitions, 50% weight for 24 repetitions, 25% weight for 50 repetitions.
    a. 4 upper body exercises: 1 pull-down back exercise, 1 reverse curl, 1 forearm, one chest
    b. 3 lower body exercises: lunges, leg quadriceps press, squats
    c. 2 core: abdominal crunches, leg scissor crosses
28. Aerobic exercise for 20 minutes

Week 4: Advanced Session #3 with ABCT 1 through 4

29. Resistance exercise for 40 minutes with ABCT 1–4: Use maximum weight for 12 repetitions, 75% weight for 18 repetitions, 50-% weight for 24 repetitions, 25-% weight for 50 repetitions.
    a. 4 upper body exercises: 1 biceps front curl with reverse curl, 1 chest, 1 deltoid, 1 triceps
    b. 3 lower body exercises: hamstring press, lunges with weights, squats with weights
    c. 2 core: Lay on back and do leg extensions from chest, supine "bicycle" touching opposite elbow to knee
30. Aerobic exercise for 20 minutes

Week 4: Advanced Session #4 with ABCT 1 through 4

31. Resistance exercise for 40 minutes with ABCT 1–4: Use maximum weight for 12 repetitions, 75% weight for 18 repetitions, 50% weight for 24 repetitions, 25% weight for 50 repetitions.
    a. 4 upper body exercises: 1 forearm, 1 biceps, 1 upper shoulder trapezius, 1 pull-down back exercise

    b. 3 lower body exercises: lunges with weights, squats with weights, quadriceps leg press.
    c. 2 core exercises: leg lifts, sit-ups
32. Aerobic exercise for 20 minutes

Week 5 and Beyond: Professional Sessions with ABCT 1 through 5.

33. Resistance exercise for 40 minutes with ABCT 1–5: Use maximum weight for 12 repetitions, 75% for 18 repetitions, 50% weight for 24 repetitions, 25% weight for 50 repetitions, maximum weight for an additional 12 repetitions.
    a. 5 upper body exercises with selection from the following: 1 biceps curl, 1 upper shoulder pull-up, 1 triceps, 1 forward with reverse biceps curl, 1 deltoid, 1 forearm/wrist curl/extension, 1 back pull-down exercise, 1 forearm reverse curl, 1 neck exercise,
    b. 4 lower body exercises with selection from the following: squats, lunges, quadriceps press, hamstring press.
    c. 2–3 core exercises with selection from the following: sit-ups, crunches, leg lifts, leg scissor crosses, leg extensions to chest.
34. Aerobic exercise for 20 minutes

16.14.2 Chest Exercises

Push-up – Position yourself like a plank, on your hands and toes. The hands should be in alignment with the chest, fingers pointing straight forward, with the hands spaced a little wider than shoulder-width apart. The tummy is tucked in, and the butt muscle is down and straight, in alignment with the back. To work different areas of the muscles, the hands can be moved further apart (more chest) or closer together (more triceps).

Primary areas worked: chest

Secondary areas worked: triceps, shoulders

Bench Press – This uses the same movement as a push-up, except you lie on your back and push a weight up instead of raising the body. It can be done with dumbbells, a barbell, or on a machine. It can also be done in an incline or decline position.

Primary areas worked: chest

Secondary areas worked: triceps, shoulders

Dip – Best done on a "dipping bar," where the body is suspended and supported only by the arms. In the beginning position, the legs hang down, the body leans slightly forward, and the arms are fully extended. The elbows bend, and the arms lower the body down, then straighten to raise the body back to the starting position.

Primary areas worked: chest

Secondary areas worked: triceps, shoulders

Chest Fly – Can be performed using either dumbbells or a fly machine. Lie on your back on a bench with your arms out to the sides holding weights (or gripping the machine bars). Arc your arms up and in from the outstretched position until they are pressed together above the chest, with arms straight out and up. Keep a slight bend in the elbows the entire time. Get a good stretch at the bottom of the movement and a good squeeze at the top.

Primary areas worked: chest

Secondary areas worked: front deltoid

Cable Chest Fly – Done on a cable machine, standing, which each hand gripping a handle. Stand with one leg in front of the other, leaning slightly forward, the arms outstretched and back, with elbows slightly bent. The arms are then pulled forward until they are aligned directly in front of the chest.

Primary areas worked: chest

Secondary areas worked: front deltoid

Back Exercises

Back Row – Done with dumbbells (one or two), a barbell, or machines. Starting lying face down on a bench, with the arms hanging down straight and gripping the weights or the machine bars. The goal is to pull weight up toward the body. There are many variations, including close-grip rows performed on a pulley machine and the one-arm version done while leaning over a bench.

Primary areas worked: latissimi, rhomboids, trapezii

Secondary areas worked: biceps, rear deltoid

Pullover – Begin lying faceup on a bench, with the arms extended beyond the head and down, holding the weight. Keeping the arms close together and elbows slightly bent, bring them up over the head in an arcing motion, then lower them back to the starting position. This is usually done with one dumbbell, although there are variations using a barbell, two dumbbells, or a pullover machine.

Primary areas worked: latissimi

Secondary areas worked: triceps, chest

Lat Pull-Down – Done using a weight machine. While sitting on the bench, reach up to grasp the bar and pull it down the top of the upper chest or upper back.

Primary areas worked: latissimi

Secondary areas worked: biceps

Dickerson – Done using either a lateral pull-down machine or a pulley system. Begin with the arms straight out in front of the body, slightly elevated to forehead level. Grasp the vertical bar. Keeping the arms stiff, elbows slightly bent and shoulder width (or a little wider apart), pull the bar down to just above the hips.

Primary areas worked: latissimi

Secondary areas worked: triceps

Pull-Up – This exercise uses body weight only. It is done hanging from a bar and pulling yourself up, or using a machine with a counterbalanced weight bar you stand on for a little help. This is ideal for those not yet strong enough to lift their own body weight.

Primary areas worked: latissimi

Secondary areas worked: biceps

Shrug – Standing and holding on to barbells or dumbbells, "shrug" your shoulders up toward your ears to pull the weight up. Arms remain straight the whole time.

Primary areas worked: trapezii

Secondary areas worked: none, or very minor shoulder action

Shoulder Exercises

Shoulder Press – The goal of this exercise is to push a weight up over the head. It can be done with dumbbells or barbells, or using a weight machine. Hand position can be varied. If a barbell or machine is used, the hands can be placed closer or farther apart on the bar. If dumbbells are used, the palms can be facing out (forward) or each other, or changed from one position to the other as the arms are raised.

Primary areas worked: deltoids

Secondary areas worked: triceps

Lateral Raise – Done with dumbbells, one held in each hand, arms hanging down to the sides, with the weights slightly in front of the body. The arms are raised to the side until the elbows reach just above the shoulder level, then are lowered back down. This exercise can be varied by keeping the elbows slightly bent, which makes it a bit harder, or completely bent, which is easier and safer for the shoulder joint.

Primary areas worked: side deltoids

Secondary areas worked: trapezii

Front Raise – Similar to the lateral raise, performed with dumbbells or a barbell. Begin with the weight(s) held in the hands, arms straight down in front of body. The arms are lifted straight out and up in front of the body in an arcing movement, stopping just above shoulder level.

Primary areas worked: front deltoids

Secondary areas worked: trapezii, chest

Rear Fly – Performed with dumbbells, with the body leaning over the legs. It can be done either seated or standing with knees bent and leaning over. Start with weights hanging straight down from the body, level with the abdominal muscles. The weight is then lifted out to the side of the body, keeping a slight bend in the elbows.

Primary areas worked: rear deltoids

Secondary areas worked: rhomboids

Upright Row – Done with a barbell or two dumbbells. Begin standing, with the arms hanging down and weights in front of the body, palms facing in toward the body. The weight is lifted up to just below chin level, with the elbows kept high through the motion.

Primary areas worked: front deltoids

Secondary areas worked: trapezii

Arm Exercises

Biceps Curl – This exercise involves lifting a weight held in the hand by bending the elbow to bring the hands up toward the shoulders. There are many variations, including using dumbbells, a barbell, or a machine; you can stand or be seated; and the palms may be facing out, in, or rotating through the movement.

Primary areas worked: biceps

Secondary areas worked: front deltoid

Triceps Extension – The "reverse" of the biceps curl, with the goal being to straighten a bent arm while holding a weight, then releasing it back into the starting position. If you're using a dumbbell, begin leaning over a bench, supporting yourself with one hand, holding a dumbbell in the other, with the dumbbell arm pulled back and its elbow bent at a 90° angle. Keeping the upper arm stationary, extend the arm straight out so that the dumbbell moves backward and up. This can also be done using a pulley.

Primary areas worked: triceps

Secondary areas worked: shoulder, latissimi

Bench Dip – Similar to the dip but performed using a weight bench to support the upper body and with the feet on the ground. Begin with your hands on the edge of the bench, palms down and supporting your weight, with your rear end hanging just off the bench and your legs straight out in front, angling down to the floor so that your heels are resting on the floor. The fingers should be facing the body and the elbows close together. The arms are then bent, lowering the body toward the floor, then straightened so the body is raised.

Primary areas worked: triceps

Secondary areas worked: shoulders, chest

Leg Exercises

Squat – The goal of this exercise is to "sit" and stand back up while holding a weight. Starting in a standing position, push the gluteus muscles backwards and lower yourself as if you are going to sit in a chair until you are in a squatting position. The upper body leans slightly forward, toes are pointed straight out in front, feet are slightly wider than shoulder-width apart. This exercise can be done with a barbell held across the back, or using a squat machine, a Smith machine, a hack squat machine, or a Smith ball on the wall.

Primary areas worked: quadriceps, gluteals, hamstrings

Secondary areas worked: back

Leg Press – Similar to a bench press, but it works the leg rather than the chest muscles. Sit or lie down in a leg press machine, with knees bent toward the chest and feet against the weight platform. Push hard with the legs against the platform until the legs straighten but not entirely; the knees should be slightly bent.

Primary areas worked: quadriceps, gluteals, hamstrings

Secondary areas worked: back

Leg Extension – Done on a machine while sitting up, with the legs down and the ankles pressing up against a padded bar. The legs are lifted with the feet rising up in an arc, pushing the bar up, until the legs are straight out in front of the body.

Primary areas worked: quadriceps

Secondary areas worked: none, or minor hip flexor action

Leg Curl – The "reverse" of the leg extension, performed lying facedown on a bench with the Achilles tendons pressed up into a padded bar or sitting up, legs straight out in front, with the Achilles tendons resting on a padded bar. The legs are flexed, pushing against the bar until the knees are bent, with the heel toward the gluteals.

Primary areas worked: hamstrings

Secondary areas worked: none, or slight lower back action

Calf Raise – The goal is to stand up on tiptoes against resistance. This can be done various ways. The simplest is to stand straight up, feet flat on the ground, holding dumbbells by the sides. Stand up on tiptoes, then descend back to feet flat on the ground.

Primary areas worked: calves

Other benefit: full body stabilization

Lunge – The idea is to "dip" one leg, knee bent, similar to the way a fencer does when lunging with the foil. Begin standing. Keeping the upper body erect, step forward so that one leg is in front of the body and one is behind. Lower the back knee toward the ground, bending the front leg as well, until the front leg is bent in a perfect 90-degree angle at the knee. The upper body is kept erect. There are many variations of this exercise, including holding the lunge while moving up and down, stepping out and pushing back, and walking. It can be done with dumbbells, barbells, and using a machine such as the Smith machine.

Primary areas worked: gluteals, quadriceps, hamstrings

Secondary areas worked: low back, abductors, adductors

Step-up – Holding dumbbells at the sides or a barbell across the back, step up onto a step or low bench (as long as it is very secure and safe) and then back down. It can be done working one leg at a time and then the other, or with alternating legs.

Primary areas worked: gluteals, hamstrings, quadriceps

Secondary areas worked: low back, abductors, and adductors

Abductor and Adductor Toners – Performed with machines, these exercises work the "outside" and "inside" of the thighs. To work the muscles on the outsides of your thighs (abductors), you sit in the machine, legs straight forward and resting on pads attached to weights, then spread them out to the sides. To work the muscles on the insides of your thighs (adductors), you do the reverse, beginning in a seated position, legs straight out in front but spread, then squeeze them together.

Primary areas worked: abductors, adductors

Secondary areas worked: none

Dead Lift – Performed with dumbbells or barbells. Begin in a kneeling position, with the butt pushed back, upper body leaning forward, and the toes pointed straight out. The back is kept in alignment, without rounding. Hands grip the weights, which rest on the floor. Stand up, using only the legs, with the arms and hands acting only as hooking and carrying mechanisms. After reaching the standing position, lower the weight in the same fashion.

Primary areas worked: trapezius, latissimi, erector spinae, gluteals, hamstrings, quadriceps, and psoas

16.15 ABCT SUMMARY

- Exercise in the morning on an empty stomach after an 8–12-hour fast.
- Drink 6 oz of water mixed with 10 g of whey protein before starting warm-up or do any exercise.
- Warm up for 5 minutes with stretching, flexing, and extension exercises of the upper and lower body.
- Start the resistance portion of ABCT based on one's present exercise level, time commitment, and desired intensity of workout. Pick ABCT 1, 2, 3, 4, or 5, with varied mixing and matching to accomplish the goals of bulk, contour, and tone. Do the intense exercise to the muscle burn. Alternate muscle groups each day for both upper and lower body, and do core exercises.
- Exercise two or three upper body and two or three lower body muscle groups per session and increase the number of muscle groups exercised with your desired intensity and training time. Do two or three core exercises with some flexibility and balance work as well.

- Ten minutes into the resistance workout, start drinking 4 oz of the ABCT Energy Shake at intervals after each exercise set. Rest 60 seconds between each repetition unless doing supersets or taking minimal rest periods.
- Take 3-second rests as needed to combat muscle fatigue.
- After completing the resistance exercises, start the aerobic program, utilizing cross-training.
- Keep the ratio of RT to aerobic exercise at 2:1.
- Exercise at least 6 times per week, but daily is best with 1 day off every week if necessary.
- Compress the exercise time and increase training intensity by doing core exercises or other lower intensity exercises during the 60-second rest periods. Alternatively, you can do the core exercises as part of the resistance exercise session.
- Eat the recommended post-exercise breakfast.

16.16 CONCLUSION

Optimal exercise with the ABCT combined AE and RT, with proper nutrition and the energy drink, result in numerous health benefits, lowers blood pressure, reduces cardiovascular disease and slows aging. Skeletal muscle is an endocrine organ that secretes over 400 myokines, hormones, and mediators that result in gene expression patterns and intracellular and extracellular signaling to reduce inflammation, oxidative stress, and modulate immune function during chronic adaptive training. An understanding of the nutrient-gene-muscle interconnections, as it relates to proteomics and metabolomics, will allow for a more scientific recommendation for the types and duration of exercise coupled with nutritional support to enhance good health outcomes, reduce morbidity, and mortality.

Here are the main elements of ABCT:

- RT – Weight lifting modified to encourage the muscles to "talk" to the body in such a way as to encourage better heart and full-body health. ABCT uses graduated weights and variable repetitions. In brief, lift the heaviest weight you can 12 times to get the burn, then decrease the weight with each subsequent set – but keep increasing the number of times you lift that weight. This is done using FIVE variable weights and repetitions as follows:
- For example, if you do a bench press at 100 lb. for 12 repetitions then do the following sequence with a 60 second rest between each set
- 75% of first weight or 75 lb. for 18 reps
- 50% of first weight or 50 lb. for 24 reps
- 25% of first weight or 25 lb. for 50 reps

100% of first weight or 100 lb. for 12 reps

This maximizes post-exercise oxygen consumption, depletes glycogen, and increases the production of lactic acid to achieve all the muscle-, hormone-, cytokine-, and interleukin-stimulating effects that lead to the health benefits of exercise.

- Aerobic Training in Intervals – Jogging, swimming, biking, and other forms of continual movement that set the heart beating at an elevated rate and keep it there for a predetermined amount of time. However, the standard approach – keeping the heart beating at a certain elevated rate for 20, 30, or even 60 minutes – is faulty. The best technique is aerobic interval training, which consists of short periods ranging from 20 to 60 seconds of "burst" aerobic training at 80 to 90% of your MAC or heart rate for your age then dropping to 50% of the MAC or heart rate for three times the length of the initial burst of activity. You then repeat this six times. The length of your burst of activity and resting period will depend on your present level of exercise conditioning. For example, if you run for 20 seconds at 80% MAC then you would do 60 seconds at 50% MAC. This more closely mimics the natural activities we evolved to perform and benefit from and strings together several periods of intense and semi-intense activity into a single, longer exercise period that still burns calories and builds endurance.
- Proper Ratio of Aerobic Training to RT – The optimal ratio of resistance to interval aerobic training should be 2:1. For example, during a 60-minute workout, you would perform 40 minutes of RT and 20 minutes of interval aerobics, with the aerobics coming after the RT. This should be done at least 4 days/week but daily is the best to achieve cardiovascular conditioning and optimal body composition with increases in lean muscle mass and reduction in body fat.

REFERENCES

ON EXERCISE

1. Houston Mark C. What Your Doctor May Not Tell You About Heart Disease. The Revolutionary Book that Reveals the Truth Behind Coronary Illness—and How You Can Fight Them. In Grand Central Life and Style. Hachette Book Group, New York, NY, 2012.
2. Vina J, Sanchis-Gomar F, Martinez-Bello V, Gomez-Cabrera MC. Exercise acts a drug; the pharmacological benefits of exercise Br J Pharmacol. 2012;167(1):1–12.
3. Meka N, Katragadda S, Cherian B. Arora RR Endurance exercise and resistance training in cardiovascular disease. Ther Adv Cardiovasc Dis. 2008;2(2):115–121.
4. Coffey VG, Hawley JA. The molecular bases of training adaptation. Sports Med. 2007;37(9):737–763.
5. McCall GE, Byrnes WC, Dickinson A, Pattany PM, Fleck SJ. Muscle fiber hypertrophy, hyperplasia, and capillary density in college men after resistance training. J Appl Physiol. 1996;81(5):2004–2012.
6. Radom-Aizik S, Hayek S, Shahar I, Rechavi G, Kaminski N, Ben-Dov I. Effects of aerobic training on gene expression in skeletal muscle of elderly men Med Sci Sports Exerc. 2005;37(10):1680–1696.
7. Ostrowski K, Schjerling P, Pedersen BK. Physical activity and plasma interleukin-6 in humans–effect of intensity of exercise Eur J Appl Physiol. 2000;83(6):512–515.
8. Pedersen BK, Ostrowski K, Rohde T, Bruunsgaard H, Can J. The cytokine response to strenuous exercise. Physiol Pharmacol. 1998;76(5):505–511.
9. Steensberg A The role of IL-6 in exercise-induced immune changes and metabolism. Exerc Immunol Rev. 2003;9:40–47.

10. Petersen AM, Pedersen BK. The anti-inflammatory effect of exercise J Appl Physiol. 2005;98(4):1154–1162.
11. Bruunsgaard H. Physical activity and modulation of systemic low-level inflammation. J Leukoc Biol. 2005;78(4):819–835.
12. Scott JP, Sale C, Greeves JP, Casey A, Dutton J, Fraser WD. Cytokine response to acute running in recreationally-active and endurance-trained men. Eur J Appl Physiol. 2013;113:1871–1882.
13. Welc SS, Clanton TL. The regulation of interleukin-6 implicates skeletal muscle as an integrative stress sensor and endocrine organ. Exp Physiol. 2013;98(2):359–371.
14. Pratley R, Nicklas B, Rubin M, Miller J, Smith A, Smith M, Hurley B, Goldberg A. Strength training increases resting metabolic rate and norepinephrine levels in healthy 50- to 65-yr-old men. J Appl Physiol. 1994;76(1):133–137.
15. Anton MM, Cortez-Cooper MY, DeVan AE, Neidre DB, Cook JN, Tanaka H. Resistance training increases basal limb blood flow and vascular conductance in aging humans. J Appl Physiol. 2006;101(5):1351–1355.
16. Okamoto T. Combined aerobic and resistance training and vascular function: effect of aerobic exercise before and after resistance training J Appl Physiol. 2007;103(5):1655–1661.
17. McCartney N, McKelvie RS, Haslam DR, Jones NL. Usefulness of weight lifting training in improving strength and maximal power output in coronary artery disease. Am J Cardiol. 1991;67(11):939–945.
18. Morra EA, Zaniqueli D, Rodrigues SL, El-Aourar LM, Lunz W, Mill JG, Carletti L. Long-term intense resistance training in men is associated with preserved cardiac structure/function, decreased aortic stiffness, and lower central augmentation pressure. J Hyperten. 2014;32:286–293.
19. Pu CT, Johnson MT, Forman DE, Hausdorff JM, Roubenoff R, Foldvari M, Fielding RA, Singh MA. Randomized trial of progressive resistance training to counteract the myopathy of chronic heart failure. J Appl Physiol. 2001;90(6):2341–2350.
20. Church TS, Blair SN, Cocreham S, Johannsen N, Johnson W, Kramer K, Mikus CR, Myers V, Nauta M, Rodarte RQ, Sparks L, Thompson A, Earnest CP. Effects of aerobic and resistance training on hemoglobin A1c levels in patients with type 2 diabetes: a randomized controlled trial. JAMA. 2010;304(20):2253–2262.
21. Mujica V, Urzúa A, Leiva E, Díaz N, Moore-Carrasco R, Vásquez M, Rojas E, Icaza G, Toro C, Orrego R, Palomo IJ. Intervention with education and exercise reverses the metabolic syndrome in adults. Am Soc Hypertens. 2010;4(3):148–153.
22. Warner SO, Linden MA, Liu Y, Harvey BR, Thyfault JP, Whaley-Connell AT, Chockalingam A, Hinton PS, Dellsperger KC, Thomas TR. The effects of resistance training on metabolic health with weight regain J Clin Hypertens (Greenwich). 2010;12(1):64–72.
23. Lamina S. Effects of continuous and interval trainingprograms in the management of hypertension: a randomized controlled trial. J Clin Hypertens (Greenwich). 2010;12(11):841–849.
24. Marzolini S, Oh PI. Brooks D Effect of combined aerobic and resistance training versus aerobic training alone in individuals with coronary artery disease: a meta-analysis. Eur J Prev Cardiol. 2012;19(1):81–94
25. Rossi A, Dikareva A, Bacon SL, Daskalopoulou SS. The impact of physical activity on mortality in patients with high blood pressure: a systematic review. J Hypertens. 2012;30(7):1277–1288.
26. Sesso HD, Paffenbarger RS Jr, Lee IM. Physical activity and coronary heart disease in men: the Harvard Alumni Health Study. Circulation. 2000;102(9):975–980.
27. Hawley JA, Burke LM, Phillips SM, Spriet LL. Nutritional modulation of training-induced skeletal muscle adaptations. J Appl Physiol. 2011;110(3):834–845.

28. Pennings B, Koopman R, Beelen M, Senden JM, Saris WH, van Loon LJ. Exercising before protein intake allows for greater use of dietary protein-derived amino acids for de novo muscle protein synthesis in both young and elderly men. Am J Clin Nutr. 2011;93(2):322–331
29. Lecoultre V, Benoit R, Carrel G, Schutz Y, Millet GP, Tappy L, Schneiter P. Fructose and glucose co-ingestion during prolonged exercise increases lactate and glucose fluxes and oxidation compared with an equimolar intake of glucose. Am J Clin Nutr. 2010;92(5):1071–1079
30. Stephens BR, Braun B. Impact of nutrient intake timing on the metabolic response to exercise. Nutr Rev. 2008;66(8):473–476.
31. Peake JM, Suzuki K, Coombes JS. The influence of antioxidant supplementation on markers of inflammation and the relationship to oxidative stress after exercise. J Nutr Biochem. 2007;18(6):357–371.
32. Fukuda DH, Smith AE, Kendall KL, Stout JR. The possible combinatory effects of acute consumption of caffeine, creatine, and amino acids on the improvement of anaerobic running performance in humans. Nutr Res. 2010;30(9):607–614.
33. Wray DW, Uberoi A, Lawrenson L, Bailey DM, Richardson RS. Oral antioxidants and cardiovascular health in the exercise-trained and untrained elderly: a radically different outcome. Clin Sci (Lond). 2009;116(5):433–441
34. Panza VS, Wazlawik E, Ricardo Schütz G, Comin L, Hecht KC, da Silva EL. Consumption of green tea favorably affects oxidative stress markers in weight-trained men. Nutrition. 2008;24(5):433–442
35. Karanth J, Jeevaratnam K. Effect of carnitine supplementation on mitochondrial enzymes in liver and skeletal muscle of rat after dietary lipid manipulation and physical activity. Indian J Exp Biol. 2010;48(5):503–510.
36. Huang A, Owen K. Role of supplementary L carnitine in exercise and exercise recovery. Med Sport Sci. 2012;59:135–142.
37. Broad EM, Maughan RJ, Galloway SDR. Effects of exercise intensity and altered substrate availability on cardiovascular and metabolic responses to exercise after oral carnitine supplementation in athletes. Int J Sport Nutr Exerc Metab. 2011;21(5):385–397
38. Addis P, Shecterle LM, St Cyr JA. Cellular protection during oxidative stress: a potential role for D-ribose and antioxidants. J Diet Suppl. 2012;9(3):178–182.
39. Cramer JT, Housh TJ, Johnson GO, Coburn JW, Stout JR. Effects of a carbohydrate-, protein-, and ribose-containing repletion drink during 8 weeks of endurance training on aerobic capacity, endurance performance, and body composition. J Strength Cond Res. 2012;26(8):2234–2242.
40. Seifert JG, Subudhi AW, Fu MX, Riska KL, John JC, Shecterle LM, St Cyr JA. The role of ribose on oxidative stress during hypoxic exercise: a pilot study. J Med Food. 2009;12(3):690–693.
41. Hoffman JR, Williams DR, Emerson NS, Hoffman MW, Wells AJ, McVeigh DM, McCormack WP, Mangine GT, Gonzalez AM, Fragala MS. L-Alanyl-L-glutamine ingestion maintains performance during a competitive basketball game J Int Soc Sports Nutr. 2012;9(1):4
42. Rowlands DS, Clarke J, Green JG, Shi X. L-Arginine but not L-glutamine likely increases exogenous carbohydrate oxidation during endurance exercise. Eur J Appl Physiol. 2012;112(7):2443–2453.
43. Ra SG, Miyazaki T, Ishikura K, Nagayama H, Suzuki T, Maeda S, Ito M, Matsuzaki Y, Ohmori H. Additional effects of taurine on the benefits of BCAA intake for the delayed-onset muscle soreness and muscle damage induced by high-intensity eccentric exercise. Adv Exp Med Biol. 2013;776:179–187.
44. Tang FC, Chan CC, Kuo PL. Contribution of creatine to protein homeostasis in athletes after endurance and sprint running. Eur J Nutr. 2013;53:61–71.

45. Howatson G, Hoad M, Goodall S, Tallent J, Bell PG, French DN. Exercise-induced muscle damage is reduced in resistance-trained males bybranched chain amino acids: a randomized, double-blind, placebo controlled study. J Int Soc Sports Nutr. 2012;9(1):20. [Epub ahead of print].
46. Breen L, Phillips SM. Nutrient interaction for optimal protein anabolism in resistance exercise. Curr Opin Clin Nutr Metab Care. 2012;15(3):226–232.
47. Pasiakos SM, McClung HL, McClung JP, Margolis LM, Andersen NE, Cloutier GJ, Pikosky MA, Rood JC, Fielding RA, Young AJ. Leucine-enriched essential amino acid supplementation during moderate steady state exercise enhances postexercise muscle protein synthesis. Am J Clin Nutr. 2011;94(3):809–818
48. Chen S, Li Z, Krochmal R, Abrazado M, Kim W, Cooper CBJ. Effect of Cs-4 (Cordyceps sinensis) on exercise performance in healthy older subjects: a double-blind, placebo-controlled trial. Altern Complement Med. 2010;16(5):585–590
49. Kumar R, Negi PS, Singh B, Ilavazhagan G, Bhargava K, Sethy NK. Cordyceps sinensis promotes exercise endurance capacity of rats by activating skeletal muscle metabolic regulators. J Ethnopharmacol. 2011;136(1):260–266
50. Noreen EE, Buckley JG, Lewis SL, Brandauer J, Stuempfle KJ. The effects of an acute dose of *Rhodiola rosea* on endurance exercise [erformance. J Strength Cond Res. 2013;27(3):839–847
51. Xu J, Li Y. Effects of salidroside on exhaustive exercise-induced oxidative stress in rats. Mol Med Rep. 2012;6(5):1195–1198
52. Noreen EE, Buckley JG, Lewis SL, Brandauer J, Stuempfle KJ. The effects of an acute dose of *Rhodiola rosea* on endurance exercise performance. J Strength Cond Res. 2012;27(3):839-847
53. Parisi A, Tranchita E, Duranti G, Ciminelli E, Quaranta F, Ceci R, Cerulli C, Borrione P, Sabatini S. Effects of chronic *Rhodiola rosea* supplementation on sport performance and antioxidant capacity in trained male: preliminary results. J Sports Med Phys Fitness. 2010;50(1):57–63.
54. Evdokimov VG. Effect of cryopowder *Rhodiola rosae* L. on cardiorespiratory parameters and physical performance of humans. Aviakosm Ekolog Med. 2009;43(6):52–56
55. Churchward-Venne TA, Breen L, Di Donato DM, Hector AJ, Mitchell CJ, Moore DR, Stellingwerff T, Breuille D, Offord EA, Baker SK, Phillips SM. Leucine supplementation of a low-protein mixed macronutrient beverage enhances myofibrillar protein synthesis in young men: a double-blind, randomized trial. Am J Clin Nutr. 2014;99(2):276–286.
56. Osterberg KL, Melby CL. Effect of acute resistance exercise on postexercise oxygen consumption and resting metabolic rate in young women. Int J Sport Nutr Exerc Metab. 2000;10(1):71–81.

16.17 WEIGHT AND BODY FAT REDUCTION

Obesity by itself is a well-known risk factor of hypertension, and losing the weight and body fat will help to lower your blood pressure and other cardiovascular risks. Total body fat, especially visceral or belly fat produces over 45 chemicals, called *adipokines* that can elevate blood pressure, cause inflammation, oxidative stress, cardiovascular disease, and diabetes mellitus. About 60% of hypertensive patients are at least 20% over ideal body weight. A weight loss of about 10–12 lb. will result in a reduction in blood pressure of 7/5 mm Hg in obese and nonobese patients. Weight loss also potentiates the effects of other lifestyle modifications and drug therapy.

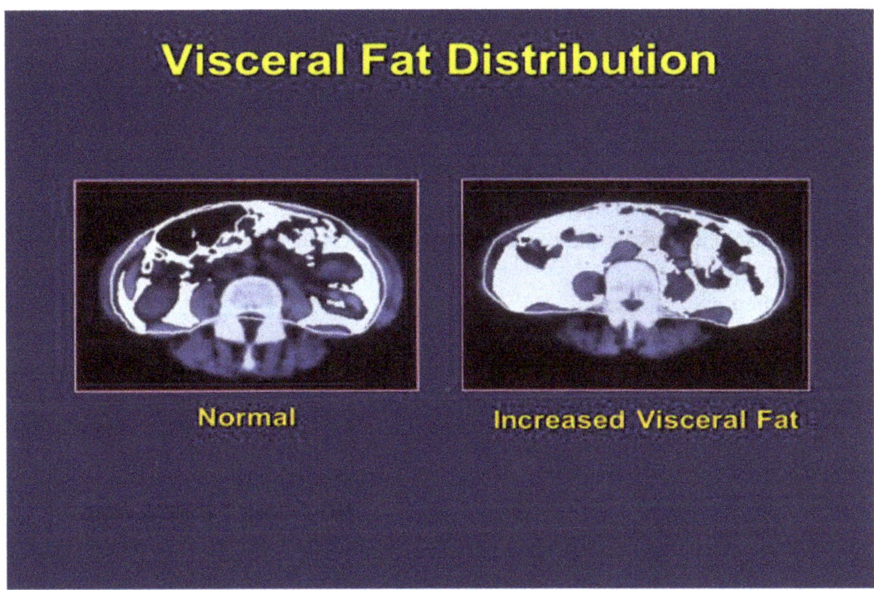

FIGURE 16.1 Visceral or belly fat is shown in the normal and the obese patient. The white represents the visceral fat.

Weight reduction should decrease adipose tissue, not lean muscle mass. Reduction in visceral obesity which is measured by the waist circumference and by a machine called body impedence analysis is particularly important in reducing blood pressure and cardiovascular risk. (Figure 16.1) Weight loss with fat loss improves the output of the heart, decreases blood volume, sodium and water retention, and swelling in the legs (edema). In addition weight and fat loss reduce insulin levels, improve insulin sensitivity, lower adrenalin levels, dilate the arteries, and reduce the sympathetic nervous system activity, plasma renin activity, and serum aldosterone levels. Weight and fat loss reduce inflammation and oxidative stress. Here are some important and practical points about weight and body fat reduction (1–14).

1. It is not safe to lose over 3.3 lb./week and the preferred weight loss is 1–2 lb./week.
2. Body fat is more important than body weight.
   Males should be <15% body fat
   Females should be <22% body fat
3. The number of calories needed per day to maintain the same weight is your weight in pounds times 10.
   i.e., 160 lb. = 1600 calories.
   1600 calories is your BMR (basal metabolic rate).
4. It takes a 3500 calorie deficit to lose 1 lb.
5. If the body mass index is over 27, there is a danger of developing significant health problems.

6. Four major factors contribute to obesity:
   - Genetics
   - Metabolic factors
   - Diet
   - Physical inactivity
7. Waist circumference over the value indicated next is associated with a high risk of disease and may be the single best predictor of obesity-related cardiovascular disease and overall morbidity and mortality:
   Men over 40 in.
   Women over 35 in.
8. Neck circumference also correlates with high disease risk.
   Men over 15.6 in.
   Women over 14.4 in.
9. Obesity will increase the risk of morbidity and mortality of the following diseases:
   - Hypertension
   - Dyslipidemia
   - Type II diabetes and insulin resistance
   - Coronary heart disease and heart attack
   - Stroke
   - Gallbladder disease
   - Osteoarthritis
   - Sleep apnea
   - Respiratory problems
   - Cancer of breast, prostate, colon, and endometrium
   - Chronic kidney disease
   - Microalbuminuria and proteinuria
10. The ideal body weight calculation: (Depends on the body frame size)
    - Women: 100 lb. first 5 ft, then 5 lb. for each additional inch of height
    - Men: 106 lb. first 5 ft, then 6 lb. for each additional inch of height
    - 10% is added for large frame and you delete 10% for a small frame

The Hypertension Institute Nutrition Program outlined in Chapters 14 and 15 is very effective in safely reducing body weight, body fat, visceral (belly) fat, preserving lean muscle mass, lowering blood pressure, decreasing blood glucose and cholesterol and other cardiovascular and general health risks. Many of our patients have been able to reduce or stop blood pressure diabetes and cholesterol medications on the Hypertension Institute Nutrition Program over 6–12 months.

REFERENCES

Obesity and High Blood Pressure

1. Whelton PK et al ACC/AHA/AAPA/ABC/ACPM/AGS/APhA/ASH/ASPC/NMA/PCNA Guideline for the prevention, detection, evaluation, and management of high blood pressure in adults: a report of the American College of Cardiology/American Heart Association Task Force on Clinical Practice Guidelines. Hypertension. 2018;71(6):e13-e115.

2. Houston M. The role of nutrition and nutraceutical supplements in the treatment of hypertension. World J Cardiol. 2014;6(2): 38–66.
3. Houston M. Nutrition and nutraceutical supplements for the treatment of hypertension: Part 1. J Clin Hypertens. 2013;15:752–757.
4. Houston M. Nutrition and nutraceutical supplements for the treatment of hypertension: Part II. J Clin Hypertens. 2013;15:845–851.
5. Houston M. Nutrition and nutraceutical supplements for the treatment of hypertension: Part III. J Clin Hypertens. 2013;15:931–937.
6. Borghi C, Cicero AF. Nutraceuticals with a clinically detectable blood pressure-lowering effect: a review of available randomized clinical trials and their meta-analyses. Br J Clin Pharmacol. 2017;83(1):163–171.
7. Sirtori CR, Arnoldi A, Cicero AF. Nutraceuticals for blood pressure control. Review. Ann Med. 2015;47(6):447–456.
8. Cicero AF, Colletti A. Nutraceuticals and blood pressure control: results from clinical trials and meta-analyses. High Blood Press Cardiovasc Prev. 2015;22(3):203–213.
9. Turner JM, Spatz ES. Nutritional supplements for the treatment of hypertension: a practical guide for clinicians. Curr Cardiol Rep. 2016;18(12):126. Review
10. Caligiuri SP, Pierce GN. A review of the relative efficacy of dietary, nutritional supplements, lifestyle and drug therapies in the management of hypertension. Crit Rev Food Sci Nutr. 2016 Nov 2;57(16):3508–3527.
11. Houston MC, Fox B, Taylor N. What Your Doctor May Not Tell You About Hypertension. The Revolutionary Nutrition and Lifestyle Program to Help Fight High Blood Pressure. AOL Time Warner, Warner Books, New York, NY, 2003.
12. Houston M. Treatment of hypertension with nutrition and nutraceutical supplement: Part 1. Altern Compliment Med. 2019;24:260–275
13. Houston M. Treatment of hypertension with nutrition and nutraceutical supplement: Part 2. Altern Compliment Med. 2019;25:23–36
14. Sinatra S, Houston M, Editors. Nutrition and Integrative Strategies in Cardiovascular Medicine. CRC Press, Boca Raton, London, New York 2015.

16.18 SMOKING AND TOBACCO PRODUCTS

Smoking is a major risk factor for heart attack, coronary heart disease, congestive heart failure, stroke, COPD (chronic obstructive lung disease), and lung cancer (1–6). Smoking accounts for over 500,000 deaths per year in the United States. Smoking is very addictive, so you must seek your doctor's help in stopping this very bad habit. Secondhand smoke, e-cigarettes, vaping, and other forms of tobacco should also be stopped. It is never too late to quit! **Discontinuation of smoking** will reduce vasoconstriction, improve endothelial function, and lower blood pressure. Stopping smoking also decreases sympathetic nervous system activity, norepinephrine (NE) levels, RAAS activity, carbon monoxide levels, platelet stickiness, clotting risk, oxidative stress, and inflammation. Here are some encouraging facts to help you quit smoking.

- Quitting smoking decreases cardiovascular risk. At about 1 year after quitting smoking, your risk for a heart attack drops dramatically.
- Within 2–5 years after quitting smoking, your risk for stroke may fall to that of a nonsmoker.

- If you stop smoking, your risks for cancers of the mouth, throat, esophagus, and bladder drop by 50% within 5 years.
- Ten years after you discontinue smoking, your risk for dying from lung cancer drops by 50%.

REFERENCES

Smoking

1. U.S. Department of Health and Human Services. The Health Consequences of Smoking—50 Years of Progress: A Report of the Surgeon General. U.S. Department of Health and Human Services, Centers for Disease Control and Prevention, National Center for Chronic Disease Prevention and Health Promotion, Office on Smoking and Health, Atlanta, 2014
2. U.S. Department of Health and Human Services. How Tobacco Smoke Causes Disease: What It Means to You. U.S. Department of Health and Human Services, Centers for Disease Control and Prevention, National Center for Chronic Disease Prevention and Health Promotion, Office on Smoking and Health, Atlanta, 2010
3. Centers for Disease Control and Prevention. Quick stats: number of deaths from 10 leading causes—national vital statistics system, United States, 2010. Morbidity Mortality Wkly Rep. 2013;62(08):155.
4. Mokdad AH, Marks JS, Stroup DF, Gerberding JL. Actual causes of death in the United States. JAMA. 2004;291(10):1238–1245.
5. U.S. Department of Health and Human Services. Women and Smoking: A Report of the Surgeon General. U.S. Department of Health and Human Services, Public Health Service, Office of the Surgeon General, Rockville, MD, 2001 [accessed 2017 Apr 20].
6. U.S. Department of Health and Human Services. Reducing the Health Consequences of Smoking: 25 Years of Progress. A Report of the Surgeon General External. U.S. Department of Health and Human Services, Public Health Service, Centers for Disease Control, National Center for Chronic Disease Prevention and Health Promotion, Office on Smoking and Health, Rockville, MD, 1989.

16.19 CAFFEINE

Caffeine is a chemical found in coffee, tea, cola, guarana, chocolate, and other products. The daily consumption of caffeine containing beverages such as coffee and tea is a "mixed story" when it comes to high blood pressure and cardiovascular disease (1–13). Your ability to metabolize caffeine in your liver is determined by your genetics. About 50% of people in the United States are slow metabolizers of caffeine and 50% are fast metabolizers. The primary gene for caffeine metabolism is **CYP1A2.** This genetic profile can be evaluated with the *Cardia X genetic test from Vibrant Labs of America* (see sources section).

Here are some important facts about caffeine, blood pressure, cardiovascular disease, and heart attack.

- **Cytochrome P-450 – CYP1A2 gene** modifies the association between caffeinated coffee intake and the risk of hypertension and cardiovascular disease in a linear relationship. Caffeine is exclusively metabolized by CYP1A2 to other less active compounds such as paraxanthine, theobromine, and theophylline.

- Rapid metabolizers of caffeinated coffee **IA/IA gene type (allele)** have lower blood pressure and lower risk of heart attack.
- Slow metabolizers of caffeine **IF/IA or the IF/IF gene type (allele)** have higher blood pressure by about 8/6 mm Hg lasting over 3 hours after consumption of coffee with caffeine, an increased risk of heart attack by 56%, fast heart rate (tachycardia), increased aortic stiffness, and increased catecholamines.
- The number of cups of caffeinated coffee consumed per day and your age determine your risk for high blood pressure and heart attack if you are a slow metabolizer. More caffeinated coffee and an age over 59 years increase the risk.

Discontinuation of caffeine is important if you have this CYP1A2 gene. Here are a few tips on how to slowly taper your caffeine and avoid any withdrawal symptoms.

1. **Pay attention** to how much caffeine you're getting from foods and beverages, including energy drinks by reading labels carefully.
2. **Go decaffeinated.** Most decaffeinated beverages look and taste the same as their caffeinated counterparts. However, some decaffeinated beverages may not be safe.
3. **Go herbal.** Herbal teas can be used as they do not have caffeine.
4. **Check the bottle.** Some over-the-counter pain relievers contain caffeine – as much as 130 mg or more of caffeine in one dose. Look for caffeine-free pain relievers instead.

REFERENCES

Caffeine

1. Houston M. The role of nutrition and nutraceutical supplements in the treatment of hypertension. World J Cardiol. 2014;6(2): 38–66.
2. Houston M. Nutrition and nutraceutical supplements for the treatment of hypertension: Part 1. J Clin Hypertens. 2013;15:752–757.
3. Houston M. Nutrition and nutraceutical supplements for the treatment of hypertension: Part II. J Clin Hypertens. 2013;15:845–851.
4. Houston M. Nutrition and nutraceutical supplements for the treatment of hypertension: Part III J Clin Hyperten. 2013;15:931–937.
5. Borghi C, Cicero AF. Nutraceuticals with a clinically detectable blood pressure-lowering effect: a review of available randomized clinical trials and their meta-analyses. Br J Clin Pharmacol. 2017;83(1):163–171.
6. Sirtori CR, Arnoldi A, Cicero AF. Nutraceuticals for blood pressure control. Review. Ann Med. 2015;47(6):447–456.
7. Cicero AF, Colletti A. Nutraceuticals and blood pressure control: results from clinical trials and meta-analyses. High Blood Press Cardiovasc Prev. 2015; 22(3):203–213.
8. Turner JM, Spatz ES. Nutritional supplements for the treatment of hypertension: a practical guide for clinicians. Curr Cardiol Rep. 2016;18(12):126. Review
9. Caligiuri SP, Pierce GN. A review of the relative efficacy of dietary, nutritional supplements, lifestyle and drug therapies in the management of hypertension. Crit Rev Food Sci Nutr. 2016 Nov 2;57(16):3508–3527.

10. Houston MC, Fox B, Taylor N. What Your Doctor May Not Tell You About Hypertension. The Revolutionary Nutrition and Lifestyle Program to Help Fight High Blood Pressure. AOL Time Warner, Warner Books, New York, NY, 2003.
11. Houston M. Treatment of hypertension with nutrition and nutraceutical supplement: Part 1. Altern Compliment Med. 2019;24:260–275
12. Houston M. Treatment of hypertension with nutrition and nutraceutical supplement: Part 2. Altern Compliment Med. 2019;25:23–36
13. Sinatra S, Houston M, Editors. Nutrition and Integrative Strategies in Cardiovascular Medicine. CRC Press, Boca Raton, London, New York 2015.

16.20 ALCOHOL

Limitation of alcohol: More than 1 drink/day such as 5–6 oz of wine, 1–2 oz of hard liquor or 24 oz of beer elevates blood pressure. Women can only consume 50% of these amounts, as they do not metabolize alcohol as well as men. There appears to be a "U-Shaped" curve for alcohol consumption and blood pressure levels as well as cardiovascular risk. Alcohol consumption should be kept below 20 g/day (1–13). Here are some important facts about alcohol.

- Acute and chronic over-ingestion of alcohol will increase blood pressure, heart attack, and stroke risk, but smaller consumption may decrease those risks if less than 20 g/day. The risk of hypertension and cardiovascular disease is a "U"-shaped curve. Risk reduction is proportional to intake up to the 20 g/day amount.
- 20 g/day or more increases blood pressure. This amount for various forms of alcohol is shown as follows:
  - Wine (Red): 5–6 oz for men and 3 oz for women (best)
  - Beer: 12–24 oz for men and 6–12 oz for women
  - Hard liquor: 1.5 oz for men and 0.75 oz for women
  - Reducing alcohol intake will reduce blood pressure and your total calorie intake.
  - 20 g/day in men and 10 g/day in women or less reduces cardiovascular risk by 31–43%

REFERENCES

Alcohol

1. Houston M. The role of nutrition and nutraceutical supplements in the treatment of hypertension. World J Cardiol. 2014;6(2):38–66.
2. Houston M. Nutrition and nutraceutical supplements for the treatment of hypertension: Part 1. J Clin Hypertens. 2013;15:752–757.
3. Houston M. Nutrition and nutraceutical supplements for the treatment of hypertension: Part II. J Clin Hypertens 2013;15:845–851.
4. Houston M. Nutrition and nutraceutical supplements for the treatment of hypertension: Part III. J Clin Hypertens 2013;15:931–937.
5. Borghi C, Cicero AF. Nutraceuticals with a clinically detectable blood pressure-lowering effect: a review of available randomized clinical trials and their meta-analyses. Br J Clin Pharmacol. 2017;83(1):163–171.

6. SirtoriCR, Arnoldi A, Cicero AF. Nutraceuticals for blood pressure control. Review. Ann Med. 2015;47(6):447–456.
7. Cicero AF, Colletti A. Nutraceuticals and blood pressure control: results from clinical trials and meta-analyses. High Blood Press Cardiovasc Prev. 2015;22(3):203–213.
8. Turner JM, Spatz ES. Nutritional supplements for the treatment of hypertension: a practical guide for clinicians. Curr Cardiol Rep. 2016;18(12):126. Review
9. Caligiuri SP, Pierce GN. A review of the relative efficacy of dietary, nutritional supplements, lifestyle and drug therapies in the management of hypertension. Crit Rev Food Sci Nutr. 2016 Nov 2;57(16):3508–3527.
10. Houston MC, Fox B, Taylor N. What Your Doctor May Not Tell You About Hypertension. The Revolutionary Nutrition and Lifestyle Program to Help Fight High Blood Pressure. AOL Time Warner, Warner Books, New York, NY, 2003.
11. Houston M. Treatment of hypertension with nutrition and nutraceutical supplement: Part 1. Altern Compliment Med. 2019;24:260–275
12. Houston M. Treatment of hypertension with nutrition and nutraceutical supplement: Part 2. Altern Compliment Med. 2019;25:23–36
13. Sinatra S, Houston M, Editors. Nutrition and Integrative Strategies in Cardiovascular Medicine. CRC Press, Boca Raton, London, New York 2015.

16.21 DE-STRESS YOUR LIFE (1–6)

Stress, anxiety, and depression can increase blood pressure and elevate your cardiovascular risk. Under these conditions, your sympathetic nervous system is activated, which increases vasoconstriction, blood pressure, heart rate, and risk for blood clotting. Acute stress can be life-saving, but chronic stress is bad for your overall health and your blood pressure. Evaluate your stress level, consult with your doctors, and try some effective means to lower it. Some behavioral modifications for stress management include biofeedback, relaxation programs, breathing exercises, yoga, Pilates, psychotherapy, hypnosis, transcendental meditation, spirituality, and religion. Reducing anxiety, stress, and treating depression will go a long way helping to lower your blood pressure along with all of the suggestions listed in this book.

REFERENCES

Stress, Anxiety and Depression and Blood Pressure

1. Cohen S, Janicki-Deverts D, Miller GE. Psychological stress and disease. JAMA. 2007;298:1685
2. Sparrenberger F, Cichelero FT, Ascoli AM, et al. Does psychosocial stress cause hypertension? A systematic review of observational studies. J Hum Hypertens. 2009;23:12–19.
3. Schwartz JE, Pickering TG, Landsbergis PA. Work-related stress and blood pressure: current theoretical models and considerations from a behavioral medicine perspective. J Occup Health Psychol. 1996;1:287–310.
4. Vrijkotte TGM, van Doornen LJP, de Geus EJC. Effects of work stress on ambulatory blood pressure, heart rate, and heart rate variability. Hypertension. 2000;35:880–886.
5. Markovitz JH, Matthews KA, Whooley M, et al. Increases in job strain are associated with incident hypertension in the CARDIA Study. Ann Behav Med. 2004;28:4–9.
6. Nilsson PM. Job strain in men, but not in women, predicts a significant rise in blood pressure after 6.5 years of follow-up. J Hypertens. 2007;25:525–531.

16.22 SLEEP

A short sleep duration, interrupted sleep, and obstructive sleep apnea (OSA) are independent risk factors for hypertension, silent small strokes, future stroke events, coronary heart disease, heart attacks, abnormal heart rhythms such as atrial fibrillation, obesity, and diabetes mellitus. Less than 6 hours of sleep is associated with all of these medical problems. Prolonged sleep over 10 hours increases stroke risk. Eight hours of good sleep appears to be the perfect sleep duration for most people to prevent the cardiovascular events and reduce blood pressure. OSA is one of the leading secondary causes of hypertension in the United States. This can be evaluated in a sleep lab or with some new outpatient testing called *WatchPat*. Treatment with continuous positive airway pressure is effective. Correcting OSA will often drop the blood pressure to near normal levels (1–10).

REFERENCES

SLEEP

1. Young T, Palta M, Dempsey J, Skatrud J, Weber S, Badr S. The occurrence of sleep-disordered breathing among middle-aged adults. N Engl J Med. 1993;328:1230–1235.
2. Peppard PE, Young T, Barnet JH, Palta M, Hagen EW, Hla KM. Increased prevalence of sleep-disordered breathing in adults. Am J Epidemiol. 2013;177:1006–1014.
3. Somers VK, White DP, Amin R, Abraham WT, Costa F, Culebras A, Daniels S, Floras JS, Hunt CE, Olson LJ, et al. Sleep apnea and cardiovascular disease. An American Heart Association/American College of Cardiology Foundation scientific statement from the American Heart Association Council for High Blood Pressure Research Professional Education Committee, Council on Clinical Cardiology, Stroke Council, and Council on Cardiovascular Nursing Council. Circulation. 2008;118:1080–1111.
4. Young T, Palta M, Dempsey J, Peppard PE, Nieto FJ, Hla KM. Burden of sleep apnea: rationale, design, and major findings of the Wisconsin Sleep Cohort study. WMJ. 2009;108:246–249.
5. Kronholm E, Partonen T, Laatikainen T, et al.. Trends in self-reported sleep duration and insomnia-related symptoms in Finland from 1972 to 2005: a comparative review and re-analysis of Finnish population samples. J Sleep Res. 2008;17:54–62.
6. Hoffstein V, Chan CK, Slutsky AS. Sleep apnea and systemic hypertension: a causal association review. Am J Med. 1991;91:190–196. [PubMed]
7. National Sleep Foundation. Sleep in America Poll 2005: Summary of Findings. National Sleep Foundation, Washington, DC, 2005.
8. Cao M, Guilleminault C. Acute and chronic sleep loss: implications on age-related neurocognitive impairment. Sleep. 2012;35:901–902.
9. Jackson ML, Gunzelmann G, Whitney P, et al. Deconstructing and reconstructing cognitive performance in sleep deprivation. Sleep Med Rev. 2013;17:215–225.
10. Abedelmalek S, Chtourou H, Aloui A, Aouichaoui C, Souissi N, Tabka Z. Effect of time of day and partial sleep deprivation on plasma concentrations of IL-6 during a short-term maximal performance. Eur J Appl Physiol. 2013;113:241–248
11. Dixit A, Thawani R, Goyal A, Vaney N. Psychomotor performance of medical students: effect of 24 hours of sleep deprivation. Indian J Psychol Med. 2012;34:129–132.
12. Ayas NT, White DP, Manson JE, et al. A prospective study of sleep duration and coronary heart disease in women. Arch Intern Med. 2003;163:205–209.

13. Ayas NT, White DP, Al-Delaimy WK, et al. A prospective study of self-reported sleep duration and incident diabetes in women. Diabetes Care. 2003;26:380–384.
14. Cappuccio FP, Stranges S, Kandala NB, et al. Gender-specific associations of short sleep duration with prevalent and incident hypertension: the Whitehall II Study. Hypertension. 2007;50:693–700.16.23

16.23 SUMMARY AND KEY TAKEAWAY POINTS

1. Aerobic and resistance exercise training will lower blood pressure by 11/8 mm Hg once you have achieved optimal cardiovascular conditioning using the ABCT exercise program.
2. Obesity, especially visceral fat, produces many adipokines that elevate blood pressure, cause inflammation and oxidative stress. As body weight and visceral fat decrease, the blood pressure will fall.
3. Smoking and other tobacco products increase blood pressure. Discontinuation will lower the blood pressure
4. Caffeine will increase blood pressure, heart rate, and risk of heart attack if you are a slow metabolizer of caffeine with the CYP 1 A2 gene. These risks are related to the amount of caffeine consumed and your age.
5. Alcohol will elevate blood pressure in men that consume over 20 g/day and in women who consume over 10 g/day.
6. Stress, anxiety, and depression will increase blood pressure both acutely and chronically.
7. Sleeping less than 8 hours/night chronically, poor quality or interrupted sleep, and obstructive sleep apnea will increase blood pressure.

17 Pharmacologic (Drug) Treatment for Hypertension

17.1 INTRODUCTION

If it is necessary for you to take medications to lower your blood pressure, there is some good news. Many of the newer blood pressure medications have very few side effects, are very effective in reducing your blood pressure, decrease your risk of cardiovascular risks and complications based on a large amount of published clinical trials, and their cost is reasonable and usually covered by your health insurance. If we all followed the Hypertension Institute program then about 70% or more patients could have their blood pressure controlled, especially those with milder forms of high blood pressure (less than 160/90 mm Hg). However, many patients will not follow all of these suggestions, and in this situation, the medications can be life-saving and avoid cardiovascular complications and events. The choice to start a blood pressure medication is made between you and your doctor based on many criteria such as the level of your blood pressure, your risk factors for cardiovascular disease, other medical problems such as diabetes mellitus or high cholesterol, your previous medical history of any cardiovascular event, and the presence of known cardiovascular disease. You must play it safe and do what is best for you to stay healthy. In this chapter, we will review the various classes of drugs, how they work and their side effects.

17.2 DIURETICS

Diuretics are often referred to as "water pills". The mechanism of action is to inhibit sodium chloride (NaCl) reabsorption in the kidney tubules. There is an initial reduction in the cardiac output secondary to reduction in blood volume, but the constriction in the arteries is reduced with long-term therapy (after 4–8 weeks), and volume reduction reverses to near normal over the same time frame. (1–5)

Diuretics are used as monotherapy (single drugs) to treat mild-to-moderate hypertension or as an adjunct to other antihypertensive agents. The major differences among the diuretics are related to duration and site of action as well as potency of diuretic action. The adverse effects are similar, particularly among the thiazide diuretics. Lower doses of diuretics are recommended. However, hydrochlorothiazide (HCTZ 12.5–25 mg/day) that was previously recommended has fallen out of favor due to adverse effects and lack of reduction in heart attack in particular and a suboptimal reduction in stroke. (1–5) Thiazide-type diuretics (except indapamide) generally lose their effectiveness in patients with serum creatinine levels in excess of 1.7 mg/dl or a creatinine clearance of less than 30 cm^3/min (both of these are measures of kidney function). Chlorthalidone is a second-line diuretic to indapamide but superior to HCTZ. Indapamide is now considered the best and first line diuretic. Indapamide has better reductions in heart attack and stroke, fewer side effects, and remains effective in patients with moderate-to-severe chronic kidney disease. Indapamide offers many advantages over other diuretics. It is more potent than other diuretics in reducing blood pressure and has mild calcium channel blocking effects and mild alpha blocking effects, which may make it the diuretic of choice in treating hypertension (1–5). Indapamide has a better metabolic profile and does not increase cholesterol, LDL cholesterol, and triglycerides or lower HDL cholesterol. Indapamide has minimal to no effect on blood sugar or insulin resistance and demonstrates less reduction in potassium and magnesium. It is also less likely to damage the kidneys compared to thiazide and thiazide-like diuretics. Indapamide also reduces heart enlargement (left ventricular hypertrophy) and platelet stickiness or aggregation. Indapamide is also effective in the presence of poorly functioning kidneys. Indapamide has been used in many blood pressure clinical studies with significant reductions in all cardiovascular and cerebrovascular events.

17.3 CENTRAL ALPHA-AGONISTS

The central alpha-agonists all stimulate a central receptor in the brain stem, which reduces sympathetic nervous system activity to the body that lowers epinephrine and norepinephrine. These effects result in a reduction in arterial resistance and blood pressure. These agents are infrequently used now due to their side effects and lack of reduction in cardiovascular disease or events in any clinical trials. (1–4)

Common side effects are sedation and dry mouth, which are minimized with low-dose long-term therapy. Concern about withdrawal syndrome has been reported with all these drugs, particularly clonidine. When low doses are used, the frequency of withdrawal syndrome is minimal and probably less than that with beta-blockers. However, duration of treatment, dose, individual variability, and concomitant medical diseases will determine the severity and frequency of a withdrawal syndrome. Therefore, it is prudent to always taper any of the central alpha agonists over at least 2–4 weeks to avoid any potential adverse effects. (1–4)

Antihypertensive efficacy is excellent and similar with all of the central alpha-agonists. Selection of therapy depends more on some of the unique side effects, duration of action, and cost. (1–4) Clonidine and methyldopa are safe to use during pregnancy. The available drugs in this class are as follows:

1. Clonidine (Catapres): oral and transdermal patch.
2. Guanabenz (Wytensin).
3. Guanfacine (Tenex).
4. Methyldopa (Aldomet).

17.4 BETA-BLOCKERS

The older beta blockers are not presently recommended for the treatment of hypertension with the exception of carvedilol (Coreg) and nebivolol (Bystolic). The older beta blockers do not reduce cardiovascular events such as heart attack or stroke. Their use is reserved for other medical indications such as heart failure, after a heart attack, after a heart stent or a bypass graft, and to control electrical problems of the heart with extra heart beats, fast heart rate, and atrial fibrillation (arrhythmias) (1–4).

The beta blockers will do the following:

a. Slow the heart rate.
b. Reduce of cardiac contraction and heart output.
c. Increase in arterial constriction.
d. Sympathetic activity is reduced.
e. Antioxidant activity (Carvedilol).
f. Increase nitric oxide (Nebivolol).
g. Bronchoconstriction (constricts the lung airways and may cause shortness of breath).
h. Fatigue.
i. Depression.
j. Erectile dysfunction.
k. Elevated blood sugar.
l. Elevated triglycerides and reduction in HDL cholesterol.
m. Insomnia.
n. Cold hands and feet.

17.5 DIRECT VASODILATORS

The direct vasodilators have a potent relaxation effect on the vascular smooth muscle of arteries, reducing arterial constriction, which lowers blood pressure by the vasodilation. They all increase heart contraction, heart rate, and blood volume. They require the concomitant use of either beta-blockers and diuretics to control these side effects. The direct vasodilators hydralazine and minoxidil therefore should not be used alone to treat chronic hypertension. Minoxidil is much more potent than hydralazine. These agents are reserved for specific cardiovascular problems and are not commonly used due to the side effects.

17.6 ALPHA1-BLOCKERS

The alpha1-blockers (indirect vasodilators) prazosin, doxazosin, and terazosin block the peripheral nerve receptor called the alpha1-adrenergic receptor and reduce arterial constriction, dilate the artery, and lower the blood pressure, but usually do not cause reflex increase in heart rate, the heart contractility is preserved or increased, and the blood volume is usually unchanged. However, the alpha blockers are not generally recommended for antihypertensive drug therapy since the publication of the ALLHAT trial.

Patients may have dizziness, syncope (pass out), low blood pressure, and fatigue. The alpha blockers are useful in prostate enlargement (1–4).

17.7 ANGIOTENSIN-CONVERTING ENZYME INHIBITORS (ACEIS)

These agents inhibit an enzyme called angiotensin-converting enzyme (ACE) that converts angiotensin I to angiotensin II, thus interrupting the renin-angiotensin-aldosterone system, decreasing the arterial constriction, dilating the arteries, lowering the blood pressure, and reducing the blood volume slightly. (1–4)

Angiotensin-II (A-II) is a potent vasoconstrictor, growth promoter in vascular and heart muscles, and is thrombogenic (clots) prooxidant, proinflammatory, and an atherogenic hormone. ACE inhibitors (ACEIs) may be as initial therapy, used alone or in combination with other antihypertensive agents to enhance their effect. Side effects are minor and infrequent, and most patients tolerate these agents well. Cough occurs in 10–15% of patients and is more common in women. Patients who cough tend to have the best antihypertensive effect. They may also decrease taste in some patients. They are effective in African-Americans, Whites, elderly, or young patients. Higher doses are often needed in the African-American patient to achieve equal blood pressure reduction. (1–4) ACEIs also have a favorable effect in preserving kidney function in both nondiabetic and diabetic hypertensives and in diabetic patients without hypertension who have proteinuria to reduce the degree of proteinuria.

17.8 CALCIUM CHANNEL BLOCKERS (CCBs)

Calcium channel blockers (CCBs inhibit the movement of calcium into vascular smooth muscle of the arteries and cause them to relax which will lower the blood pressure. These agents are useful in the treatment of all degrees of hypertension (mild, moderate, or severe). (1–4)

1. The higher the blood pressure, the greater the reduction.
2. Low-renin hypertensive patients (volume-dependent patients) have the best response (75–80% response rate as monotherapy), but most patients respond well.
3. African-Americans and elderly patients also respond well (75–80% with monotherapy).
4. Mild edema in the absence of weight gain may be seen with long-term use. ACEI and angiotensin II receptor blocker (ARB) will counteract this edema. Diuretics are not effective treatment for CCB-induced edema, whereas the ARBs and ACEIs are the best treatment for this type of edema.
5. Their antihypertensive effect is enhanced by most other antihypertensive agents.
6. The effect on lipids is neutral or favorable. No adverse effect is seen on potassium, magnesium, glucose, uric acid, homocysteine, or other metabolic parameters.
7. There is a low adverse effect profile but may they may cause headache, constipation, dizziness, palpitations, flushing, and edema of the legs.

8. CCBs are very effective as monotherapy.
9. CCBs have been shown to reduce the incidence of vascular dementia, heart attack, and stroke.
10. Amlodipine and other CCBs in numerous clinical studies may reduce CVA better than any other antihypertensive drug classes. Amlodipine is the preferred CCB.

17.9 ANGIOTENSIN II RECEPTOR BLOCKERS (ARBs)

Ang-II receptor blockers, like ACEIs, interfere with the renin-angiotensin-aldosterone system. ARBs block the binding of Ang-II to one of its receptor sites called the AT1 receptor. Blockade of the AT1 receptor induces vasodilation and other beneficial vascular effects and lowers the blood pressure. In addition, there is an increase in nitric oxide production.

Ang-II receptor blockers have almost no side effects and generally have a more favorable safety and tolerability profile than ACEIs. They do not cause the adverse effects, such as cough and angioedema. (1–4)

17.10 RENIN INHIBITORS

The direct renin inhibitor (aliskiren, Tekturna) decreases plasma renin activity and inhibits the conversion of angiotensinogen to angiotensin I. This results in a decrease in angiotensin I and angiotensin II levels in the blood. There are significant reductions in both systolic and diastolic blood pressure and additive effects are seen with virtually all other classes of antihypertensive agents except with ARB's, and ACEI's. They have very few side effects, but no clinical trials have been published that proves they reduce cardiovascular events. (1–4)

17.11 THE CLASSES OF ANTIHYPERTENSIVE DRUGS AND THEIR NAMES

- Diuretics and serum aldosterone receptor antagonists (SARAs).
- Beta-blockers.
- ACEIs.
- ARBs.
- CCBs.
- Alpha blockers.
- Alpha-2 receptor agonists.
- Combined alpha and beta-blockers.
- Central agonists.
- Peripheral adrenergic inhibitors.
- Vasodilators.
- Renin inhibitors.

17.11.1 Diuretics

Generic Name	Common Brand Names
Thiazide diuretics and thiazide-like diuretics	
Chlorthalidone	Hygroton*
Chlorothiazide	Diuril*
Hydrochlorothiazide	Esidrix*, Hydrodiuril*, Microzide*
Indapamide	Lozol*
Metolazone	Mykrox*, Zaroxolyn*
Potassium-sparing diuretics	
Amiloride hydrochloride	Midamar*
Spironolactone (SARA)	Aldactone*
Triamterene	Dyrenium*
Eplerenone (SARA)	Inspra
Loop diuretic	
Furosemide	Lasix*
Bumetanide	Bumex*
Combination diuretics	
Amiloride hydrochloride + hydrochlorothiazide	Moduretic*
Spironolactone + hydrochlorothiazide	Aldactazide*
Triamterene + hydrochlorothiazide	Dyazide*, Maxzide*

17.11.2 Beta-blockers

Generic Name	Common Brand Names
Acebutolol	Sectral*
Atenolol	Tenormin*
Betaxolol	Kerlone*
Bisoprolol fumarate	Zebeta*
Carteolol hydrochloride	Cartrol*
Metoprolol tartrate	Lopressor*
Metoprolol succinate	Toprol-XL*
Nadolol	Corgard*
Penbutolol sulfate	Levatol*
Pindolol*	Visken*
Propranolol hydrochloride*	Inderal*
Solotol hydrochloride	Betapace*
Timolol maleate*	Blocadren*
Carvedilol	Coreg
Nebivolol	Bystolic
Combination beta-blocker/diuretic	
Hydrochlorothiazide and bisoprolol	Ziac*

17.11.3 ACE Inhibitors

Angiotensin is a chemical that causes the arteries to become narrow, especially in the kidneys but also throughout the body. ACE stands for angiotensin-converting enzyme. ACEIs help the body produce less angiotensin, which helps the blood vessels relax and open up, which, in turn, lowers blood pressure.

Generic Name	Common Brand Names
Benazepril hydrochloride	Lotensin*
Captopril	Capoten*
Enalapril maleate	Vasotec*
Fosinopril sodium	Monopril*
Lisinopril	Prinivil*, Zestril*
Moexipril	Univasc*
Perindopril	Aceon*
Quinapril hydrochloride	Accupril*
Ramipril	Altace*
Trandolapril	Mavik*

17.11.4 Angiotensin II Receptor Blockers

Generic Name	Common Brand Names
Candesartan	Atacand*
Eprosartan mesylate	Teveten*
Irbesartan	Avapro*
Losartan potassium	Cozaar*
Telmisartan	Micardis*
Valsartan	Diovan*
Olmesartan	Benicar
Azilsartan medoxomil	Edarbi

17.11.5 Calcium Channel Blockers

Generic Name	Common Brand Names
Amlodipine besylate	Norvasc*, Lotrel*
Bepridil	Vascor*
Diltiazem hydrochloride	Cardizem CD*, Cardizem SR*, Dilacor XR*, Tiazac*
Felodipine	Plendil*
Isradipine	DynaCirc*, DynaCirc CR*
Nicardipine	Cardene SR*
Nifedipine	Adalat CC*, Procardia XL*
Nisoldipine	Sular*
Verapamil hydrochloride	Calan SR*, Covera HS*, Isoptin SR*, Verelan*

17.11.6 Alpha Blockers

Generic Name	Common Brand Names
Doxazosin mesylate	Cardura*
Prazosin hydrochloride	Minipress*
Terazosin hydrochloride	Hytrin*

17.11.7 Combined Alpha and Beta-blockers

Generic Name	Common Brand Names
Carvedilol	Coreg*
Labetalol hydrochloride	Normodyne*, Trandate*

17.11.8 Central Alpha Agonists

Generic Name	Common Brand Names
Alpha methyldopa	Aldomet*
Clonidine hydrochloride	Catapres*
Guanabenz acetate	Wytensin*
Guanfacine hydrochloride	Tenex*

17.11.9 Peripheral Adrenergic Inhibitors

These medications reduce blood pressure by blocking neurotransmitters in the brain. This blocks the smooth muscles from getting the "message" to constrict. These drugs are rarely used.

Generic Name	Common Brand Names
Guanadrel	Hylorel*
Guanethidine monosulfate	Ismelin*
Reserpine	Serpasil*

17.11.10 Blood Vessel Dilators (Vasodilators)

Blood vessel dilators, or vasodilators, can cause the muscle in the walls of the blood vessels (especially the arterioles) to relax, allowing the vessel to dilate (widen). This allows blood to flow through better.

Generic Name	Common Brand Names
Hydralazine hydrochloride	Apresoline*
Minoxidil	Loniten*†

- Hydralazine (Apresoline)* may cause headaches, swelling around the eyes, heart palpitations, or aches and pains in the joints. Usually none of these symptoms are severe, and most will go away after a few weeks of treatment. This drug is not usually used by itself.
- Minoxidil (Loniten)* is a potent drug that is usually used only in resistant cases of severe high blood pressure. It may cause fluid retention (marked weight gain) or excessive hair growth.

17.12 SUMMARY AND TAKEAWAY POINTS

The preferred drugs to lower blood pressure are ACEI, ARB, CCB (amlodipine), indapamide, Bystolic, Coreg, and spironolactone. The older beta blockers excluding Bystolic and Coreg should not be used for hypertension. HCTZ should no longer be used alone or in combination with other agents to lower blood pressure. Indapamide is the preferred diuretic, and chlorthalidone would be the second. Various and rational combinations are used depending on the severity of the blood pressure and other clinical indications. The side effects of all of these medications is low, and the cost is reasonable and usually covered by most insurance companies. Your doctor will monitor various labs when prescribing these drugs.

REFERENCES

1. Whelton PK, et al. ACC/AHA/AAPA/ABC/ACPM/AGS/APhA/ASH/ASPC/NMA/PCNA Guideline for the prevention, detection, evaluation, and management of high blood pressure in adults: a report of the American College of Cardiology/American Heart Association Task Force on Clinical Practice Guidelines. Hypertension. 2018 Jun;71(6):e13–e115.
2. ESH/ESC Task Force for the Management of Arterial Hypertension. 2013 Practice guidelines for the management of arterial hypertension of the European Society of Hypertension (ESH) and the European Society of Cardiology (ESC): ESH/ESC Task Force for the Management of Arterial Hypertension. J Hypertens. 2013;31:1925–1938.
3. Flack JM, Calhoun D, Schiffrin EL. The new ACC/AHA hypertension guidelines for the prevention, detection, evaluation, and management of high blood pressure in adults. Am J Hypertens. 2018;31(2):133–135.
4. Houston MC. Handbook of Hypertension. Wiley Blackwell, 2009.
5. Burnier M, Bakris G, Williams B. Redefining diuretics use in hypertension: why select a thiazide-like diuretic? J Hypertens. 2019 Aug;37(8):1574–1586.

18 Workbook
What is Your Risk for Hypertension?

18.1 TAKE A LOOK AT THE LIST BELOW TO FIND OUT WHAT YOUR RISK OF HIGH BLOOD PRESSURE MAY BE AND TOTAL YOUR POINTS

Score 15 or more is a high risk for having or developing high blood pressure
Score 8–15 is a moderate risk for having or developing high blood pressure
Score 0–7 is a low risk for having or developing high blood pressure
Your Score ______________________

If your score is a moderate-to-high risk (8 or higher), have your blood pressure checked by your doctor.

18.2 PREDICTORS OF NEW ONSET HYPERTENSION

If you do not yet have hypertension but are concerned that you may be at risk, there are some clinical clues and lab tests that will help predict that risk:

- Genetics: if one of your parents had high blood pressure, you have a 25% chance of developing high blood pressure yourself. If both parents had high blood pressure, then the risk is 50% that you will have high blood pressure. If your parents or a sibling developed high blood pressure before the age of 50 years, then your risk is even higher to develop hypertension but also at an earlier age. SCORE POINTS FOR ONE PARENT ________3________
  POINTS FOR BOTH PARENTS ________6________
  POINTS FOR PARENT OF SIBLING WITH HYPERTENSION BEFORE AGE 50 ________7________
- Race: African-American or Hispanic POINTS ________2________
  Caucasians, Asian, Indian, Native American: POINTS ________1________
- Gender: Male: 2 POINTS__________ FEMALE: 1 POINT__________
- Age: over 60: 1 POINT ____________
- Resting heart rate over 80 beats/min at rest: 1 POINT ____________
- Abnormal blood glucose such as fasting or post meal glucose or hemoglobin A1c (HbA1c,) or fasting serum insulin: 1 POINT ________________
- Kidney disease and loss of protein and albumin in the urine: 2 POINTS_____
- Overweight or obese: 2 POINTS__________

- Hypertensive response to exercise. A systolic blood pressure over 200 mm Hg: 2 POINTS ________________
- White coat hypertension (WCH): your blood pressure is elevated in the doctor's office but is normal at home out of the doctor's office: 1 POINT_______
- Masked hypertension (MH): your blood pressure is elevated at home out of the doctor's office but is normal in the doctor's office: 1 POINT ___________
- Alcohol abuse: excessive alcohol consumption of over 20 g/day in men and 10 g/day in women: 2 POINTS________________
- Medications and drug abuse: see **Table I** for a list of these: 1 POINT _______
- Tobacco use of any kind and smoking: 1 POINT ________________
- Poor diet with high sodium, low potassium, low magnesium, not enough fruits and vegetables, not enough quality protein, too much trans fats and certain saturated fat, too much sugar, refined carbohydrates and starches and possibly caffeine: 3 POINTS ________________
- Too much emotional stress, anxiety, hostility, or depression: 2 POINTS_____
- Low income: 1 POINT________________
- Less education: 1 POINT________________

19 Grand Summary and Conclusions

High blood pressure is one of the most common diseases that effects the US population and is associated with a high incidence of cardiovascular events and early death. The causes of high blood pressure include genetics and environment and the underlying physiology is a diseased artery that has inflammation, oxidative stress, and immune vascular dysfunction. Early detection, proper awareness of the risks for high blood pressure, complete testing for arterial and heart damage, and aggressive treatment with lifestyle such as optimal nutrition, exercise, body fat and weight loss, stress reduction, and stopping all tobacco products coupled with scientifically proven nutrition supplements and new and better drugs that lower blood pressure will reduce the cardiovascular complications and improve survival. The Hypertension Institute Program as outlined in the following will give you the best chance of controlling your blood pressure and living a health life.

1. Determine the blood pressure level and other important measurements using a 24-hour ambulatory blood pressure monitoring device (24-hour ABPM) in conjunction with regular office blood pressures measured correctly using the AHA criteria and instruct the patient in the proper use of home blood pressure readings with the best validated blood pressure monitors.
2. Measure in the blood your micronutrient and macronutrient status and optimally replace all of those deficiencies with proper nutrition and supplements, antioxidants, and minerals. We recommend the **Spectracell Labs Micronutrient Test (MNT), Houston, TX.** for nutrient testing **(see Sources section).**
3. Measure blood tests that determine the type of hypertension that is present. The two forms are called **high-renin hypertension and low-renin hypertension**. The blood tests include a plasma renin activity or PRA (a hormone that controls blood pressure) and aldosterone (a hormone that controls blood pressure and blood volume). This will be discussed in detail later in this book.
4. Measure the genetics that determines your blood pressure and risk for coronary heart disease, heart attack, blood pressure, diabetes mellitus, cholesterol, and other blood fats. We recommend **Vibrant America Labs in San Francisco for the CardiaX cardiovascular genomic profile (see Sources section).**
5. Assess the presence and severity of the artery function, structure and damage, artery elasticity and stiffness, endothelial function, glycocalyx function, nitric oxide levels, heart function and stiffness, heart size (enlargement), risk for coronary heart disease, coronary artery calcification, rest

and exercise blood pressure, heart rate and its variability, the function of your nervous system and how it relates to blood pressure, and your overall cardiovascular risk with various noninvasive cardiovascular testing.

6. Exclude all of the secondary causes of hypertension.
7. Assess all of the new and emerging blood and urine tests, which are called cardiovascular risk factors, in addition to the usual measured risk factors such as blood fats and cholesterol, blood sugar (diabetes mellitus), homocysteine, and inflammation markers.
8. Properly measure obesity, total and regional body fat with a special machine called **body impedance analysis (BIA).** Maintain your ideal body weight, BMI, and body fat.
9. Determine the need for early and aggressive control of blood pressure based on the information listed previously.
10. Start the Hypertension Institute blood pressure nutrition program.
11. Use specific blood pressure lowering nutritional supplements.
12. Exercise regularly with both resistance and aerobic exercises using guidelines that are recommended in this book (ABCT) and by your physician.
13. De-stress your life with meditation, relaxation, breathing exercises, and more.
14. Stop all tobacco products.
15. Reduce or stop alcohol.
16. Stop caffeine if your genetics show that you cannot break down caffeine rapidly (slow metabolizer).
17. Stop or reduce all medications, if possible, that may increase your blood pressure.
18. Use the best medications to lower blood pressure, improve arterial function and structure, and decrease cardiovascular events.

Sources

General Hypertension Education and Information Hypertension Institute: www.hypertensioninstitute.com

RECOMMENDED NUTRITIONAL SUPPLEMENT COMPANIES

Company name: Biotics Research Corporation
Phone number: 800-231-5777
Email: biotics@bioticsresearch.com
Website: www.bioticsresearch.com

Company name: Designs for Health
Phone number: 860-623-6314
Email: info@designsforhealth.com
Website: www.designsforheath.com

Company name: Metagenics and Metagenics Institute
Website: Metagenics.com and MetagenicsInstitute.com (nonbranded educational content)
Email: (email for Metagenics is sent through a website) and for MI it is info@metagenicsinstitute.com
Phone number: 800-692-9400

Company name: Human N
Phone number: 512-488-4477
Email: Professional@humann.com
Website: https://humannpro.com/drhouston

Company name: AC Grace Company
Phone number: 800-833-4368 or 903-636-4368
Email: Info@acgrace.com
Website: www.acgrace.com

Company name: Ortho Molecular Products
Phone number: 800-332-2351
Email: contactus@ompimail.com
Website: www.orthomolecularproducts.com

Company: Calroy Health Sciences, LLC
Product: Arterosil HP
Website: arterosil.com
Email: support@arterosil.com
Phone: 800-609-6409

Company name: MitoQ Ltd.
Phone number: +649-379-8222
Email: customerservice@mitoq.com
Website: www.mitoq.com

ADDITIONAL NUTRITIONAL SUPPLEMENT COMPANIES
Xymogen
Carlson Labs
Douglas Labs
Dr. Sinatra
Pure Encapsulations
Standard Process
Swanson
Klaire Labs
Juice Plus (NSA)

LAB TESTING COMPANIES, CARDIOVASCULAR TESTING, AND MEDICAL EQUIPMENT COMPANIES
Company name: SpectraCell Laboratories, Inc.
Phone number: 800-227-5227
Email: support@spectracell.com
Website: www.spectracell.com

Company name: Vibrant America Clinical Lab
Phone number: 866-364-0963
Email: support@vibrant-america.com
Website: www.vibrant- america.com

Company name: AtCor Medical (Cardiovascular and blood pressure testing company)
Phone number: +1 (630) 228-8871
Email: info@atcormedical.com
Website: www.atcormedical.com

Predictive Health Diagnostics, Inc: Puls Test
www.pulstest.com
Info@pulstest.com
Phone: 866-299-8998
Fax: 888-424-7505

Company name: Salveo Diagnostics (Laboratory testing company)
Phone number: 844-725-8365
Email: info@salveodiagnostics.com
Website: salveodiagnostics.com

Index

Note: Locators in *italics* represent figures and **bold** indicate tables in the text.

B

C

D

E

F

O

P

Q

R

S

W

Z

For Product Safety Concerns and Information please contact our EU
representative GPSR@taylorandfrancis.com
Taylor & Francis Verlag GmbH, Kaufingerstraße 24, 80331 München, Germany

www.ingramcontent.com/pod-product-compliance
Lightning Source LLC
Chambersburg PA
CBHW060338220326
41598CB00023B/2743
9780367647797